Oral Microbiology

Fifth Edition

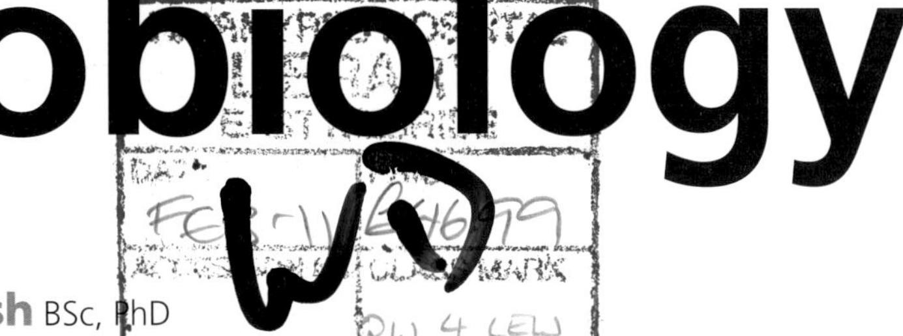

Professor Philip D Marsh BSc, PhD

Programme Leader, Health Protection Agency, Centre for Emergency Preparedness & Response, Salisbury, UK, and Professor of Oral Microbiology, Leeds Dental Institute, Leeds, UK

and

Dr Michael V Martin MBE, BDS, BA, PhD, FRCPath, FFGDP (UK)

Formerly Senior Lecturer and Consultant Microbiologist to Liverpool Dental Hospital and School, Liverpool, UK

with contributions by

Professor Michael A O Lewis PhD, BDS, FDSRCPS, FDSRCS (Ed&Eng), FRCPath, FHEA, FFGDP (UK)

Professor of Oral Medicine, School of Dentistry, Cardiff University, Cardiff, UK, and Dean of the Dental Faculty, Royal College of Physicians and Surgeons of Glasgow, UK

and

Dr David W Williams, BSc (Hons), PhD

Reader in Oral Microbiology, School of Dentistry, Cardiff University, Cardiff, UK

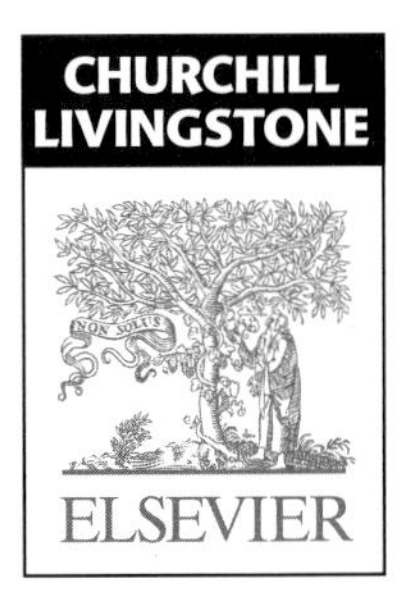

Edinburgh London New York Oxford Philadelphia St Louis Sydney Toronto 2009

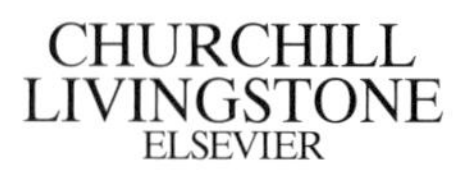

First Edition 1980
Second Edition 1984
Third Edition 1992
Fourth Edition 1999
Fifth Edition 2009
Reprinted 2009, 2010

ISBN 978-0-443-10144-1

British Library Cataloguing in Publication Data
A catalogue record for this book is available from the British Library

Library of Congress Cataloging in Publication Data
A catalog record for this book is available from the Library of Congress

Notice

Knowledge and best practice in this field are constantly changing. As new research and experience broaden our knowledge, changes in practice, treatment and drug therapy may become necessary or appropriate. Readers are advised to check the most current information provided (i) on procedures featured or (ii) by the manufacturer of each product to be administered, to verify the recommended dose or formula, the method and duration of administration, and contraindications. It is the responsibility of the practitioner, relying on their own experience and knowledge of the patient, to make diagnoses, to determine dosages and the best treatment for each individual patient, and to take all appropriate safety precautions. To the fullest extent of the law, neither the Publisher nor the Authors assumes any liability for any injury and/or damage to persons or property arising out of or related to any use of the material contained in this book.

The Publisher

Printed in China

Contents

Preface

The aim of the latest Edition of this successful textbook continues to be to describe the complex relationship between the resident oral microflora and the host in health and disease. The Fifth Edition has been completely rewritten and enlarged, while retaining and extending its philosophy of explaining this relationship in ecological terms. This approach is of benefit to the reader by providing a clear set of principles to explain the underlying issues that determine whether the microflora will have a beneficial or an adverse relationship with the host at a particular site. This information provides a foundation that can be exploited by research workers or health professionals to understand, prevent or control disease.

In the decade since the Fourth Edition was first published there have been huge advances in the field of oral microbiology. To reflect these advances, two new authors (Professor Mike Lewis and Dr David Williams, Cardiff) have been recruited to provide additional inputs especially on viral and fungal pathogens, and on the role of oral microbes in acute and chronic infections.

This new Edition reflects the impact that the genomic era has had on the subject area. The application of molecular biology techniques has revolutionized our knowledge of the richness and diversity of the microbes that can be found in the mouth, and highlighted that even with the most sophisticated of techniques only around 50% of the microflora can be cultured in the laboratory. These molecular approaches have also implicated the involvement of even more complex consortia of microorganisms in the aetiology of a number of oral diseases. This Edition also highlights the biological and clinical significance of the existence of the oral microflora in the form of a biofilm on dental and mucosal surfaces. Contemporary views on therapeutic and prophylactic antibiotic use, infection control, and the relationships between oral and general health are also discussed.

This new Edition builds on the success of previous ones, and provides an even more comprehensive coverage of the field of oral microbiology. The book will be suitable for undergraduate and postgraduate students, research workers, and a wide range of clinical dental professionals.

P D Marsh
M V Martin
M A O Lewis
D W Williams

Acknowledgements

We would like to thank the many colleagues who have provided information and permission to reproduce certain Figures, especially Bob ten Cate, Mike Curtis, Sónia da Silva, Deirdre Devine, Andrew Featherstone, Matthias Hannig, Tony Hayes, Mike Hill, Annette Moter, Bente Nyvad, Cleber Overney, Joel Rudney, William Wade, Rob Whiley and Egija Zaura. Particular thanks also go to our families who have supported us throughout the preparation of this Edition, and the publishers for their helpful contributions.

Note on cover images

The main front cover image is a confocal laser scanning microscopy view of *Candida parapsilosis*. The top right inserted image is a plaque sample stained to show live (green) and dead (red) bacteria. The centre right image shows *Candida albicans* stained with calcofluor white. The bottom right image is a view of subgingival plaque taken from a site with periodontal disease stained with probes to show general bacteria (green) and TM7 bacteria (blue).

With thanks to the Listerine Clinical Programme for Schools of Dentistry, Dental Therapy and Dental Hygiene for contribution of the top right image which was derived from the 2008 Resource Tool Kit.

The bottom right image is published with kind permission of CC Ouverney, GC Armitage, DA Relman and the American Society for Microbiology.

Chapter 1

Introduction

The mouth is the gateway of the body to the external world and represents one of the most biologically complex and significant sites in the body. This is where the first stages of the digestive process take place and, consequently, the mouth is richly endowed with sensory functions (taste, smell, temperature and texture). It also plays a critical role in communication, whether by speech or via facial expressions, and makes a significant contribution to our appearance. Recent studies have re-affirmed an earlier concept that oral health is inextricably linked to general health, and vice versa. Maintaining a healthy mouth, therefore, is of vital importance for a person's self-esteem and general well-being.

The mouth is an easily accessible part of the body and so can provide health care workers with a window into a person's oral and general health. Disease that is localized elsewhere in the body can be reflected in the mouth and, as a result, saliva is becoming increasingly recognized as a key diagnostic fluid. For example, oral candidosis (Ch. 9) in previously healthy young adults can be the first sign of HIV infection, while antibodies against a range of viruses can be detected in saliva. Risk factors for general health, such as tobacco habits, alcohol abuse and an inadequate diet, can also have a deleterious effect on oral health while, in an analogous manner, oral disease can also have an impact on the overall health of the individual. Recent studies suggest that severe periodontal disease in some populations might be a risk factor for premature or low birth weight babies, ischaemic heart disease, pulmonary disease and diabetes mellitus (see later, and Ch. 6).

The mouth is one of the key interfaces between the body and the external environment, and can act as a site of entry for some microbial pathogens, especially from the air or via ingestion from the diet. Therefore, it is equipped with a comprehensive array of defence strategies that includes elements of both the innate and adaptive immune system (see Ch. 2). Indeed, the ability of the host to recognise and respond to invading pathogens while simultaneously tolerating a diverse resident microflora (see Ch. 3) remains one of the most remarkable feats of evolution, and the precise mechanisms that permit this level of discrimination are still not fully understood.

THE HUMAN MICROFLORA

It has been estimated that the human body is made up of over 10^{14} cells of which only around 10% are mammalian. The remainder are the microorganisms that comprise the resident microflora of the host. This resident microflora does not have merely a passive relationship with its host, but contributes directly and indirectly to the normal development of the physiology, nutrition and defence systems of the organism. In general, these natural microfloras live in harmony with humans and animals and, indeed, all parties benefit from the association. Loss or perturbation of this resident microflora can lead to colonization by exogenous (and often pathogenic) microorganisms, thereby predisposing sites to disease.

The microbial colonization of all environmentally accessible surfaces of the body (both external and internal) begins at birth. Such surfaces are exposed to a wide range of microorganisms derived from the environment and from other persons. Each surface, however, because of its physical and biological properties, is suitable for colonization by only a proportion of these microbes. This results in the acquisition, selection and natural development of a diverse but characteristic microflora at distinct sites (Fig. 1.1). For example, staphylococci and micrococci predominate on the skin surface but rarely become established in significant numbers in the mouth of a healthy person. Similarly, less than 30 out of over 700 types of microorganism found in the mouth were able to colonize the gastrointestinal tract, despite the continual passage of these microbes through the gut. Furthermore, the predominant species of bacteria can differ markedly at distinct surfaces in the mouth despite these organisms having equal opportunities to colonize each site, and this is due again to subtle variations in key parameters than influence microbial growth and competitiveness (see Ch. 4).

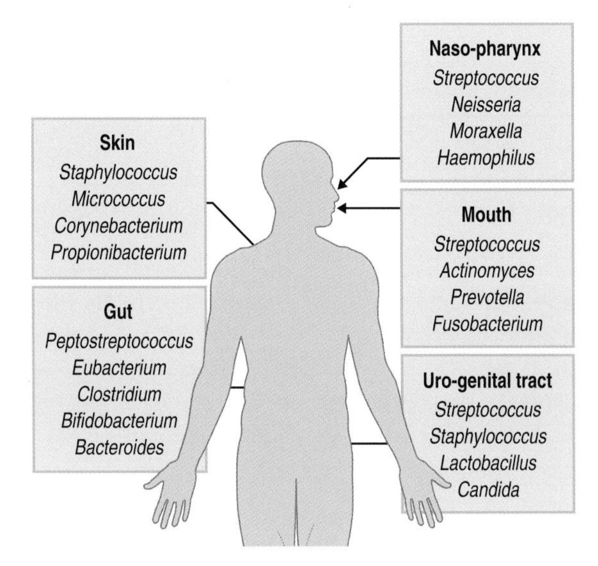

Fig. 1.1 Distribution of the resident human microflora. The predominant groups of microorganism at some distinct anatomical sites are listed.

THE ORAL MICROFLORA IN HEALTH AND DISEASE

The mouth is similar to other sites in the body in having a natural microflora with a characteristic composition and existing, for the most part, in a harmonious relationship with the host. This microflora is described in Chapter 3 and its intra-oral distribution is presented in Chapter 4. Perhaps more commonly than elsewhere in the body, this relationship can break down in the mouth and disease can occur. This is usually associated with:

- major changes to the biology of the mouth from exogenous sources (examples include: antibiotic treatment or the frequent intake of fermentable carbohydrates in the diet) or from endogenous changes such as alterations in the integrity of the host defences following drug therapy, which perturb the natural stability of the microflora, or
- the presence of microorganisms at sites not normally accessible to them; for example, when oral bacteria enter the blood stream following tooth extraction or other traumas and are disseminated to distant organs, where they can cause abscesses or endocarditis.

Bacteria with the potential to cause disease in this way are termed '**opportunistic pathogens**', and many oral microorganisms have the capacity to behave in this manner. Indeed, most individuals suffer at some time in their life from localized episodes of disease in the mouth caused by imbalances in the composition of their resident oral microflora. The commonest clinical manifestations of such imbalances are dental caries and periodontal diseases (see Ch. 6), both of which are highly prevalent in industrialized societies and are now on the increase in developing countries; other acute and chronic infections occur but less frequently (see Ch. 7). Dental caries is the dissolution of enamel or root surfaces (demineralization) by acid produced primarily from the metabolism of fermentable carbohydrates in the diet by bacteria colonizing the tooth surface (dental plaque). Dental plaque is also associated with the aetiology of periodontal diseases in which the host mounts an inappropriate inflammatory response to an increased microbial load (due to plaque accumulation) around the gingivae, resulting in damage to the supporting tissues of the teeth.

Caries and periodontal diseases pose distinct challenges when it comes to determining their microbial aetiology. These diseases occur at sites with a pre-existing diverse, natural resident microflora, while even more complex but distinct consortia of micro-organisms are implicated with pathology. It is necessary, therefore, to determine which microbial species are implicated directly in active disease, which are present as a result of disease and which are merely innocent bystanders. Numerous studies have shown that these common diseases are caused by shifts in the balance of the resident microflora, in which some minor components of dental plaque become predominant due to a change in local environmental conditions. These shifts in dental plaque composition in caries and periodontal disease are described in detail in Chapter 6.

THE SCALE OF ORAL DISEASES

Although rarely life-threatening, oral diseases are a problem for health service providers in developed countries because of their high prevalence within the general population and the huge costs associated with their treatment. These costs are increased still further by the treatment of a range of acute infections (predominantly dentoalveolar abscesses) and chronic conditions such as actinomycosis and fungal infections; these are described in Chapters 7 and 9. For example, the National Health Service in the United Kingdom spends over £1.6 billion per annum on dental treatment, and this figure increases to over £2.6 billion when the burgeoning private sector costs are included, while in the USA, there were 500 million dental care visits at a cost of $94 billion in 2006.

In general, dental health in developing countries is improving due to better oral hygiene, the use of more effective oral care products, and a greater awareness of dental disease among the general population. As a result, the incidence of dental caries has been falling in children over the past few decades. The World Health Organization (WHO) goal for 50% of 5-year-old children to have no caries has already been achieved by many countries. This has been accompanied by an increase in the number of people who retain their teeth into later life. In Europe, 80% of older adults now have some natural teeth, and the average number of teeth retained by these individuals has also risen. In the UK, 30% of adults were edentulous in 1978 but this figure had reduced to 13% by 1998. However, these trends should not induce a feeling of complacency – the increase in the number of teeth being kept means that susceptible sites and surfaces are at risk of dental disease (including caries) throughout the life of an individual. Children who at present are enjoying low levels of decay will need to develop a lifestyle that embraces good oral hygiene, an appropriate diet and regular visits to dental professionals if they are to avoid problems later in life due to periodontal diseases or root surface caries. Currently, over half of adults in the UK have periodontal pockets with a depth of four millimetres or greater, and two thirds had an average of six teeth with exposed, decayed or treated root surfaces. The incidence of periodontal diseases and root surface caries increases with age; over 80% of adults aged 65 years or over have pocketing of four millimetres or more, compared to only 40% of individuals in the 35–44 year age group, while about 60% of individuals aged over 60 years now have root caries or dental restorations.

Profound disparities in oral health exist within a population due to differences in socio-economic status (SES) and race or ethnicity. In Europe, surveys have shown that around 80% of childhood caries is found in <20% of children. In the USA, Mexican-American children have more caries than non-Hispanic black communities, with non-Hispanic white populations having the least decay; this difference is further accentuated by low SES. A similar situation exists with periodontal disease, where non-Hispanic black and poor people in the USA have more periodontal disease than other groups in each age band. There is also evidence of a gradual increase in dental caries in urban areas of developing countries, probably as a result of changing dietary habits. For example, the number of decayed, missing and filled teeth (DMFT) in 12-year-old children in Thailand was 0.4 in 1960 but had increased to 1.6 by 2000–01. Three quarters of adults in some parts of the developing world have been found to suffer from periodontal disease. Few individuals in these communities take remedial action due to a general lack of awareness of the presence or consequence of such diseases. Advances in prevention could lead to a major reduction in the prevalence of these diseases, with the potential for massive savings in health care budgets.

Dental diseases (including caries and periodontal diseases) result from a complex interaction of environmental triggers (primarily, the nature of the diet and exposure to antimicrobial agents), the resident

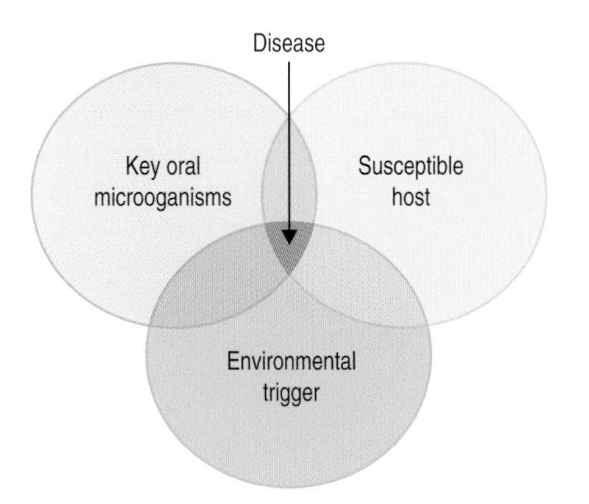

Fig. 1.2 The inter-relationships that lead to oral disease. Environmental triggers include a high sugar diet and antibiotic therapy, while host susceptibility might increase due to reduced saliva flow or immunosuppression.

microflora, and the host (Fig. 1.2). In order to determine the aetiology and biological mechanisms behind these diseases it is necessary to understand the factors that influence these interactions. This requires an appreciation of the principles of microbial ecology. In this book, the relationships among oral microorganisms, and between these microorganisms and the host, will be examined. The general composition of the oral microflora is well characterized, but much less is known about how the properties of the mouth influence the composition and metabolism of the resident microflora in health and disease. The oral microflora is in dynamic equilibrium with the host, and a change in a key parameter that influences microbial growth can perturb this equilibrium and determine whether the microflora will have a commensal or pathogenic relationship with the host at a site. An understanding of these inter-relationships (oral microbial ecology) is fundamental to developing appropriate treatment strategies.

SUMMARY

Dental diseases are highly prevalent and are a huge economic burden to health care providers. Diseases such as caries and periodontal diseases are a consequence of imbalances in the normal oral microflora. Therefore, understanding the dynamic relationships that exist between the host, the local environment and the oral microflora is fundamental to educating patients and preventing disease, and can identify the risk factors that drive these deleterious changes in the microflora.

MICROBIAL ECOLOGY

The philosophy of this text-book is that the key to a more complete understanding of the role of microorganisms in dental disease depends on a paradigm shift away from concepts that have been derived from studies of diseases with a simple and specific (single species) aetiology to an appreciation of ecological principles. Most diseases of the mouth have a polymicrobial (multiple species) aetiology. The ability of consortia of bacteria to cause disease depends on the outcome of various interactions both among the microbes themselves, and between these microorganisms and the host. It may be necessary, therefore, to take a more holistic approach when relating the oral microflora to disease. The activity and behaviour of these microbes is intimately linked to other biological systems in the mouth (Figs 1.2 and 1.3). Thus, the composition and metabolism of bacteria at a site will be influenced by the flow rate and properties of saliva, the life-style of an individual (in particular, the presence of a tobacco habit, the nature of the diet, and exposure to medication), and the integrity of the host defences. For example, caries may occur not only because of the frequent intake of fermentable carbohydrates in the diet, but also as a consequence of long-term medication for an unrelated medical

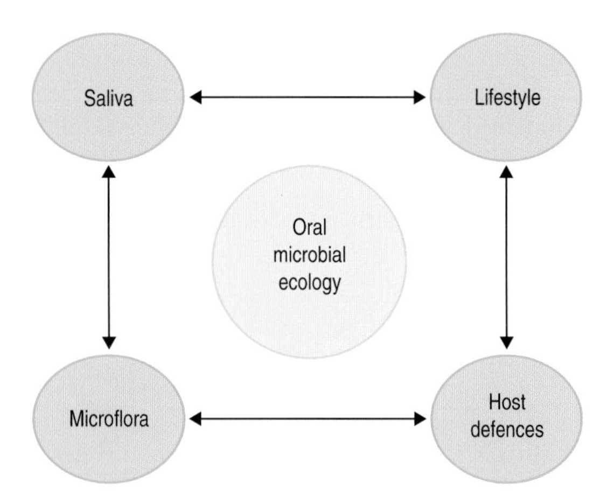

Fig. 1.3 The inter-relationships that influence the microbial ecology of the mouth in health and disease. The predominant microorganisms in the mouth might alter due to changes in saliva flow, life-style (e.g. tobacco habit, diet) or to changes in the integrity of the host defences. These changes may predispose sites to disease.

complaint since a side-effect of such treatment can often be a reduced saliva flow. A common adverse effect of certain drugs is a reduction in the production of saliva, which in turn reduces its protective properties. Similarly, smoking tobacco can impair the functioning of the host defences, leading to a failure to control the growth of potentially pathogenic microorganisms. Oral fungal infections arise following the wearing of dentures, suppression of the host defences, or antibiotic therapy that removes competing indigenous bacteria. Acceptance of such ecological principles can more readily explain the transition of the oral microflora from having a commensal to a pathogenic relationship with the host, and also open up new opportunities for prevention, treatment and control.

Much of the terminology used in this book to describe events in microbial ecology will be as defined by Alexander (1971). The site where microorganisms grow is the **habitat**. The microorganisms growing in a particular habitat constitute a **microbial community** made up of populations of individual species or less well-defined groups (taxa); alternative terms are **microbiota** or **microflora**. The growth of microbial communities on surfaces is termed a **biofilm** (see Ch. 5). The microbial community in a specific habitat together with the biotic and abiotic surroundings with which these organisms are associated is known as the **ecosystem**. The **niche** is defined here as the *function* of an organism in a particular habitat. Thus, the niche is not the physical location of an organism but is its *role* within the community. This role is dictated by the biological properties of each microbial population. Species with identical functions in a particular habitat will compete for the same niche, while the co-existence of many species in a habitat is due to each population having a different role (niche) and thus avoiding competition.

A number of terms have been used to describe the characteristic mixtures of microorganisms associated with a site. These include the normal, indigenous, or commensal microflora, but some difficulties in nomenclature arise if some of the organisms are associated with disease on occasions. Alexander (1971) proposed that species found characteristically in a particular habitat should be termed **autochthonous** microorganisms. These multiply and persist at a site and contribute to the metabolism of a microbial community (with no distinction made regarding disease potential), and can be contrasted with **allochthonous** organisms which originate from elsewhere and are generally unable to colonize successfully unless the ecosystem is severely perturbed. Alternatively, a simple approach has been to use the term **'resident microflora'** to include any organism that is regularly isolated from a site; again, no distinction concerning disease potential is made. Microorganisms that have the potential to cause disease are termed **pathogens**. As stated earlier, those that cause disease only under exceptional circumstances are described as **opportunistic pathogens**, and can be distinguished from **true** or **overt pathogens** which are consistently associated with a particular disease.

THE ORAL MICROFLORA AND GENERAL HEALTH

The significance of oral diseases is generally considered only in the context of the health of the mouth, but evidence is accumulating that suggests that they can also have an impact on the general health of an individual. In periodontal diseases, for example, large numbers of Gram negative bacteria accumulate around the roots of the teeth, and produce virulence factors such as lipopolysaccharide (LPS), cytotoxic metabolites, and immunoreactive molecules. The host mounts an inflammatory response to the microbial 'insult', and prostaglandins and pro-inflammatory cytokines are produced. These bacterial and host factors can enter the blood stream due to the high vascularity of the periodontium and are now believed to affect distant sites in the body.

Some recent human epidemiological studies and animal experiments have demonstrated that periodontal diseases represent a previously unrecognised and clinically significant risk factor for preterm low birth weight babies, either as a direct consequence of pre-term labour or to premature rupture of membranes, although this has not been confirmed in all population groups. Furthermore, inflammatory changes associated with periodontal microorganisms can predispose to diabetes or affect glycaemic control. Additionally, oral microorganisms, including periodontal pathogens, can enter the blood stream during transient bacteraemias, where they may play a role in the development and progression of atherosclerosis, thereby increasing the risk for coronary heart disease.

The mouth may also affect general health by acting as a reservoir for opportunistic pathogens. Oral hygiene is poor among patients in intensive care, and dental plaque from these patients contains large numbers of potential respiratory pathogens. Aspiration of these pathogens (and bacteria implicated in periodontal disease; Ch. 6) into the lower respiratory tract can increase the likelihood of serious lung infection, especially in immunocompromised or elderly people. *Helicobacter pylori* is also detected in dental plaque on occasions, and this organism is strongly associated with chronic gastritis and peptic ulcers, and is a risk factor for gastric cancer. *Helicobacter pylori* is not a normal bacterial inhabitant of the mouth, and its presence may be associated with gastro-oesophagal reflux. Its intermittent persistence in the mouth is linked with the presence of deep periodontal pockets, and this carriage may aid its transmission from person-to-person. This pathogen may be retained in dental plaque by selective adherence to already attached bacteria, namely *Fusobacterium* spp., by a process called coadherence or coaggregation (see Ch. 5). Cystic fibrosis (CF) is often accompanied by lung infection caused by opportunistic pathogens such as *Pseudomonas aeruginosa, Haemophilus influenzae, Burkolderia cepacia* and staphylococci. CF patients have fewer dental health problems, probably as a consequence of their long-term intensive antibiotic therapy. Studies have shown that a number of oral sites in CF patients can be colonised by *P. aeruginosa*, suggesting that the mouth could act as reservoir for this organism. Evidence of transfer of these bacteria to dental equipment has been reported, which highlights the need for effective cross-infection control strategies (Ch. 12).

The properties of the mouth that influence its function as a microbial habitat together with the major groups of microorganisms that reside there will be described in the next two chapters. Subsequent chapters will describe the acquisition and development of the oral microflora (Ch. 4), especially dental plaque (Ch. 5). The remainder of the book will consider the role of the oral microflora in disease, including infections in the mouth due to exogenous microbes, and will describe strategies for infection control in the dental surgery.

SUMMARY

Oral microorganisms can have an impact on the general health of an individual. Periodontal pathogens, together with the host's inflammatory response to subgingival bacteria, may be risk factors for cardiovascular disease, preterm or low birth weight babies, or diabetes. Oral bacteria can act as opportunistic pathogens at distant sites in the body, e.g. following entry to the blood stream (bacteraemia) or aspiration into the lungs.
The mouth may also act as a reservoir for pathogenic bacteria such as *Pseudomonas aeruginosa* and *Helicobacter pylori*, emphasizing the need for effective infection control strategies in the dental surgery.

CHAPTER SUMMARY

The mouth has a resident microflora with a characteristic composition that exists, for the most part, in harmony with the host. This microflora is of benefit to the host and contributes to the normal development of the physiology and host defences of animals and humans. Components of this microflora can act as opportunistic pathogens when the habitat is disturbed or when microorganisms are found at sites not normally accessible to them. Dental diseases, caused by imbalances in the resident microflora, are highly prevalent and extremely costly to treat. Dental diseases may also act as risk factors for more serious medical conditions, such as heart and pulmonary disease; the mouth can also act as a reservoir for exogenous pathogens such as *Helicobacter pylori* and *Pseudomonas aeruginosa*, emphasising the need for effective infection control strategies. Oral health has a strong influence on the quality of life of an individual, and is more than merely preserving the integrity of the teeth and their supporting tissues. An understanding of the relationship between the oral microflora and the host, and how this relationship can be perturbed by exogenous and endogenous factors, is critical to understanding oral diseases and in developing new preventative strategies.

FURTHER READING

Alexander M 1971 Microbial ecology. John Wiley, New York.

Dowsett SA, Kowolik MJ 2003 Oral *Helicobacter pylori*: can we stomach it? Crit Rev Oral Biol Med 14:226-233.

Hobdell M, Petersen PE, Clarkson J et al 2003 Global goals for oral health 2020. Int Dent J 53:285-288.

Marsh PD 2003 Are dental diseases examples of ecological catastrophes? Microbiol 149:279-294.

Ruby J, Goldner M 2007 Nature of symbiosis in oral disease. J Dent Res 86:8-11.

Scannapieco FA 2005 Systemic effects of periodontal diseases. Dent Clin North Am 49:533-550.

Socransky SS, Haffajee AD 2005 Periodontal microbial ecology. Periodontology 2000 38:135-187.

Taylor GW, Borgnakke WS 2008 Periodontal disease: associations with diabetes, glycemic control and complications. Oral Dis 14:191-203.

Wilson M 2005 Microbial inhabitants of humans. Their ecology and role in health and disease. Cambridge University Press, Cambridge.

Xiong X, Buekens P, Fraser WD et al 2006 Periodontal disease and adverse pregnancy outcomes: a systematic review. BJOG 113: 135-143.

Chapter | 2 |

The mouth as a microbial habitat

THE MOUTH AS A MICROBIAL HABITAT

The properties of the mouth make it ecologically distinct from all other surfaces of the body, and dictate the types of microbe able to persist, so that not all of the microorganisms that enter the mouth are able to colonize. Moreover, distinct habitats exist even within the mouth, each of which will support the growth of a characteristic microbial community because of their particular biological features. Habitats that provide obviously different ecological conditions include **mucosal surfaces** (such as the lips, cheek, palate, and tongue) and **teeth** (Table 2.1). The properties of the mouth as a microbial habitat are dynamic, and will change during the life of an individual. During the first few months of life the mouth consists only of mucosal surfaces for microbial colonization. The eruption of teeth provides a unique, hard non-shedding surface which enables much larger masses of microorganisms (dental plaque) to accumulate as biofilms; in addition, gingival crevicular fluid (GCF) is produced which can provide additional nutrients for subgingival microorganisms. The ecology of the mouth will change over time due to the eruption or extraction of teeth, the insertion of orthodontic bands or dentures, and any dental treatment including scaling and restorations. Transient fluctuations in the stability of the oral ecosystem may be induced by the frequency and type of food ingested, variations in saliva flow (for example, certain medications impair saliva flow), and courses of antibiotic therapy.

Four features that help to make the oral cavity distinct from other areas of the body are: specialized mucosal surfaces, teeth, saliva and gingival crevicular fluid. These will be considered now in more detail.

Mucosal surfaces

The mouth is similar to other ecosystems in the digestive tract in having mucosal surfaces for microbial colonization. The microbial load is relatively low on

Table 2.1 Distinct microbial habitats within the mouth

Habitat	Comment
Lips, cheek, palate	• biomass restricted by desquamation • some surfaces have specialized host cell types
Tongue	• highly papillated surface • acts as a reservoir for obligate anaerobes
Teeth	• non-shedding surface enabling large masses of microbes to accumulate (dental plaque biofilms) • teeth have distinct surfaces for microbial colonization; each surface (e.g. fissures, smooth surfaces, approximal, gingival crevice) will support a distinct microflora because of their intrinsic biological properties.

such surfaces due to desquamation. However, the oral cavity does have specialized surfaces which contribute to the diversity of the microflora at certain sites. The papillary structure of the dorsum of the tongue provides refuge for many microorganisms which would otherwise be removed by mastication and the flow of saliva. Such sites on the tongue can also have a low redox potential (see later), which enable obligately anaerobic bacteria to grow. Indeed, the tongue can act as a reservoir for some of the Gram negative anaerobes that are implicated in the aetiology of periodontal diseases (Ch. 6), and are responsible for malodour (Ch. 4). The mouth also contains keratinized (as in the palate) as well as non-keratinized stratified squamous epithelium which may influence the intra-oral distribution of some microorganisms.

Teeth

The mouth is the only normally-accessible site in the body that has hard non-shedding surfaces for microbial colonization. Teeth do not appear in the mouth until after the first few months of life. The primary dentition is usually complete by the age of 3 years, and around 6 years the permanent teeth begin to erupt; this process is complete by about 12 years of age. Local ecological conditions will vary during these periods of change, which will in turn influence the composition of the resident microbial community at a site.

Teeth (and dentures) allow the accumulation of large masses of microorganisms (predominantly bacteria) and their extracellular products, termed dental plaque. Plaque is an example of a biofilm (Ch. 5) and, while it is found naturally in health, it is also associated with dental caries and periodontal disease. In disease, there is a shift in the composition of the plaque microflora away from the species that predominate in health (Ch. 6).

Each tooth is composed of four tissues – **pulp, dentine, cementum** and **enamel** (Fig. 2.1). The pulp receives nerve signals and blood supplies from the tissues of the jaw via the roots. Thus the pulp is able to nourish the dentine and act as a sensory organ by detecting pain. Dentine makes up the bulk of the tooth and functions by supporting the enamel and protecting the pulp. Dentine is composed of bundles of collagen filaments surrounded by mineral crystals. Tubules run continuously through the body of the dentine from the pulp to the dentine–enamel and to the dentine–cementum junctions. Enamel is the most highly calcified tissue in the body and is normally the only part of the tooth exposed to the environment. Cementum is a specialized calcified connective tissue that covers and protects the roots of the tooth. Cementum is important for the anchorage of the tooth; embedded in the cementum are the fibres of the periodontal ligament which anchor each tooth to the periodontal bone of the jaw. With ageing, recession of the gingival tissues can expose cementum to microbial colonization and disease (root surface caries; Ch. 6).

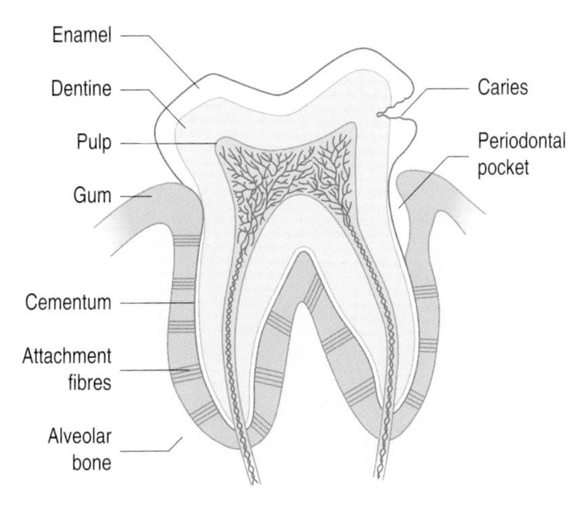

Fig. 2.1 Tooth structure in health and disease.

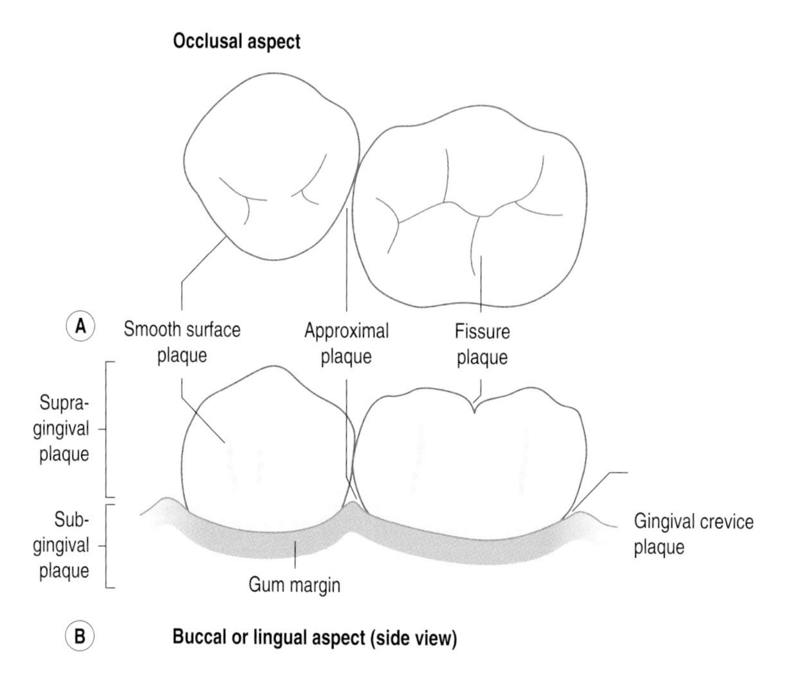

Fig. 2.2 Diagram illustrating the different surfaces of a tooth, and the terminology used to describe dental plaque sampling sites.

The ecological complexity of the mouth is increased still further by the range of habitats found on the tooth. Teeth do not provide a uniform habitat but possess several distinct surfaces (Table 2.1, Fig. 2.2), each of which is optimal for colonization and growth by different populations of microorganism. This is due to the physical nature of the particular surface and the resulting biological properties of the area. The stagnant areas between adjacent teeth (approximal) and in the gingival crevice afford most protection to colonizing microorganisms from the adverse conditions in the mouth. Both sites are also anaerobic and, in addition, the gingival crevice region is bathed in the nutritionally-rich gingival crevicular fluid (GCF; see later), particularly during inflammation, resulting in these areas supporting a more diverse microbial community. Smooth surfaces are more exposed to the environment and can only be colonized by a limited number of bacterial species adapted to such extreme conditions. The properties of a smooth surface will differ according to whether it faces the cheek (buccal surface) or the inside (lingual surface) of the mouth. Pits and fissures of the biting (occlusal) surfaces of the teeth also offer protection from oral removal forces such as saliva flow, and can contain impacted food debris. Such protected areas are associated with the largest microbial communities and, in general, the most disease.

The relationship between the environment and the microbial community is not unidirectional. Although the properties of the environment dictate which microorganisms can occupy a given site, the metabolism of the microbial community will modify the physical and chemical properties of their surroundings, for example, by consuming oxygen and releasing carbon dioxide and hydrogen to create a more anaerobic environment. Environmental conditions on the tooth also vary in health and disease (Fig. 2.1). For example, as caries progresses, the advancing front of the lesion penetrates the dentine. The nutritional sources will change and local conditions may become acidic and more anaerobic due to the accumulation of products of bacterial metabolism. Similarly, in disease, the gingival crevice develops into a periodontal pocket and the production of GCF is increased. These new environments will select the microbial community most adapted to the prevailing conditions. This is a dynamic relationship, with each change in the local environment invoking a new response by the resident microorganisms, and possibly resulting in a shift in the composition and metabolism of the microflora.

Saliva

The mouth is kept moist and lubricated by saliva which flows to form a thin film (approximately 0.1 mm deep) over all the internal surfaces of the oral cavity. Saliva enters the oral cavity via ducts from the major paired parotid, submandibular and sublingual glands as well as from the minor glands of the oral mucosa (labial, lingual, buccal and palatal glands) where it is produced. There are differences in the chemical composition of the secretions from each gland, but the complex mixture is termed 'whole saliva' (Table 2.2). Saliva plays a major role in maintaining the integrity of teeth by clearing food and by buffering the potentially damaging acids produced by dental plaque following the metabolism of dietary carbohydrates. Bicarbonate is the major buffering system in saliva, but phosphates, peptides and proteins are also involved. The mean pH of saliva is between pH 6.75 and 7.25, although the pH and buffering capacity will vary with the flow rate. Within a mouth, the flow rate and the concentration of components such as proteins, calcium and phosphate have circadian rhythms, with the slowest flow of saliva occurring during sleep. Thus, it is important to avoid consuming sugary foods or drinks before sleeping because the protective functions of saliva are reduced.

The major organic constituents of saliva are proteins and glycoproteins, such as mucin, and they influence the oral microflora by:

- adsorbing to the tooth surface to form a conditioning film (the acquired pellicle), which determines which microorganisms are able to attach (Chs 4 and 5),
- acting as primary sources of nutrients (carbohydrates and proteins) for the resident microflora,
- aggregating exogenous microorganisms, thereby facilitating their clearance from the mouth by swallowing, and
- inhibiting the growth of some exogenous microorganisms.

Table 2.2 The mean concentration (mg/100 ml) of selected constituents of whole saliva and gingival crevicular fluid (GCF) from humans

Constituent	Whole saliva		GCF
	Resting	**Stimulated**	
Protein	220	280	7×10^3
IgA	19		110*
IgG	1		350*
IgM	<1		25*
C_3	tr	tr	40
Amylase	38		–
Lysozyme	22	11	+
Albumin	tr	tr	+
Sodium	15	60	204
Potassium	80	80	70
Calcium	6	6	20
Magnesium	<1	<1	1
Phosphate	17	12	4
Bicarbonate	31	200	–

tr = trace amounts.
*determined in GCF samples from patients with periodontitis.

Other nitrogenous compounds provided by saliva include urea and numerous amino acids. Oral microorganisms require amino acids for growth, but not all of these are present free in saliva, and are obtained from salivary proteins and peptides by the action of microbial proteases and peptidases. The concentration of free carbohydrates is low in saliva, and most oral bacteria produce glycosidases to degrade the side-chains of host glycoproteins (Fig. 5.13). The metabolism of amino acids, peptides, proteins and urea can lead to the net production of alkali, which contributes to the rise in pH following acid production after the dietary intake of fermentable carbohydrates (Fig. 2.3).

Antimicrobial factors, including lysozyme, lactoferrin, and the sialoperoxidase system, are present in saliva (Table 2.3) and play a key role in controlling bacterial and fungal colonization of the mouth. Antibodies have been detected, with secretory IgA (sIgA) being the predominant class of immunoglobulin; IgG and IgM are also present but in lower concentrations. A range of peptides with antimicrobial activity, including histidine-rich polypeptides (histatins), cystatins and defensins are also present in saliva. A fuller description of these factors, and a discussion of their role in controlling the resident oral microflora are discussed later in this chapter. The properties of saliva are fundamental to the maintenance of a healthy mouth; consequently, it is often referred to as the 'defender of the oral cavity'.

Gingival crevicular fluid (GCF)

Serum components can reach the mouth by the flow of a serum-like fluid through the junctional epithelium of the gingivae (Fig. 2.6). The flow of this gingival crevicular fluid (GCF) is relatively slow at healthy sites, but increases by 147% in gingivitis and by up to 30-fold in advanced periodontal diseases, as part of the inflammatory response to the accumulation of plaque around the gingival margin. GCF can influence the microbial ecology of the site in a number of ways. Its flow will

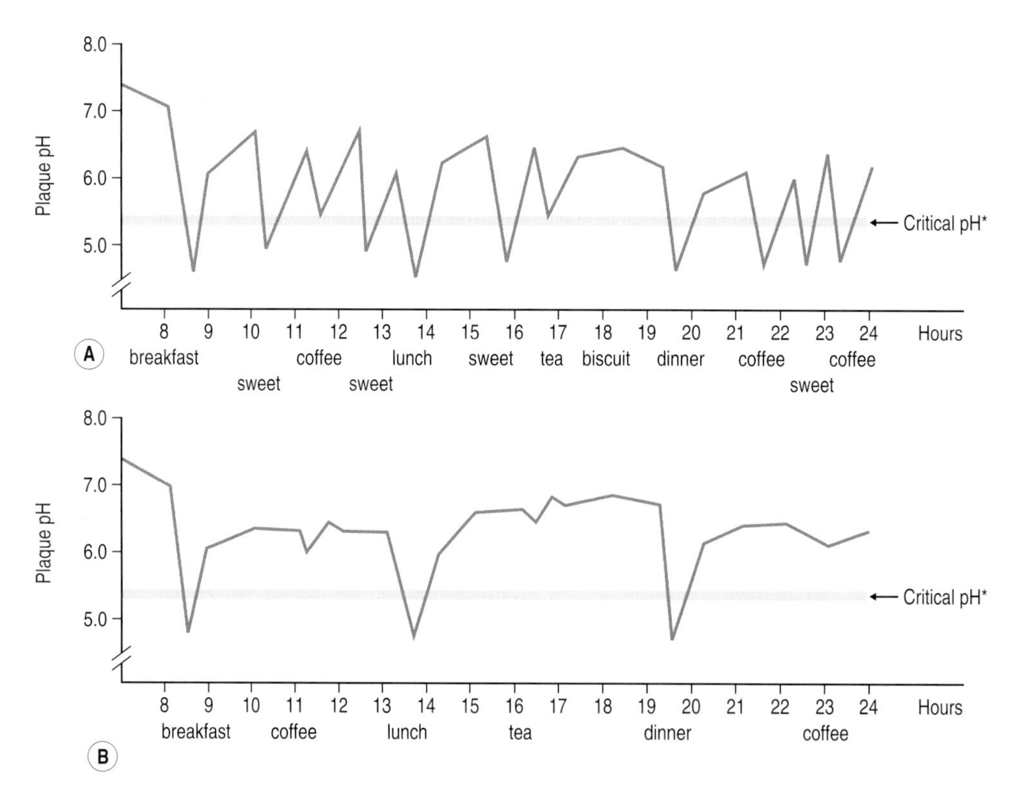

Fig. 2.3 Schematic representation of the changes in plaque pH in an individual who (A) has frequent intakes of fermentable carbohydrate during the day, or (B) limits their carbohydrate intake to main meals only. The critical pH is the pH below which demineralization of enamel is enhanced.

Table 2.3 Specific and non-specific host defence factors of the mouth

Defence factor	Main function
Non-specific:	
Saliva flow	Physical removal of microorganisms
Mucin/agglutinins	Physical removal of microorganisms
Lysozyme-protease-anion	Cell lysis
Lactoferrin	Iron sequestration
Apo-lactoferrin	Cell killing
Sialoperoxidase system	Hypothiocyanite production (neutral pH) Hypocyanous acid production (low pH)
Histatins	Antifungal with some antibacterial activity
Defensins (α- & β-)	Antimicrobial & immunomodulatory activity
Cystatins, SLPI & TIMP	Cysteine, serine & metallo-protease inhibitors
Chitinase & chromogranin	Antifungal
Cathelicidin	Antimicrobial
Calprotectin	Antimicrobial
Specific:	
Intra-epithelial lymphocytes & Langerhans cells	Cellular barrier to penetrating bacteria and/or antigens
sIgA	Prevents microbial adhesion & metabolism
IgG, IgA, IgM	Prevent microbial adhesion; opsonins; complement activators
Complement	Activates neutrophils
Neutrophils/macrophages	Phagocytosis

remove non-adherent microbial cells, and will also introduce components of the host defences, especially IgG and neutrophils. GCF can also act as an additional and novel source of nutrients for the resident microorganisms (Table 2.2). Many bacteria from subgingival plaque are proteolytic and interact synergistically to break down the host proteins and glycoproteins to provide peptides, amino acids and carbohydrates for growth. Essential cofactors for growth, including haemin for black-pigmented anaerobes, can also be obtained from the degradation of haeme-containing molecules such as transferrin, haemopexin, and haemoglobin.

The increased production of gingival crevicular fluid during disease is associated with a rise in the pH of the periodontal pocket. The mean pH during health is approximately 6.90 and this can rise during inflammation in gingivitis and periodontal disease to between pH 7.25 and 7.75. Even such a modest change in pH can alter the competitiveness of individual bacteria, which can affect the proportions of bacteria, especially as some of the putative periodontal pathogens are favoured by an alkaline environment (Fig. 2.4). Also, the activity of some proteases associated with the virulence of these opportunistic pathogens is enhanced at alkaline pH (pH 7.5–8.0).

GCF contains components of the host defences (Tables 2.2 and 2.3) which play an important role in regulating the microflora of the gingival crevice in health and disease. In contrast to saliva, IgG is

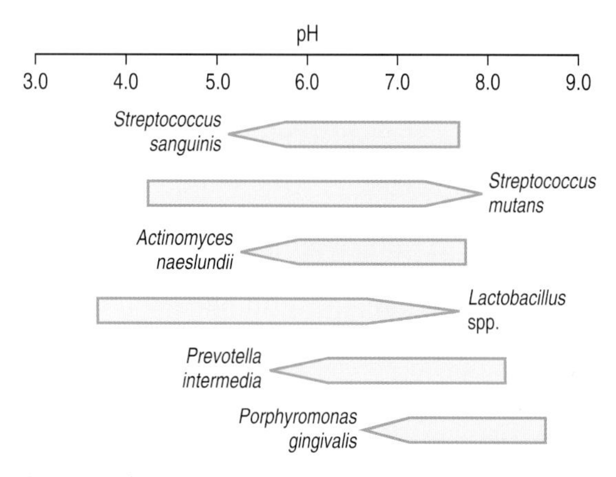

Fig. 2.4 A diagrammatic representation of the pH range for growth of some oral bacterial species.

the predominant immunoglobulin; IgM and IgA are also present, as is complement. GCF contains leukocytes, of which 95% are neutrophils, the remainder being lymphocytes and monocytes. The neutrophils in GCF are viable and can phagocytose bacteria within the crevice. A number of enzymes can be detected in GCF, including collagenase and elastase, which are derived both from phagocytic host cells and subgingival bacteria. These enzymes can degrade host tissues and thereby contribute to the destructive processes associated with periodontal diseases (Ch. 6). Several of these enzymes are under evaluation as potential diagnostic markers of active periodontal breakdown for use in the clinic as chairside kits.

SUMMARY

The properties of the mouth that make it distinct from other microbial habitats in the body include the presence of teeth, saliva and gingival crevicular fluid (GCF). Teeth are unique because they are non-shedding surfaces thereby permitting the accumulation of large masses of microorganisms and their products (dental plaque), especially at stagnant sites that offer protection from oral removal forces. Saliva and GCF provide components of the host defences, and are also important sources of nutrients for microorganisms, while saliva also acts as a buffer to maintain a favourable pH for oral health.

FACTORS AFFECTING THE GROWTH OF MICROORGANISMS IN THE ORAL CAVITY

Many factors influence the growth of microorganisms; some of particular relevance to the oral cavity will be considered in the following sections.

Temperature

The human mouth is kept at a relatively constant temperature (35–36 °C) which provides stable conditions suitable for the growth of a wide range of microorganisms. Periodontal pockets with active disease (inflammation) have a higher temperature (up to 39 °C) compared with healthy sites. Even such relatively small rises in temperature can significantly alter bacterial gene expression, and possibly the competitiveness of individual species. A rise in temperature down-regulated expression of some of the major proteases as well as the gene coding for the major subunit protein of fimbriae (these surface structures mediate attachment of the bacterium to host cells) in the periodontal pathogen, *Porphyromonas gingivalis*, and up-regulated synthesis of superoxide dismutase, which is involved in the neutralization of toxic oxygen metabolites.

Redox potential/anaerobiosis

Despite the accessibility of the mouth to air with an oxygen concentration of approximately 20%, the oral microflora comprises few, if any, truly aerobic (oxygen-requiring) species. The majority of organisms are either facultatively anaerobic (can grow in the presence or absence of oxygen) or obligately anaerobic (require reduced conditions, where oxygen can be toxic to these organisms). In addition, there are some capnophilic (CO_2-requiring) and microaerophilic species (requiring low concentrations of oxygen for growth). Anaerobiosis is frequently described in rigid terms, and oral microorganisms are separated into aerobes and anaerobes on their ability to grow in the presence or absence of oxygen. However, a wide spectrum of oxygen tolerances exist among these organisms and sharp distinctions cannot be made between these groups.

Oxygen concentration is the main factor limiting the growth of obligately anaerobic bacteria. It is the commonest and most readily reduced electron acceptor in the majority of microbial habitats, and its presence results in the oxidation of the environment. Anaerobic species require reduced conditions for their normal metabolism; therefore, it is the degree of oxidation–reduction at a site that governs the survival and relative growth of these organisms. This oxidation–reduction level is usually expressed as the redox potential (Eh). Oxygen is only one of the many interacting components influencing the Eh of a habitat and its inhibitory action is usually attributed to its ability to raise the redox potential. Even if oxygen is totally excluded from the environment some anaerobes will not grow if the redox potential is too high. Similarly, some strains can tolerate increased concentrations of oxygen if the Eh is maintained at low levels. In general, the distribution of anaerobes in the mouth will be related to the redox potential at a particular site, although some survive at overtly aerobic habitats by existing in close partnership with oxygen-consuming species. Obligate anaerobes also possess specific molecular defence mechanisms which enable them to cope with low levels of oxygen; these will be described in Chapter 4.

The degree of anaerobiosis has been determined in various areas of the mouth. The oxygen tension of the anterior surface of the tongue was 16.4%, the posterior surface 12.4%, and the buccal folds of the upper and lower jaw only 0.3–0.4%. Microelectrodes have enabled the redox potential to be measured at specific sites in the oral cavity. The redox potential has been shown to fall during plaque development on a clean enamel surface from an initial Eh of over +200 mV (highly oxidized) to −141 mV (highly reduced) after 7 days. The development of plaque in this way is associated with a specific succession of colonizing microorganisms (Chs 4 and 5). Early colonizers will utilize O_2 and produce CO_2; later colonizers may produce H_2 and other reducing agents such as sulphur-containing compounds and volatile fermentation products. Thus, as the Eh is gradually lowered, sites become suitable for the survival and growth of a changing pattern of organisms, and particularly obligate anaerobes.

The Eh of the gingival crevice is normally around +70 mV but falls during inflammation to around −50 mV in gingivitis, while even lower values will occur in advanced periodontal disease (ca. −300 mV). This is to be expected since highly anaerobic organisms, such as oral spirochaetes, can be isolated from sites with advanced disease. Approximal areas (between teeth) are also likely to have a low Eh, since again many obligate anaerobes grow successfully at these sites.

Gradients of O_2 concentration and Eh will exist in the oral cavity, particularly in thick biofilms, and so dental plaque will be suitable for the growth of bacteria with a range of oxygen tolerances. The redox potential at various depths will be influenced by the metabolism of the organisms present and the ability of gases to diffuse in and out of plaque. The metabolism or properties of particular bacteria will be influenced by the Eh of the environment. For example, the activity of intracellular glycolytic enzymes and the pattern of fermentation products of *Streptococcus mutans* varies under strictly anaerobic conditions. Therefore, the perturbation of the redox potential at a site could have a significant impact on the composition and metabolism of the microbial community. This approach is being actively pursued as a strategy to control subgingival plaque in periodontal disease, for example, by using redox agents to raise the Eh and make conditions unfavourable for strictly anaerobic bacteria (Ch. 6).

pH

Many microorganisms require a pH around neutrality for growth, and are sensitive to extremes of acid or alkali. The pH of most surfaces of the mouth is regulated by saliva (the mean pH for unstimulated whole saliva is between 6.75 and 7.25) so that, in general, optimal pH values for microbial growth will be provided at sites bathed by this fluid. The palate has a mean pH of 7.34, while the mean pH of the tongue, the floor of the mouth and the buccal mucosa is 6.8, 6.5 and 6.3, respectively.

Shifts in the proportions of bacteria within dental plaque can occur following fluctuations in environmental pH. After sugar consumption, the pH in plaque can fall rapidly to below pH 5.0 by the production of acids (predominantly lactic acid) by bacterial metabolism (Fig. 2.3); the pH then recovers slowly to resting values. Depending on the frequency of sugar intake, the bacteria in plaque will be exposed to varying challenges of low pH. Many of the predominant plaque bacteria that are associated with healthy sites can tolerate brief conditions of low pH, but are inhibited or killed by more frequent or prolonged exposures to acidic conditions. These latter conditions are likely to occur in subjects who commonly consume sugar-containing snacks or drinks between meals (Fig. 2.3). This can result in the enhanced growth of, or colonization by, acid-tolerant (aciduric) species, especially mutans streptococci and *Lactobacillus* species (Fig. 2.4), which are normally absent or only minor components in dental plaque at healthy sites. Such a change in the bacterial composition of plaque predisposes a surface to dental caries. The acid tolerance of these bacteria is achieved by the possession of particular metabolic strategies and the induction of a specific set of stress response proteins (Ch. 4).

In contrast, the pH of the gingival crevice can become alkaline during the host inflammatory response in periodontal disease, probably as a result of bacterial metabolism, e.g. ammonia production from urea and from the deamination of amino acids. The pH of the healthy gingival crevice is approximately pH 6.90, and rises to between pH 7.2 and 7.4 during disease, with a few patients having pockets with a mean pH of around 7.8. This degree of change can alter the pattern of gene expression in subgingival bacteria, thereby increasing the competitiveness of some of the putative pathogens, for example, by favouring the growth of pathogenic anaerobes such as *P. gingivalis* that have a pH optimum for growth of around pH 7.5 (Fig. 2.4).

Nutrients

Populations within a microbial community are dependent solely on the habitat for the nutrients essential for their growth. Therefore, the association of an organism with a particular habitat is direct evidence that all of the necessary growth-requiring nutrients are present. In Chapter 3 it will become apparent that the mouth can support a microbial community of great diversity and richness, and satisfy the requirements of many nutritionally-demanding bacterial populations.

(i) Endogenous nutrients

The persistence and diversity of the resident oral microflora is due primarily to the metabolism of the endogenous nutrients provided by the host, rather than by exogenous factors in the diet. The main source of endogenous nutrients is saliva, which contains amino acids, peptides, proteins and glycoproteins (which also act as a source of sugars and amino-sugars), vitamins and gases. In addition, the gingival crevice is supplied with GCF which, in addition to delivering components of the host defences, contains novel nutrients, such as albumin and other host proteins and glycoproteins, including haeme-containing molecules (Table 2.2). The difference in source of endogenous nutrients is one of the reasons for the variation in the microflora of the gingival crevice compared with other oral sites (Chs 4 and 5).

Evidence for the importance of endogenous nutrients has also come from the observation that a relatively diverse microbial community persists in the mouth of humans and animals fed by intubation (stomach tube). The proportions of the *S. mitis*-group of bacteria increase in the saliva of children on a starvation diet prior to bone marrow transplantation; these streptococci satisfy their nutritional and energy requirements primarily from the metabolism of host glycoproteins. Also, the oral microflora of animals with dietary habits ranging from insectivores and herbivores to carnivores is broadly similar at the genus level.

Oral bacteria produce glycosidases which can release carbohydrates from the oligosaccharide side chains of salivary mucins. Similarly, organisms isolated from the gingival crevice and periodontal pocket can degrade host proteins and glycoproteins including albumin, transferrin, haemoglobin, and immunoglobulins. Oral microorganisms generally interact synergistically to break down these endogenous nutrients as few species have the full enzyme complement to independently fully catabolize these nutrients. Individual organisms possess different but overlapping patterns of enzyme activity, so that they cooperate and interact with species with complementary degradative activities to achieve complete breakdown of these substrates (Ch. 4).

(ii) Exogenous (dietary) nutrients

Superimposed upon these endogenous nutrients is the complex array of foodstuffs ingested periodically in the diet. Despite the complexity of the diet, fermentable carbohydrates are the only class of compound that markedly influence the ecology of the mouth. These carbohydrates can be broken down to acids while, additionally, sucrose can be converted by bacterial enzymes (glucosyltransferases, GTF, and fructosyltransferases, FTF) into two main classes of exopolymer (glucans and fructans) which can be used to consolidate attachment or act as extracellular nutrient storage compounds, respectively (Ch. 4).

The frequent consumption of dietary carbohydrates is associated with a shift in the proportions of the microflora of dental plaque. The levels of acid-tolerating species, especially mutans streptococci and lactobacilli, increase while the growth of acid-sensitive species (for example, some strains of *Streptococcus sanguinis* and *S. gordonii*) is inhibited, and they decrease. The metabolism of plaque changes so that the predominant fermentation product becomes lactate. Such alterations to the microflora and its metabolism can predispose a site to dental caries. Laboratory studies suggest that it is the repeated low pH generated from sugar metabolism rather than the availability of excess carbohydrate *per se* that is responsible for these perturbations to the microflora.

Dairy products (milk, cheese) have some influence on the ecology of the mouth. The ingestion of milk or milk products can protect the teeth against caries. This may be due to the buffering capacity of milk proteins or due to decarboxylation of amino acids after proteolysis since several bacterial species can metabolise casein. Milk proteins and casein derivatives can also adsorb on to the tooth surface, in exchange for albumin in the enamel pellicle, and reduce the adhesion of mutans streptococci; they can also sequester calcium phosphate and enhance remineralization. Kappa-casein can inhibit GTF adsorption into the pellicle and reduce enzyme activity, thereby suppressing glucan formation. Milk can also modify the structure of the enamel pellicle *in vivo*, producing a distinct globular structure. Cheese has been shown to increase salivary flow rates and to rapidly elevate plaque pH changes following a sucrose rinse.

Xylitol is a sugar substitute that has been added to some confectionery; it cannot be metabolized by oral bacteria and, in addition, xylitol can be inhibitory to the growth of *Streptococcus mutans*. Lower levels of this species have been reported in plaque and saliva of those that frequently consume confectionery containing this polyol. Other alternative sweeteners can also reduce the growth and metabolism of oral bacteria.

Nitrate in green vegetables may influence the oral microflora. Nitrate derived from the diet is concentrated by salivary glands so that salivary concentrations are higher than plasma. This nitrate can be rapidly converted to nitrite by bacterial nitrate reductases. At low pH, this acidified nitrite can be inhibitory to the growth of bacteria implicated in both caries and periodontal diseases, possibly by the further conversion of nitrite to nitric oxide.

Host defences

The health of the mouth is dependent on the integrity of the mucosa (and enamel) which acts as a physical barrier to prevent penetration by microorganisms or antigens (Fig. 2.5). The host has a number of additional defence mechanisms which play an essential role in maintaining the integrity of these oral surfaces, many of which have more than one function. For example, the chemical properties of salivary mucins result in the formation of hydrophilic, viscoelastic gels which function as protective barriers over the oral epithelium, as well as acting in solution as bacterial aggregating factors (the relevance of this property is described below). The host defence molecules are listed in Table 2.3 and their spheres of influence are indicated diagrammatically in Figures 2.5 and 2.6. These defences are divided into non-specific and specific factors. The former, unlike, for example, antibodies, do not require prior exposure to an organism or antigen for activity and so provide a continuous, broad spectrum of protection. An alternative terminology is for the non-specific and specific factors to be termed **innate immunity** and **adaptive immunity**, respectively.

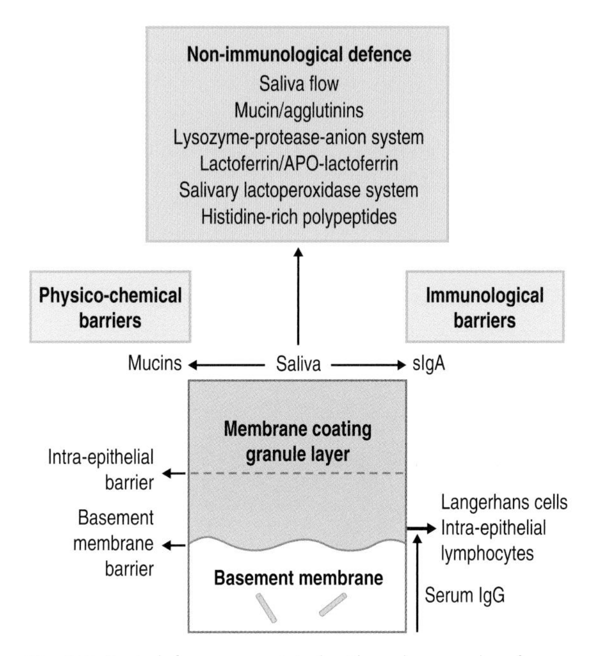

Fig. 2.5 Host defences associated with oral mucosal surfaces.

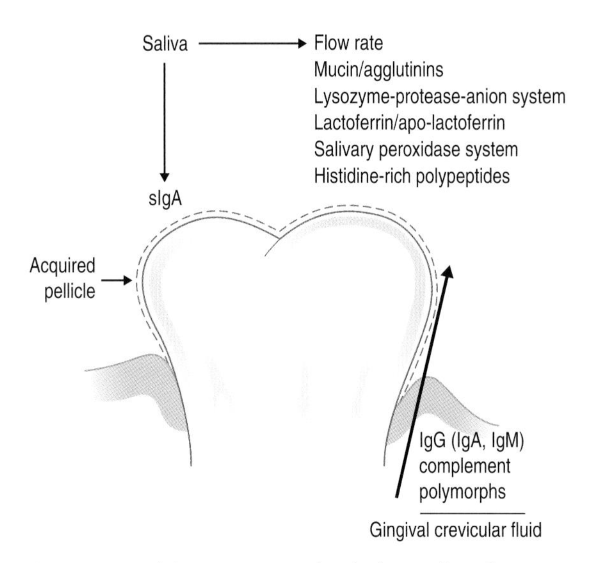

Fig. 2.6 Host defences associated with the tooth surface.

(i) Innate immunity

Microorganisms are unable to maintain themselves in saliva by cell division alone because they are lost at an even faster rate by **swallowing**. Although saliva contains between approximately 10^8 viable microorganisms ml^{-1}, these organisms are all derived from dental plaque and the oral mucosa, especially the tongue. Chewing and the natural flow of saliva (or GCF in the gingival crevice) will remove microorganisms not firmly attached to an oral surface, and their physical removal by swallowing is an important defence mechanism. When saliva flow is blocked, for example, in sedated patients in intensive care, a shift in the composition of the oral microflora can occur resulting in overgrowth by Gram negative species, and this can lead to pulmonary complications. In addition, desquamation ensures that the bacterial load on most mucosal surfaces is light. Thus, the ability of microorganisms to attach firmly to oral surfaces and evade these removal forces becomes a key survival strategy. Paradoxically, saliva also plays an important role in facilitating microbial colonization. Salivary molecules such as proline-rich peptides, statherin, and amylase, are adsorbed on to oral surfaces to form an acquired pellicle, which provides receptors to which only certain microbes are able to attach. Subsequently, salivary glycoproteins act as a nutrient source for the growth of the colonizing organisms. In these ways, saliva plays a pivotal role in determining which microorganisms form part of the resident oral microflora, and which are inhibited and removed. Microbial attachment will be described in more detail in Chapters 4 and 5.

Some salivary molecules can aggregate microbes, which also facilitates their removal from the mouth by swallowing; some of these mechanisms are calcium dependent while others are not. The molecules responsible for agglutination have been characterized. **Mucins** are high-molecular-weight glycoproteins containing >40% carbohydrate. Their protein backbone has oligosaccharide side chains of different length and composition; some of these side chains are branched and sialic acid and fucose are common terminal sugars. Two chemically distinct mucins have been identified in human saliva, and are termed mucin glycoproteins 1 and 2 (MG1 and MG2, respectively); MG1 has a molecular weight >103 kDa while MG2 is only 130–150 kDa. These mucins not only agglutinate oral bacteria, but can also interact with exogenous pathogens such as *Staphylococcus aureus* and *Pseudomonas aeruginosa*, as well as viruses including influenza virus. Mucin binding to bacteria appears to involve blood group reactive components such as *N*-acetylgalactose and sialic acid. Mucins such as MG2 may interact with other salivary components, including secretory IgA, to enhance their antimicrobial activities. A related molecule (salivary agglutinin; M.Wt. 340 kDa) is also highly glycosylated and carries blood group active antigens, and is similar to another defence glycoprotein present in the lung.

Lysozyme is a 14 kDa basic protein that can also aggregate both Gram positive bacteria (including streptococci) and Gram negative periodontal pathogens. It can also lyse bacteria by hydrolyzing peptidoglycan, which confers rigidity to their cell walls. At acidic pH, the lytic action of lysozyme is enhanced by monovalent anions (bicarbonate, fluoride, chloride, or thiocyanate) and proteases found in saliva. **Chitinase** has been detected in saliva, and may function by attacking yeast cell walls. Other non-specific factors in oral secretions include **lactoferrin** (M.Wt = 75 kDa) which is a high-affinity, iron-binding glycoprotein. Iron is essential for microbial growth, and so the host will avidly sequester this cation using iron-binding proteins. A major challenge for microbial pathogens entering the host is to scavenge sufficient iron for growth. Iron-free lactoferrin (**apo-lactoferrin**) can be bactericidal to a range of Gram positive and Gram negative bacteria, although direct binding of the protein to the cell surface is necessary. Lactoferrin is a multi-functional protein having bacteriostatic, bactericidal, fungicidal, antiviral and anti-inflammatory and immunomodulatory properties.

The salivary peroxidase enzyme system (**sialoperoxidase**) can generate hypothiocyanite at neutral pH or hypothiocyanous acid at low pH in the presence of hydrogen peroxide, and both can inhibit glycolysis by plaque bacteria. Hydrogen peroxide is generated as an end product of metabolism by several resident bacterial species, including *Streptococcus sanguinis* and *S. mitis*. Myeloperoxidase is found in polymorphonuclear (PMN) leucocytes, which migrate into the gingival crevice as part of the inflammatory host response to plaque accumulation, and may contribute to the total peroxidase activity measured in saliva.

A number of types of **antimicrobial peptide** (also referred to as **host defence peptides** because their effects can also be immunomodulatory) have been identified in saliva, including histatins and defensins. Antimicrobial peptides are small, cationic peptides (often <50 amino acids) that can act synergistically with other innate defence molecules to not only inhibit exogenous pathogens but also to provide a means by which the host can exert some control over the resident oral microflora. These peptides also bind and neutralize potentially inflammatory molecules found on the surface of microbes (such as lipopolysaccharide) and are chemotactic for host defence cells (neutrophils and lymphocytes), and in this way they play an important immunomodulatory role.

Histatins are a family of histidine-rich basic peptides found in human parotid and submandibular/sublingual gland saliva. There are numerous histatins in human saliva, the majority of which are degradation fragments of two parent molecules, histatin 1 and histatin 3. The major histatins found in saliva are histatins 1, 3 and 5. Individual histatins may have distinct roles, or may function optimally under specific conditions. For example, histatin 5 is more active than histatins 1 and 3 in terms of killing germinated yeast cells, and has the greatest antibacterial activity. In contrast, histatin 3 is a more potent inhibitor of yeast germination. Histatins 1 and 3 appear to be most effective at low pH and low ionic strength. Histatins 5 and 8 could inhibit coaggregation between certain pairs of oral bacteria, interfere with the growth of *S. mutans*, and aggregate other oral streptococci. Histatins can also inhibit host and bacterial proteases and adhesins, and prevent induction of cytokines by bacterial outer membrane proteins. Overall, these peptides have a broad spectrum of antifungal and antibacterial activity, and have properties that may serve to link the innate and the acquired immune system.

Defensins are a family of antibacterial peptides with a broad spectrum of antibacterial, antifungal and antiviral (including HIV) activity. Some are expressed constitutively (e.g. human β-defensin-1) in salivary glands (Fig. 2.7), while others are induced by bacteria and inflammatory mediators. Human β-defensins (HBDs) protect mucosal surfaces, including the gingivae, buccal mucosa and the tongue. HBDs can be associated with mucin, which may protect them from degradation and facilitate their contact with mucin-aggregated bacteria. α-defensins are found primarily (and in high concentrations) in neutrophils, and are responsible for microbial killing within granules. In contrast, β-defensins are mainly found in epithelial cells, and can be detected in monocytes and dendritic cells. HBDs have also been detected in saliva, GCF and gingival junctional epithelium, probably due to release from host phagocytic and other defence cells such as neutrophils, macrophages, monocytes and dendritic cells. The concentration of neutrophil-derived peptides increases in the mouth following inflammation. **Cathelicidin** (LL-37 peptide) is another antimicrobial peptide that is secreted by epithelial

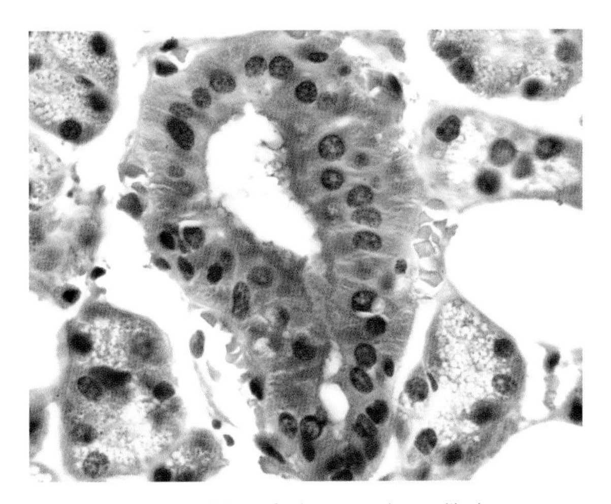

Fig. 2.7 Immunostaining of a human submandibular gland with antibodies to demonstrate the presence of the antimicrobial peptide, β-defensin.

cells and is also found in neutrophils, but is present in secondary granules, which degranulate extracellularly. Synthetic analogues of antimicrobial peptides are being investigated as a novel strategy to inhibit specific oral microbes, and as immunomodulatory therapeutics.

Other salivary proteins that can influence microbial growth include **cystatins**; these are a diverse group of cysteine protease inhibitors and at least nine are present in human saliva. They differ slightly in molecular weight (14–15 kDa), charge, and degree of phosphorylation. Their protease-inhibiting properties imply that their role includes the control of proteolytic activity, either from the host, such as proteases released during inflammation, or from microorganisms. Cystatins are also able to form complexes with mucins, which may enable them to be targeted to different oral surfaces where they may play a role in modulating de-/remineralization processes on enamel. Other inhibitory proteins include **secretory leucocyte proteinase inhibitor** (SLPI), which also has antimicrobial and antiviral properties, **tissue inhibitors of metalloproteinases** (TIMPs), calprotectin (a calcium- and zinc-binding protein which can inhibit bacterial growth), and **chromogranin A** (with anti-fungal and anti-yeast properties). Many of the innate antimicrobial factors described in this section are common to other exocrine secretions (tears, milk, seminal and vaginal secretions) thereby emphazising their fundamental role in providing protection to the host against infection.

(ii) Adaptive immunity

Components of the specific host defences (intraepithelial lymphocytes and Langerhans cells, immunoglobulins IgG and IgA) are found on and within the mucosa (Fig. 2.5), where they act as a barrier to penetrating antigens. The predominant immunoglobulin in the healthy mouth is secretory IgA (sIgA), which is produced by plasma cells in the salivary gland. sIgA is composed of IgA heavy and light chains (300 kDa), secretory component (70 kDa), and the J chain (15 kDa). The J chain connects the two IgA molecules into a dimer, while the secretory component stabilizes the molecule and reduces its susceptibility to attack by acids or general proteases. sIgA can agglutinate oral bacteria, modulate enzyme activity, and inhibit the adherence of bacteria to the buccal epithelium and to enamel. sIgA is usually considered to be a first line of defence by virtue of its local dispersal of environmental antigens. Compared with other classes of immunoglobulin, sIgA is only weakly complement-activating and opsonizing and, therefore, is less likely to cause damage to tissues by any indirect effect of an inflammatory response. Other components (IgG, IgM, IgA, and complement), can be found in saliva but are almost entirely derived from GCF (Table 2.2). GCF also contains leukocytes, of which approximately 95% are polymorphs, the remainder being lymphocytes and monocytes.

Specific antibody production can be stimulated by bacterial antigens associated with plaque at the gingival margin or on the oral mucosa. Salivary antibodies have been detected with activity against a range of oral bacteria, including streptococci, while circulating antibodies (particularly IgG) to a variety of oral microbial antigens have been reported, even in health. In the absence of inflammation, the naturally low levels of complement and polymorphs would reduce antibody-mediated phagocytosis. However, antibodies might still influence the oral microflora, either by interfering with colonization or by inhibiting metabolism. The pattern of the host response in GCF, saliva, or serum is being explored as a method of improved diagnosis of disease or as a means of recognizing at-risk individuals.

The antimicrobial factors described above do not necessarily operate in isolation. Combinations of specific and non-specific host defence factors can function synergistically so that, for example, lysozyme and sIgA can react with salivary agglutinins (mucins) and so be presented directly to immobilized cells. Other synergistic combinations include mucins or sIgA and salivary peroxidase.

Perhaps surprisingly, in spite of this rich array of antimicrobial factors, the mouth harbours a diverse collection of microorganisms. Indeed, this resident microflora confers several beneficial functions on the host. A full description of the indigenous oral microflora, together with a consideration of how it might persist in spite of the host defences, and the benefits it provides will be considered in subsequent chapters.

Host genetics

Studies of periodontal disease have suggested that gender, host genetics and ethnicity can influence disease susceptibility, and possibly also affect the microflora. The reasons for this are unknown, but may reflect some variation in the local immune response. For example, IgG2 is elevated in some forms of periodontal disease, and levels of this immunoglobulin have been related to host genetics. Genetic polymorphisms associated with interleukin-1 (IL-1), or other cytokines, can increase the likelihood of detecting certain key periodontal pathogens, and predispose individuals to periodontitis.

A wide selection of strains of *Aggregatibacter* (formerly *Actinobacillus*) *actinomycetemcomitans* (implicated in aggressive periodontitis; Ch. 6) from different geographical areas have been screened for their genetic relatedness. Strains belonging to serotype *b* were found to overproduce a particular virulence factor (a leukotoxin), and these were all isolated from individuals who could be traced to North West Africa for as yet unknown reasons. Adolescents who carried these serotype *b* strains had an 18-fold increased risk of developing localized aggressive periodontitis. In an adult periodontitis group, *P. gingivalis* and anaerobic streptococci were associated more with African-American subjects whereas *Fusobacterium nucleatum* was found more commonly in Caucasian individuals. This issue is complex, however, as highlighted by a study of young (4–16 years), healthy subjects living in California. Although there was a trend of an increased likelihood of detecting two or more periodontal pathogens (*A. actinomycetemcomitans, P. gingivalis, Tannerella forsythia, Treponema denticola*) in the saliva of Hispanic and Asian-American compared to Caucasian subjects, a more significant factor was related to the length of time their parents had lived in the USA, rather than to ethnicity *per se*. The salivary detection of these selected periodontal bacteria decreased as the number of years of parental residence in the USA increased.

The subgingival microflora of twins has also been compared. The microflora of twin children living together was more similar than that of unrelated children of the same age. Further analysis showed that the microflora of identical twins was more similar than that of fraternal twins, again suggesting some genetic influence.

Antimicrobial agents and inhibitors

In addition to the components of the host defences present in saliva and GCF, the resident oral microflora can be regularly challenged with modest concentrations of antimicrobial and antiplaque agents. Antiplaque agents can remove already attached cells, or prevent adhesion of new cells to the acquired pellicle, without necessarily killing the bacteria whereas antimicrobial agents have a direct inhibitory effect on the microorganism that can be either lethal (bactericidal) or inhibitory, but non-lethal (bacteriostatic). Both types of agent can be delivered from toothpastes (dentifrices) and mouthwashes. Toothpastes contain detergents such as sodium lauryl sulphate as a foaming agent. These are markedly bactericidal in laboratory tests and can lead to the reduction of salivary bacterial counts *in vivo*. Detergents are not usually retained in the mouth for long periods and so their effect is usually transitory. Fluoride is present in most toothpastes and although its primary beneficial anti-caries action is due to its incorporation into enamel and its influence on de- and re-mineralization (Ch. 6), it can also inhibit bacterial metabolism, particularly glycolysis, even at low concentrations especially under acidic conditions. In this way, fluoride may help prophylactically to suppress cariogenic and acid-tolerant species such as mutans streptococci under the very conditions under which they would otherwise flourish. Many toothpastes and mouthrinses are now being manufactured with proven antimicrobial agents, although formulation issues mean that not all can be used in toothpastes. Metal ions, phenolic compounds, and plant extracts have been successfully formulated into toothpastes, and their mode of action will be discussed in more detail in Chapter 6. The regular use of products containing these agents has been carefully assessed to ensure that their action is selective so that they inhibit organisms implicated with disease rather than those associated with oral health, thereby ensuring that the natural beneficial properties of the resident microflora are not irrevocably disrupted.

Other antimicrobial agents can be delivered via mouthrinses, and the most potent agent to date is chlorhexidine. This agent has proven antibacterial, antiviral and antifungal activity (Ch. 6), and it also has marked antiplaque activity, which is useful for individuals for whom oral hygiene is difficult. Other mouthrinses contain antimicrobial agents including 'essential oils' (such as thymol and menthol), Triclosan and plant extracts. Some of these agents can also combat oral malodour (halitosis).

Antibiotics given systemically or orally for problems at other sites in the body will enter the mouth via saliva or GCF and can affect the stability of the oral microflora. Within a few hours of taking prophylactic high doses of penicillins or erythromycin, the salivary microflora can be suppressed permitting overgrowth by yeasts or the emergence of antibiotic-resistant bacteria (Chs 8 and 9). These resistant bacteria can persist at significant levels for several weeks before returning to their low base-line values. The antibiotic should be changed if several courses of treatment are necessary and the interval between courses is less than one month.

Concluding remarks

Despite the potential for regular environmental perturbations in some of the host and environmental factors described above, once established at a site, the oral microflora remains relatively stable in composition and proportions over time. This stability is termed microbial homeostasis and is discussed further in Chapter 5.

SUMMARY

The mouth provides conditions suitable for the growth of a diverse collection of microorganisms, despite the presence of a complex array of components of the innate and adaptive host defences. The resident microflora is provided with a wide range of endogenous and exogenous nutrients, together with sufficient heterogeneity in pH and redox potential, to accommodate microbes with a variety of requirements.

CHAPTER SUMMARY

The mouth is not a uniform habitat for microbial growth and colonization. A variety of surfaces produce distinct habitats due to their physical nature and biological properties. These include a variety of mucosal surfaces as well as teeth; the latter are unique for microbial colonization by virtue of their being hard and non-shedding thereby providing the opportunity for substantial biofilm formation (dental plaque).

The surfaces of the mouth are lubricated by saliva, while the gingival crevice is bathed with GCF. Both fluids will remove weakly-attached microorganisms by their flushing action, and they deliver components of the innate and adaptive immune response that help regulate bacterial and fungal colonization. Saliva and GCF contribute to the acquired pellicle, and are also the primary sources of nutrients for oral microorganisms. Consortia of different bacterial species with complementary patterns of glycosidase and protease activities are required to break down host glycoproteins. In these ways, saliva and GCF play pivotal roles in the microbial ecology of the mouth. Dietary components have much less of an influence on the composition of the microflora of the mouth, although the frequent intake of fermentable carbohydrates can lead to increases in acidogenic and acid-tolerating (aciduric) organisms that are potentially cariogenic due to the low pH generated from their catabolism. Other factors that influence the growth of microorganisms in the mouth include the Eh and pH of a site, the activity of the host defences, and the presence of antimicrobial agents.

There is a dynamic interaction between the oral environment and the composition and metabolism of the resident oral microflora. Therefore, a substantial change in a key environmental parameter that affects microbial growth can disrupt the natural balance of the microflora and select for organisms that are potentially pathogenic.

FURTHER READING

Aframian DJ, Davidowitz T, Benoliel R 2006 The distribution of oral mucosal pH values in healthy saliva secretors. Oral Dis 12:420-423.

Darveau R 2000 Oral innate host defense responses: interactions with microbial communities and their role in the development of disease. In: Kuramitsu HK, Ellen RP (eds) Oral bacterial ecology. The molecular basis. Horizon Scientific Press, Wymondham, p 169-218.

Delima AJ, van Dyke TE 2000 Origin and function of the cellular components in gingival crevicular fluid. Periodontology 2000 31:55-76.

Devine DA 2003 Antimicrobial peptides in defence of the oral and respiratory tracts. Molec Immunol 40:431-443.

Devine DA, Cosseau C 2008 Antimicrobial host defense peptides in the oral cavity. Adv Appl Microbiol 63:281-322.

Lamster IB, Ahlo JK 2007 Analysis of gingival crevicular fluid as applied to the diagnosis of oral and systemic

diseases. Ann N Y Acad Sci 1098: 216-229.
Nibali L, Ready DR, Parkar M et al 2007 Gene polymorphisms and the prevalence of key periodontal pathogens. J Dent Res 86:416-420.
Nieuw Amerongen AV, Veerman ECI 2002 Saliva – the defender of the oral cavity. Oral Dis 8:12-22.
Sirinian G, Shimizu T, Sugar C et al 2002 Periodontopathic bacteria in young healthy subjects of different ethnic backgrounds in Los Angeles. J. Periodontol 73:283-288.
Uitto VJ 2003 Gingival crevicular fluid – an introduction. Periodontology 2000 31: 9-11.

Chapter 3

The resident oral microflora

The resident oral microflora is diverse and consists of a wide range of viruses, mycoplasmas, bacteria, yeasts and even, on occasions, protozoa. This diversity is due to the fact that the mouth is composed of a number of varied habitats supplied with diverse nutrients. In addition, in biofilms such as dental plaque, gradients develop in parameters of ecological significance, such as oxygen tension and pH, providing conditions suitable for the growth and survival of microorganisms with a wide spectrum of requirements. Under such conditions, no single bacterial population has a particular advantage and numerous species can co-exist. Plaque also functions as a true microbial community and numerous examples of synergistic metabolic interactions have been described. This will enable some fastidious bacteria to survive and grow as part of a mixed culture under conditions they would be unable to tolerate if in pure culture in a more homogeneous environment.

Before the microbial community at individual sites in the mouth can be considered in detail (Chs 4 and 5), the types and properties of the organisms found commonly in health and disease will be described. First, however, it may be instructive to discuss the principles of microbial classification and identification, and describe briefly some of the methods used. **Classification** is the arrangement of organisms into groups (taxa) on the basis of their similarities and differences. In contrast, **identification** is the process of determining that a new isolate belongs to a particular taxon; the aim of classification is to define these taxa at the **genus** or **species** level. Traditionally, a hierarchical system has existed for the naming of bacteria so that groups of closely-related organisms form a species, and related species are placed in a genus, etc. (Table 3.1); species are designated by Latin

Table 3.1 Hierarchical ranks in microbial classification

Taxonomic rank	Example
Kingdom	*Procaryotae*
Division	*Firmicutes*
Sub-division	low G+C content of DNA
Order	-
Family	*Streptococcaceae*
Genus	*Streptococcus*
Species	*Streptococcus mutans*
Serotype*	*Streptococcus mutans* serotype *c*
Strain*	*Streptococcus mutans* NCTC 10449**

*These ranks are not formally recognised in taxonomy, but are of great practical importance.
**NCTC = National Collection of Type Cultures.

or latinized binomials (e.g. *Streptococcus mutans*; the genus is '*Streptococcus*' and the species is '*mutans*', Table 3.1). If an isolate does not belong to an existing taxon, then a new species can be proposed. The naming of bacteria to reflect this classification (**nomenclature**) is regulated by international committees. Once an organism has been placed in a species, it may be possible to sub-type individual strains; this can be valuable in epidemiological studies investigating transmission of strains between individuals. The interrelationships between these approaches (classification, identification, strain typing) are shown in Fig. 3.1. The classification, nomenclature and identification of microorganisms is referred to as **taxonomy**, although, sometimes, the terms classification and taxonomy are used interchangeably.

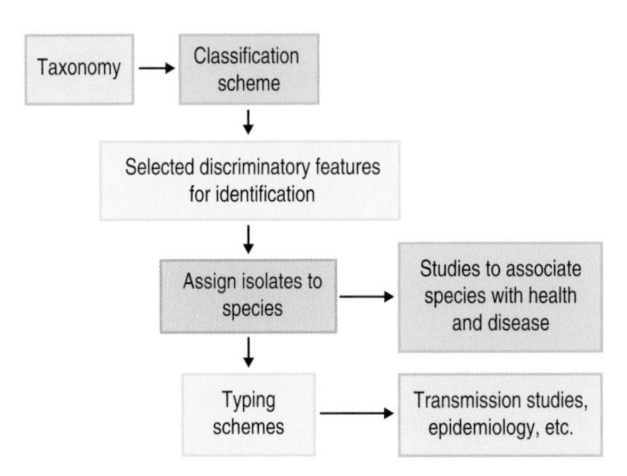

Fig. 3.1 Diagramatic representation to distinguish classification, identification and typing of bacterial strains.

PRINCIPLES OF MICROBIAL CLASSIFICATION

As stated above, the purpose of classification schemes is to develop a logical arrangement of organisms based on their similarities and relationships. This requires the determination and comparison of as many characteristics as possible, although in identification schemes, only a few key discriminatory tests may be needed to distinguish between certain organisms. Early classification schemes relied heavily on morphological and simple physiological criteria such as the shape of the cell, and the pattern of fermentation of simple sugars (Table 3.2). In effect, these approaches analysed only a fraction of the

Table 3.2 Some characteristics used in microbial classification and identification schemes

Characteristic	Examples
Cellular morphology	Shape; Gram stain reaction; flagella; spores; size
Colonial appearance	Pigment; haemolysis; shape; size
Carbohydrate fermentation	Acid or gas production
Amino acid hydrolysis	Ammonia production
Pattern of fermentation products	Butyrate; lactate; acetate
Preformed enzymes	Glycosidases (e.g. α-glucosidase)
Antigen	Monoclonal/polyclonal antibodies to cell surface proteins
Lipids	Menaquinones, long-chain fatty acids
DNA	Base composition (G + C ratio); 16S rRNA gene sequence
Enzyme profile	Presence/absence; electrophoretic mobility
Peptidoglycan	Amino acid composition e.g. lysine

components encoded by the genetic material of the cell (the **genome**). **Chemotaxonomy**, in which there is a broader analysis of more complex components of the cell (for example, the chemical composition of the cell wall or of membrane lipids, whole cell protein profiles, etc) led to major improvements in classification schemes. The structure of cells can also be compared using immunological techniques (**serology**), in which specific antibodies (polyclonal or monoclonal) are used to detect cell surface antigens.

Contemporary classification schemes are based more on determining the genetic relatedness among strains. As the properties of an organism are dictated by what is encoded by its genome, the ultimate comparison is to determine the similarity in **DNA base composition**. The mole percentage of guanine (G) plus cytosine (C) in the total DNA can be determined. Organisms with markedly different G+C contents are unrelated, while organisms that have similar G+C values are closely related, although similarity in gross DNA composition is not unequivocal proof of close relatedness because the base pairs could be organised in a different sequence. In such a situation, genotypic similarity can be confirmed by determining the degree of relatedness (**homology**) between the DNA from two strains i.e. the abilities of heat-denatured, single strands of DNA from different strains to re-anneal with each other, or to a reference strain, during slow cooling **(DNA–DNA hybridization).** A high level of homology reflects an overall similarity in the nucleotide sequences from the DNA of the two strains being compared, and hence confirms the close taxonomic relationship of the strains.

Classification is now dominated by comparisons of the sequence of **16S ribosomal RNA genes** (16S rRNA). Within the rRNA gene, some stretches of DNA sequence are conserved while other areas are highly variable and reflect evolutionary divergence. These genes are around 1500 nucleotides long, which is short enough for rapid sequencing in conventional laboratories (using automated DNA sequencing equipment) but long enough to provide valuable discriminatory information to demonstrate similarities and differences among strains. The conserved regions can be used as a template for the design of 'universal' PCR (polymerase chain reaction) oligonucleotide primers that can be used to amplify the rest of the 16S rRNA gene, which can then be sequenced to identify differences in the variable regions. The sequences can be compared with those from other microorganisms, and to sequences in nucleotide databases, so that the relationship of an isolate to known species can be determined and **evolutionary (phylogenetic) trees** can be developed. The technique is relatively rapid, and has facilitated the analysis of a far wider range of bacteria than was previously possible. Comparison of 16S rRNA gene sequences have revolutionized the field of microbial taxonomy, and has clarified the classification of many previously heterogeneous groups of oral bacteria, such as the streptococci (Table 3.3) and anaerobic Gram positive rods formerly grouped as *Eubacterium* species (Fig. 3.5). In addition to classifying unknown strains, this approach can also be used to identify isolates, and has many advantages over conventional cultural approaches (see later; Fig. 3.2).

A consequence of classification is the proposal of new species. A species represents a collection of strains that share many features in common, and which differ considerably from other strains. Once a species has been recognised, then a **type strain** is nominated that has properties representative of the species. Type strains are held in national collections,

Table 3.3 Species of oral streptococci isolated from humans

Group	Species	
mutans-group*	*S. mutans*	serotypes *c,e, f, k*
	S. sobrinus	seroype *d, g*
	S. criceti	serotype *a*
	S. ratti	serotype *b*
salivarius-group	*S. salivarius*	
	S. vestibularis	
anginosus-group	*S. constellatus*	
	S. intermedius	
	S. anginosus	
mitis-group	*S. sanguinis*	
	S. gordonii	
	S. parasanguinis	
	S. oralis	
	S. mitis	
	S. cristatus	
	S. oligofermentans	
	S. sinensis	
	S. australis	
	S. peroris	
	S. infantis	

*mutans streptococci also include *S. ferus* (isolated from rats), *S. macacae* and *S. downei* (serotype *h*) (isolated from monkeys).

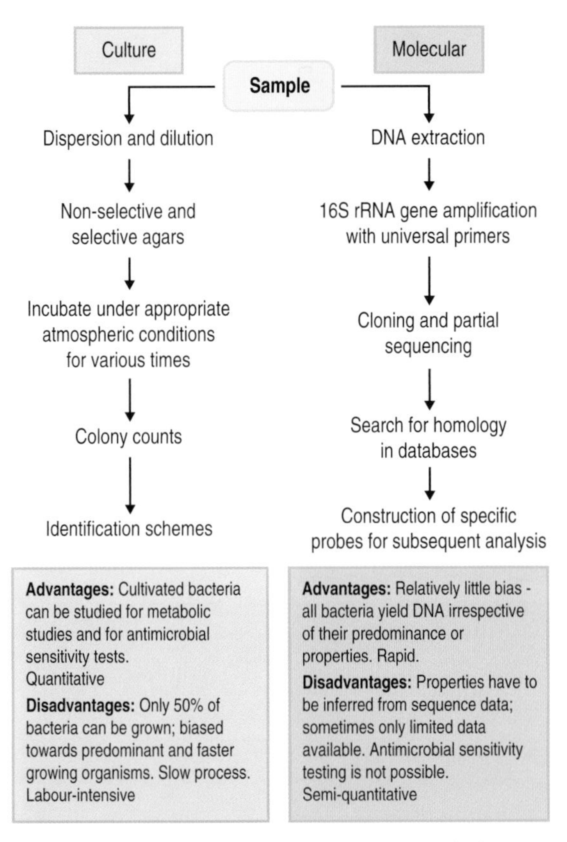

Fig. 3.2 The main stages in determining the microbial composition of the microflora of samples from the mouth using either culture or molecular approaches.

such as the American Type Culture Collection, ATCC, or the National Collection of Type Cultures, NCTC, which is located in the United Kingdom.

A species may be divided into subspecies if minor but consistent phenotypic variations can be recognised. Likewise, groups of strains within a species can sometimes be distinguished by a special characteristic. For example, strains with a special biochemical or physiological property are termed **biovars** or **biotypes**, while strains with a distinctive antigenic composition are described as **serovars** or **serotypes,** and can be recognised using appropriate antibodies. Molecular approaches can also be adapted for subtyping strains within a species. Whole genomic DNA can be digested by different restriction enzymes (**endonucleases**), which cut the nucleic acid in specific places; these digests are then electrophoresed on an agarose gel to generate a chromosomal fingerprint. Different strains generate different patterns (**restriction fragment length polymorphisms, RFLPs**), although strains that appear to give similar patterns need to be compared after digestion with more than one enzyme. This approach can yield patterns too complex to analyse. In order to overcome this problem, the restriction fragments can be blotted onto nitrocellulose or nylon membranes, and hybridized with a suitably labelled probe to give a simpler profile. A 'universal probe' can be used, based on part of the rRNA gene sequence, and this can yield different patterns within a species (**ribotyping**). Ribotyping has allowed insights to be made into the transmission of strains among family members, especially from mothers to their babies, and in demonstrating the turnover of specific ribotypes (and specific clones) at a site (Ch. 4).

PRINCIPLES OF CONVENTIONAL MICROBIAL IDENTIFICATION

Once organisms have been correctly classified using rigorous techniques, then more simple identification schemes can be devised in which only limited numbers of key discriminatory properties are compared (Fig. 3.1, Table 3.2). The first stage might involve the reaction of an organism with the Gram stain, and the determination of cellular morphology. Bacteria are then described as being, for example, Gram positive cocci or Gram negative rods, etc. Depending on the outcome of that division, simple physiological tests may be performed, such as the determination of sugar fermentation patterns, the profiles of acidic fermentation products following glucose metabolism, or selected enzyme activities. The rapid detection (ca. 4 hours) of constitutively-expressed enzymes by concentrated suspensions of bacteria has simplified the identification of some groups of bacteria. Ecologically-relevant substrates that detect enzymes such as glycosidases that cleave sugar residues from salivary mucins are now more commonly used to differentiate groups of bacteria that had previously been difficult to separate, for example, some oral streptococci. Some of these tests have been incorporated in kits and sold commercially, together with computerized databases, to facilitate identification.

Monoclonal antibodies and nucleic acid (oligonucleotide) probes have been developed for the rapid identification of some species, but primarily those associated with disease. Such antibodies and probes can be labelled with a signalling group to aid in detection; examples include fluorescent dyes (Fig. 3.3), radiolabels, or enzymes such as horseradish peroxidase. These techniques have the advantage

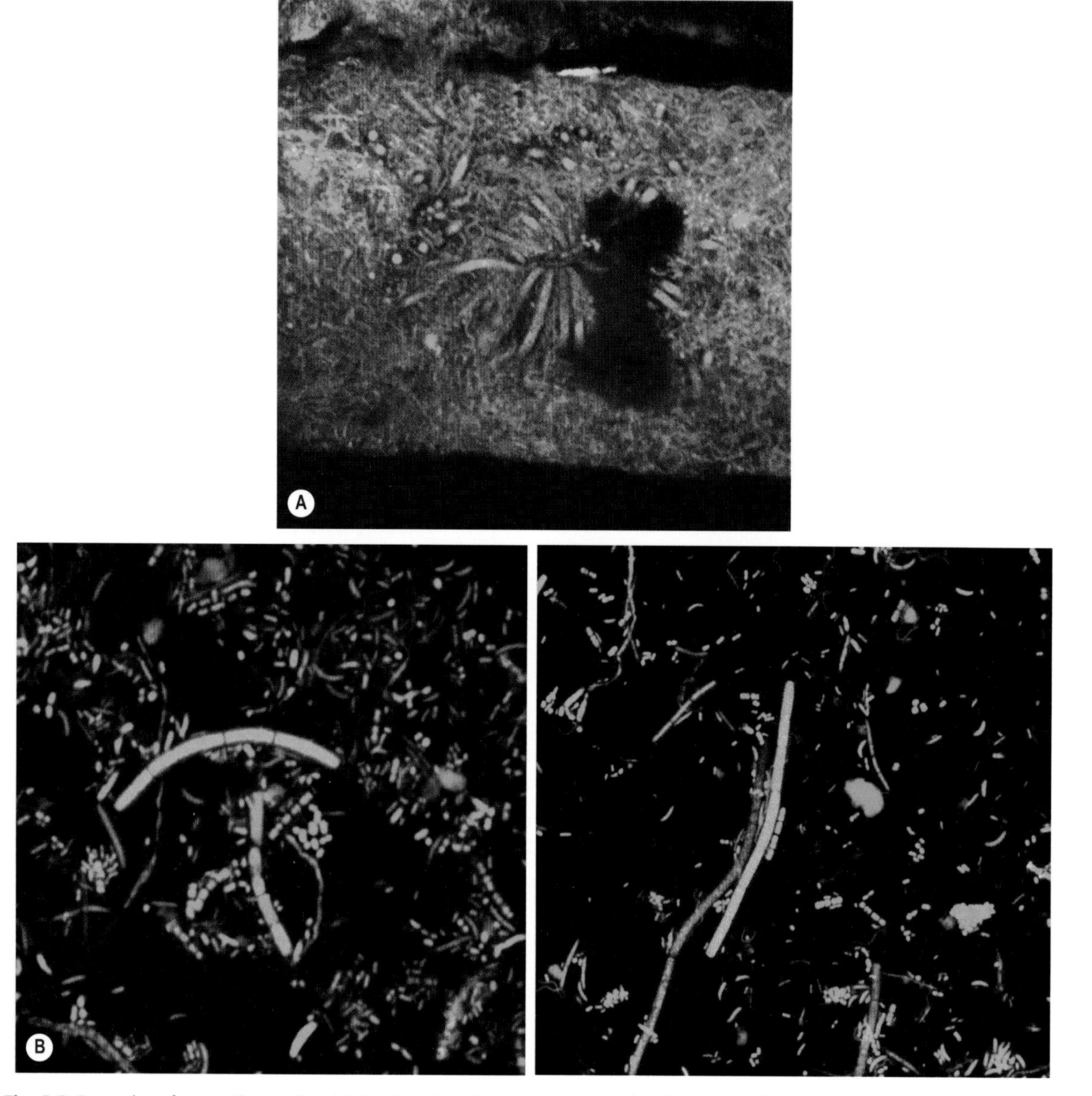

Fig. 3.3 Examples of currently unculturable bacteria in sub-gingival plaque visualized using fluorescent *in situ* hybridization (FISH) techniques. (A) 16S rRNA oligonucleotide probes were used to detect bacteria (green) and *Treponema* spp (red). Courtesy of Dr Annette Moter and produced with permission by Springer-Verlag GmbH & Co. (Norris SJ, Paster BJ, Moter A and Gobel UB, The genus *Treponema*, in The Prokaryotes, Third Edition; Springer, Berlin, 2007). (B) 16S rRNA oligonucleotide probes were used to detect bacteria (green) and members of the TM7 phylum (blue). Courtesy of Dr Cleber Ouverney and the American Society for Microbiology (see Ouverney et al Appl Environ Microbiol 2003 69:6294-6298).

that organisms can be detected directly in plaque or a clinical sample without the need for lengthy culturing, although a potential drawback is that they can detect dead as well as viable cells.

Conventional microbial identification schemes can only be used when organisms have been isolated and grown in pure culture. Inevitably, the procedure for achieving pure culture (sample dispersion and dilution, growth on selective and non-selective agar plates, incubation conditions, etc) leads to the introduction of bias towards those microorganisms that grow quickly and easily under laboratory conditions (Fig. 3.2). Alternative, culture-independent, procedures have evolved out of modern taxonomic approaches, and these are giving a more accurate picture of the diversity (richness) of the microflora from a wide range of habitats.

THE IMPACT OF MOLECULAR MICROBIAL ECOLOGY

As stated above, the genetic relatedness of microorganisms is now primarily determined by comparisons of **16S ribosomal RNA** (rRNA) **gene** sequences. The biggest impact of this approach has been in the analysis of diverse communities of microorganisms from a number of habitats (**molecular microbial ecology**), including the mouth. Comparisons of the number of cells in samples that can be observed by microscopy versus those that can be cultured in the laboratory, even when using the most advanced techniques, has shown that only a proportion of the microflora at a site can be grown. The culturable fraction can vary from less than 1% of the total cell count in some marine habitats to about 50% of the oral microflora. These organisms that cannot currently be grown are termed '**unculturable**'; the reasons for this may be ignorance of an essential nutrient or other growth requirement, or because they evolved to grow as part of a community of cells, rather than as an isolated pure culture. Molecular ecological approaches have enabled the construction of phylogenetic trees that include currently unculturable organisms, so that in many cases, a genus and species name can still be assigned. Oligonucleotide probes can also be synthesized so that the presence of these organisms can be determined relatively simply in clinical samples using rapid tests, such as the polymerase chain reaction (PCR) or by *in situ* hybridization, usually with a fluorescent label (Fig. 3.3). An important benefit of these PCR-based molecular approaches is their potential to detect organisms that are present in low numbers. Although the properties of these uncultivable organisms cannot be determined using conventional tests (such as sugar fermentation patterns or their antibiotic sensitivity profile), databases of genes exist that can be interrogated to search for homologous sequences with known functions. This can provide insights into potentially important properties of these unculturable organisms, such as their cell wall structure, their virulence attributes, and the metabolic pathways they might use.

The existence of these unculturable bacteria cannot be ignored, since their presence at a site could be highly significant; for example, the aetiological agent of syphilis is a spirochaete, *Treponema pallidum*, that still cannot be grown in the laboratory. Two large families of novel unculturable bacteria have been identified in the mouth (Fig. 3.3), and these are commonly detected in deep periodontal pockets; further details will be presented later in this Chapter. In addition, some genera contain examples of both culturable and unculturable species; for example, there are around 50 *Treponema* species that can be seen by microscopy and detected by molecular approaches but which cannot be grown (Fig. 3.3A). Similarly, the molecular analysis of the microflora associated with dento-alveolar abscesses and endodontic infections has consistently identified novel groups of bacteria that were not recognised, or were grossly under-estimated, in parallel cultural studies (Fig. 3.2).

Molecular approaches have also been developed to compare the diversity of oral microbial communities from different sites in health and disease. These approaches include microbial community profiling using denaturing gradient gel electrophoresis (DGGE). Total genomic DNA is extracted from clinical samples, amplified by PCR using universal primers for bacterial 16S rRNA genes, and products resolved on polyacrylamide gels with a denaturing gradient. DGGE profiles can be analysed using appropriate software, and novel or discriminatory bands can be excised from the gel, cloned, and sequenced, enabling a presumptive identification to be made. Alternatively, techniques based on checkerboard DNA–DNA hybridization using labelled whole genomic probes and nylon membranes can be used to simultaneously screen multiple clinical samples for around 40 different pre-selected microbial species.

These culture-independent approaches are radically changing our perception of the diversity of the resident oral microflora in health and disease. Work is underway to identify the signature DNA sequences of all of the microorganisms in the mouth (culturable and unculturable). In the future, DNA microarray chips will be available, with the ability to detect each component or specific subsets of the resident oral microflora, enabling clinicians to rapidly screen for the presence or absence of over 700 organisms, thereby leading to the promise of improved diagnostic and treatment opportunities.

SUMMARY

Knowledge of the oral microflora depends on accurate and robust classification systems from which simpler identification schemes can be developed. Both processes have been revolutionized by the advent of molecular approaches, especially those based on 16S rRNA gene sequences. Comparisons of data from culture and molecular approaches suggest that around 50% of the oral microflora is currently classed as being 'unculturable'.

DIFFICULTIES ARISING FROM RECENT ADVANCES IN MICROBIAL CLASSIFICATION

Although recent advances have led to improvements in the classification of oral bacteria, such improvements have also generated a number of difficulties when interpreting or comparing early data when a previous (and sometimes flawed) nomenclature was in use. The classification of many groups of oral bacteria has been revolutionized in a relatively short time period, with many new genera and species described. A species highlighted in an early study may now have been reclassified and hence renamed, and so new and old terminologies may coexist in the scientific literature. For example, *Streptococcus sanguis* has been reported in the literature for many decades but, as of 1989, its description became more limited and organisms that were previously included within this species are now known to be sufficiently different as to warrant a distinct species epithet, e.g. *S. gordonii*. Consequently, some strains reported in earlier studies as *S. sanguis* may not have the same properties as strains more recently identified as *S. sanguis sensu stricto*. Furthermore, the Latin name originally given to some of the oral streptococci has recently been shown to be erroneous, and so *S. sanguis* is now termed *S. sanguinis*. For similar reasons, *S. parasanguis*, *S. rattus*, *S. cricetus* and *S. crista* have been renamed as *S. parasanguinis*, *S. ratti*, *S. criceti* and *S. cristatus*, respectively. Thus, great care has to be taken when interpreting older (and not so old) scientific literature.

Microbial taxonomy is a dynamic area with existing species being reclassified due to the application of more stringent tests, together with the recognition of genuinely newly-discovered species from sites such as periodontal pockets and infected root canals. The emphasis paid to the classification and identification of the oral microflora is necessary because without valid subdivision and accurate identification of isolates, the specific association of species with particular diseases (**microbial aetiology**) cannot be determined. Likewise, it has to be accepted that further changes in microbial classification schemes will occur in the future and new genera and species will be identified. The properties of the main groups of microorganism found in the mouth will now be described.

GRAM POSITIVE COCCI

Streptococcus

Streptococci have been isolated from all sites in the mouth and comprise a large proportion of the resident cultivable oral microflora. The majority are alpha-haemolytic (partial haemolysis) on blood agar and early workers grouped them together, calling them viridans streptococci. However, haemolysis is not a reliable property in distinguishing these streptococci, and many oral species contain strains showing all 3 types of haemolysis (alpha, beta and gamma). These 'viridans'-group streptococci are now clustered into four groups (Table 3.3) and will now be described.

Mutans-group (mutans streptococci)

There is great interest in the mutans streptococci because of their role in the aetiology of dental caries. *S. mutans* was originally isolated from carious human teeth by Clarke in 1924 and, shortly afterwards, was recovered from a case of infective endocarditis (growth of bacteria on damaged heart valves). Little attention was paid to this species until the 1960s when it was demonstrated that caries could be experimentally-induced and transmitted in animals artificially-infected with strains resembling *S. mutans*. The name of this species derives from the fact that cells can lose their coccal morphology and often appear as short rods or as cocco-bacilli (Fig. 3.4A). Nine serotypes have been recognised (*a*–*h*, and *k*), based on the serological specificity of carbohydrate antigens located in the cell wall, although some serotypes are found only in animals. Subsequent work showed that sufficient differences existed between clusters of these serotypes to warrant their sub-division into seven distinct species (Table 3.3); these species are described collectively as **mutans streptococci**. Mutans streptococci are recovered almost exclusively from hard,

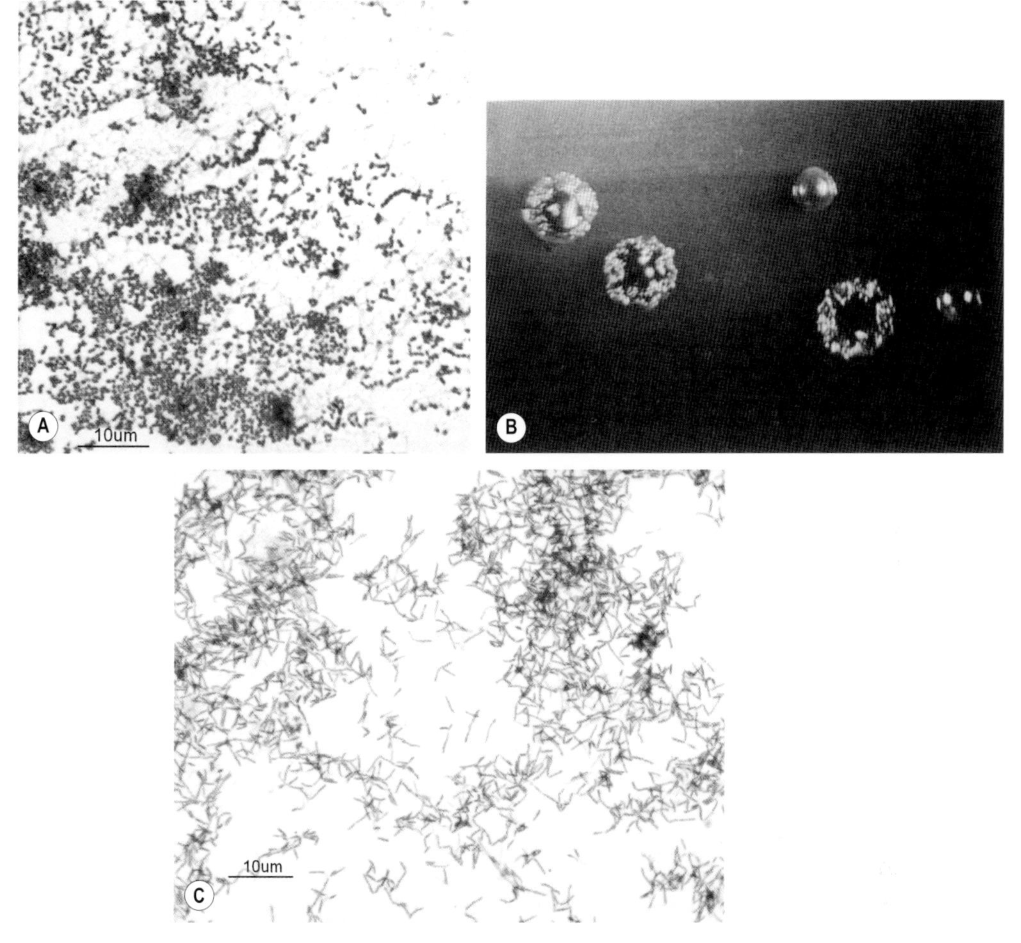

Fig. 3.4 (A) The cell morphology of *Streptococcus mutans* when viewed by light microscopy. (B) The colony morphology of *Streptococcus mutans* growing on sucrose-containing agar. (C) The cell morphology of *Actinomyces naeslundii*.

non-shedding surfaces in the mouth, such as teeth or dentures, and they can act as opportunistic pathogens, being isolated from cases of infective endocarditis (biofilms growing on damaged heart valves; Ch. 8). Mutans streptococci are regularly isolated from dental plaque at carious sites, but their prevalence is low on sound enamel.

The specific epithet, *S. mutans*, is now limited to human isolates previously belonging to serotypes *c, e, f* and *k*. This is the most commonly isolated species of mutans streptococci, and epidemiological studies have implicated *S. mutans* as the primary pathogen in the aetiology of enamel caries in children and young adults, root surface caries in the elderly, and nursing (or bottle) caries in infants (Ch. 6). The next most commonly isolated species of the mutans streptococci group is *S. sobrinus* (serotypes *d* and *g*), which has also been associated with human dental caries. Less is known about the role of *S. sobrinus* in disease because some studies do not attempt to distinguish between these species, while some commonly-used selective media for the isolation of mutans streptococci contain bacitracin which can be inhibitory to the growth of both *S. sobrinus* and *S. criceti* (formerly *S. cricetus*) (serotype *a*). *S. criceti* is recovered only rarely from humans. Some people harbour more than one species of mutans streptococci in their mouth.

The antigenic structure of mutans streptococci has been studied in detail in order to establish serological typing schemes and during the development of a prospective caries vaccine (Ch. 6). Mutans streptococci possess cell wall carbohydrate antigens, lipoteichoic acid, lipoproteins and cell wall or cell wall-associated proteins (Ch. 4). Antigen I/II (also termed antigen B, SpaP or Pac) has generated considerable interest because of its inclusion in a possible sub-unit vaccine; a similar protein is designated SpaA in *S. sobrinus*. Antigen I/II may be involved in the initial adherence of *S. mutans* to the tooth surface by interacting with components of the salivary pellicle (Chs 4 and 5).

Mutans streptococci make extracellular soluble and insoluble extracellular polysaccharides (glucan, mutan and fructan) from sucrose that are associated with plaque maturation (Chs 4 and 5) and cariogenicity (Ch. 6). The glucans and fructans are produced by glucosyl- and fructosyltransferases, respectively. Mutan is a highly insoluble glucan that is only produced by mutans streptococci, while the fructan is unusual in having an inulin-like structure. These polymers contribute to the characteristic colonial morphology of mutans streptococci when growing on sucrose-containing agar plates (Fig. 3.4B). Mutans streptococci can also synthesise intracellular polysaccharides when there is excess sugar, and these can act as carbohydrate reserves, and be converted to acid during periods when dietary carbohydrates are not available. Mutans streptococci can scavenge dietary sugars very efficiently, and rapidly convert them to acidic fermentation products (mainly lactate); significantly, they are also able to grow and survive under the acidic conditions they generate, by the induction of specific molecular stress responses (Ch. 4; Fig. 2.4). Mutans streptococci can communicate with other mutans streptococci by the release of diffusible signalling molecules that can induce genetic competence (an ability to take up extracellular DNA) and acid tolerance in neighbouring cells.

Salivarius-group

This group comprises *S. salivarius* and *S. vestibularis*. Strains of *S. salivarius* are commonly isolated from most areas of the mouth although they preferentially colonize mucosal surfaces, especially the tongue. They produce large quantities of an unusual extracellular fructan (polymer of fructose but with a levan structure) from sucrose (Ch. 4), as well as a levanase that can degrade this type of fructan. This levan gives rise to characteristically large mucoid colonies when *S. salivarius* is grown on sucrose-containing agar. *S. salivarius* also produces some extracellular soluble and insoluble glucans from sucrose. *S. salivarius* is isolated only rarely from diseased sites, and is not considered a significant opportunistic pathogen.

S. vestibularis is isolated mainly from the vestibular mucosa of the human mouth. These strains do not produce extracellular polysaccharides from sucrose, but do produce a urease (which can generate ammonia and hence raise the local pH) and hydrogen peroxide (which can contribute to the sialoperoxidase system [Ch. 2], and inhibit the growth of competing bacteria).

Anginosus-group

Representative species of this group are readily isolated from dental plaque and from mucosal surfaces, and are an important cause of serious, purulent disease in humans, including maxillo-facial infections. They are commonly found in abscesses of internal organs, especially of the brain and liver, and have also been recovered from cases of appendicitis, peritonitis, meningitis and endocarditis. Initially, these bacteria were grouped together as either *S. milleri* (in Europe) or as *S. MG-intermedius* and *S. anginosus-constellatus* (in North America). These bacteria are now differentiated into *S. constellatus*, *S. intermedius* and *S. anginosus*; *S. constellatus* is subdivided further into subspecies *constellatus* and subspecies *pharyngis*. *S. intermedius* is isolated mainly from liver and brain abscesses, while *S. anginosus* and *S. constellatus* are derived from purulent infections from a wider range of sites. *S. intermedius* strains produce a protein toxin, intermedilysin, which may affect neutrophil function and enable the cell to evade the host defences in abscess formation. No strains from this group make extracellular polysaccharides from sucrose.

Mitis-group

The recent application of molecular phylogenetic techniques (involving the determination of 16S rRNA gene sequences) has resolved many of the previous anomalies in the classification of this group, resulting in the identification of some new species.

S. sanguinis (formerly *S. sanguis*) and *S. gordonii* are early colonizers of the tooth surface, and both produce extracellular soluble and insoluble glucans (Ch. 4) from sucrose that contribute to plaque formation. Both species can generate ammonia from arginine. *S. sanguinis* produces a protease that can cleave sIgA (IgA protease) while *S. gordonii* can bind salivary α-amylase enabling these organisms to break down starch. Amylase-binding may also mask bacterial antigens and allow the organism to avoid recognition by the host defences (host mimicry). Both species are composed of several biotypes.

Two of the most common streptococcal species in the mouth are *S. mitis* and *S. oralis*. Strains of *S. oralis* produce neuraminidase (an enzyme that removes sialic acid from oligosaccharide side chains of salivary mucins) and an IgA protease, but cannot bind α-amylase. *S. mitis* is subdivided into two biotypes, and these show different distribution patterns in the mouth. Strains representing these two species are able to take up extracellular DNA (i.e. they are genetically competent), and this process is facilitated in biofilms such as dental plaque where bacteria are in close proximity to one another. Consequently, it is perhaps not surprising that there is considerable genetic and phenotypic heterogeneity when the properties of large numbers of *S. mitis* and *S. oralis* strains are compared. Some, but not all, strains from these two species are able to produce extracellular glucan from sucrose.

Other members of this group include *S. parasanguinis* (formerly *S. parasanguis*) which has been isolated from clinical specimens (throat, blood, urine). Strains can hydrolyse arginine but not urea, and can bind salivary α-amylase, but cannot produce extracellular polysaccharides from sucrose. *S. cristatus* (formerly *S. crista*) is characterised by the presence of tufts of fibrils on their cell surface (Ch. 4). More recently, new species have been described including *S.oligofermentans*, *S. sinensis* (isolated from cases of infective endocarditis), *S. australis*, *S. infantis* and *S. peroris*. The significance of some of these species to the ecology of the mouth has yet to be determined.

Members of the mitis-group are opportunistic pathogens, particularly in infective endocarditis (Ch. 8). *S. pneumoniae* can be isolated from the nasopharynx and is a significant opportunistic pathogen, and can acquire and transfer antibiotic resistance genes among other members of the mitis-group.

Other Gram positive cocci

Strains that were originally described as being nutritionally-variant streptococci (NVS) have been isolated from the mouth when appropriate isolation media are used. These have been re-classified as *Granulicatella adiacens* (previously *S. adiacens* and *Abiotrophia adiacens*) and *Abiotrophia defectiva* (previously *S. defectivus*). *G. adiacens* is common in the mouth, and is an early colonizer of the tooth surface, although it is overlooked in most studies because of the need for their isolation media to be supplemented with growth factors such as cysteine or pyridoxal. These bacteria often exhibit satellitism, an enhanced growth pattern around colonies of certain other bacteria that produce these co-factors. Other Gram positive cocci include *Gemella* spp. (*G. haemolysans* and *G. morbillorum*), although cells sometimes appear Gram negative on staining.

Anaerobic Gram positive cocci are commonly recovered from teeth, especially from carious dentine, infected pulp chambers and root canals (Ch. 6), advanced forms of periodontal disease (Ch. 6), and from dental abscesses (Ch. 7). They are also recovered from deep-seated abscesses elsewhere in the body, and are usually isolated in mixed culture (polymicrobial infections). The classification of this group of organisms is confused. Originally, strains were placed in the genus, *Peptostreptococcus*, and representative species included *P. micros*, *P. magnus* and *P. anaerobius*. However, *P. micros* and *P. magnus* have been moved to new genera as *Parvimonas micra* and *Finegoldia magna*, respectively, while oral strains of *P. anaerobius* are now designated *Peptostreptococcus stomatis*.

Enterococci have been recovered in low numbers from several oral sites when appropriate selective media have been used; the most frequently isolated species is *Enterococcus faecalis*. Enterococci can be isolated from the mouth of immuno- and medically-compromised patients, and have been isolated from periodontal pockets that fail to respond to therapy and from infected root canals. Lancefield group A streptococci (*S. pyogenes*) are not usually isolated from the mouth of healthy individuals, although they can often be cultured from the saliva of people suffering from streptococcal sore throats, and may be associated with a particularly acute form of gingivitis (Ch. 6).

Staphylococci and micrococci are also not commonly isolated in large numbers from the oral cavity although the former are found in denture plaque, as well as in immunocompromised patients and individuals suffering from a variety of oral infections (Chs 7 and 11). Although these bacteria are not usually considered to be members of the resident oral microflora, they may be present transiently, and they have been isolated from some sites with root surface caries and from some periodontal pockets that fail to respond to conventional therapy. Interestingly, this is in sharp contrast to other surfaces of the human body in close proximity to the mouth, such as the skin surface and the mucous membranes of the nose, where they are among the predominant components of the microflora. This finding emphasizes the major differences that must exist in the ecology of these particular habitats. Skin and nasal flora must be passed consistently into the mouth and yet these organisms are normally unable to colonize or compete against the resident oral microflora.

GRAM POSITIVE RODS AND FILAMENTS

Actinomyces

Actinomyces species form a major portion of the microflora of dental plaque, particularly at approximal sites and the gingival crevice. They have been associated with root surface caries and their numbers increase during gingivitis (Ch. 6). Cells of *Actinomyces* species appear as short rods, but are often pleomorphic in shape; some cells show a true branching morphology (Fig. 3.4C), while those of *A. israelii* can be filamentous. Some species (particularly *A. naeslundii*) are heavily fimbriated (cell surface structures involved in attachment), while others have relatively smooth surfaces. *Actinomyces* spp. ferment glucose to a characteristic pattern of metabolic end products, namely succinic, acetic and lactic acids, and this property is exploited in the identification of this genus. Some newly described species have been identified in a variety of clinical specimens (*A. radingae, A. neuii, A. johnsonii, A. europaeus, A. graevenitzii, A. funkei, A. dentalis* and *A. turicensis*), including infective endocarditis and abscesses, but the source and habitat of these species is not yet fully understood. *A. radicidentis* has been isolated from endodontic infections.

The most common representative in plaque is *A. naeslundii*, which was subdivided into two genospecies (*A. naeslundii* genospecies 1 and genospecies 2). *A. naeslundii* genospecies 2 is now classified as *A. oris*. Some strains of *A. naeslundii* produce an extracellular slime and a fructan from sucrose with a levan-like structure; the fructosyltransferase is produced constitutively. *A. naeslundii* strains also produce enzymes that can hydrolyse fructans with a variety of structures, including levans and inulins. Some strains also produce urease (this enzyme may have a role in modulating pH in plaque) and neuraminidase (can modify receptors in the enamel acquired pellicle). Two types of fimbriae can be found on the surface of cells of *A. naeslundii*. Each type serves a specific function, and is implicated either in cell-to-cell contact (coaggregation) or in cell-to-surface interaction (Chs 4 and 5). *A. viscosus* is a closely related species found in animals.

Actinomyces israelii can act as an opportunistic pathogen causing a chronic inflammatory condition called actinomycosis (Ch. 7). The disease is usually associated with the orofacial region, but it can disseminate to cause deep seated infections in other sites in the body such as the abdomen. Strains of *A. israelii* characteristically form 'granules' and such granules may contribute to their ability to disseminate around the body by affording cells physical protection from the environment, from the host defences, and from antibiotic treatment. *A. israelii* species have also been found in cervical smears of women using intrauterine contraceptive devices.

Following comparisons of 16S rRNA gene sequences, strains originally classified as *A. israelii* serotype II have now been designated as a separate species, *A. gerencseriae*, which is a common but minor component of the microflora of the healthy gingival crevice, although it has also been isolated from abscesses. Strains of *A. gerencseriae* can also form protective 'granules' (see previous comments on *A. israelii*). *A. georgiae* is facultatively anaerobic and is also found occasionally in the healthy gingival crevice. Other species include *A. odontolyticus*, of which about 50% of strains form colonies with a characteristic red-brown pigment. This species, together with *A. naeslundii*, are early colonizers of the mouth of infants, although *A. odontolyticus* has also been associated with the very earliest stages of enamel demineralization, and with the progression of small caries lesions. *A. meyeri* has been reported occasionally and in low numbers from the gingival crevice in health and disease, and from brain abscesses.

Eubacterium and related genera

Until recently, *Eubacterium* was a poorly defined genus that contained a variety of obligately anaerobic, filamentous bacteria that often appear Gram-variable when stained. Many strains are asaccharolytic, and therefore appear non-reactive in classification schemes. They are also difficult to cultivate and many laboratories have not isolated them from plaque while others have found numerous 'taxa' (>25) in various forms of periodontal disease. When recovered and identified, these asaccharolytic species can comprise over 50% of the anaerobic microflora of periodontal pockets and are common in dento-alveolar abscesses. The application of molecular taxonomic approaches has identified many new bacterial genera (Fig. 3.5), and oral eubacteria are now restricted to *Eubacterium saburreum, E. yurii,*

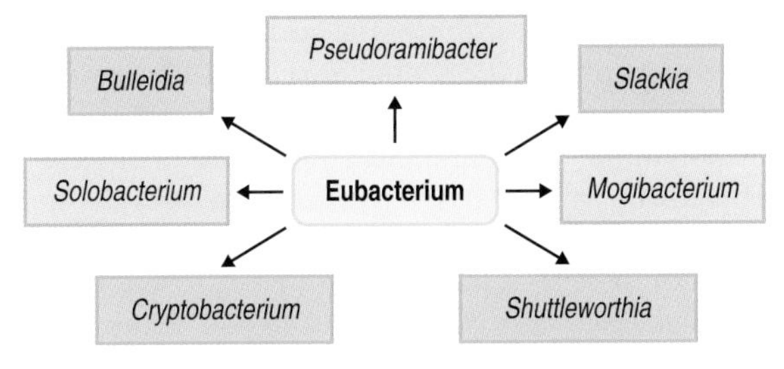

Fig. 3.5 Recent changes in the nomenclature of bacteria originally grouped together as *Eubacterium* species.

E. infirmum, *E. sulci*, *E saphenum*, *E. minutum*, *E. nodatum*, and *E. brachy*.

New genera include *Mogibacterium* (e.g. *M. timidum* [formerly *E. timidum*], *M. vescum* and *M. pumilum*), *Pseudoramibacter* (e.g. *P. alactolyticus*, formerly *E. alactolyticum*) and *Slackia* (e.g. *S. exigua*, formerly *E. exiguum*), all of which have been recovered from infected root canals. Other new genera include *Cryptobacterium* (e.g. *C. curtum*), *Shuttleworthia* (e.g. *S. satelles*), *Solobacterium* (e.g. *S. moorei*) and *Bulleidia* (e.g. *B. extructa*). Many of these bacteria have been found in periodontal pockets and/or abscesses, and some can produce butyrate and ammonia from amino acid metabolism, but the clinical significance of these organisms has yet to be determined.

Lactobacillus

Lactobacilli are commonly isolated from the oral cavity, especially dental plaque and the tongue, although they usually comprise less than 1% of the total cultivable microflora. However, their proportions and prevalence increase in advanced caries lesions both of the enamel and of the root surface. A number of homo- and hetero-fermentative species have been identified, producing either lactate or lactate and acetate, respectively, from glucose. The most common species are *L. casei*, *L. rhamnosus*, *L. fermentum*, *L. acidophilus*, *L. salivarius*, *L. plantarum*, *L. paracasei*, *L. gasseri* and *L. oris*.

Little is known of the preferred habitat of these species in the normal mouth, and most studies still merely group them as 'lactobacilli' or *Lactobacillus* spp.. They are highly acidogenic and acid tolerant, and are associated with advanced caries lesions and carious dentine. Simple tests with selective media have been designed for estimating the numbers of lactobacilli in patients' saliva to give an indication of the cariogenic potential of a mouth. Although these tests are often unreliable, they are useful for monitoring the dietary behaviour of a patient because levels of lactobacilli correlate closely with the intake of dietary carbohydrate. Some lactobacilli are being considered as possible oral probiotic strains.

Other genera

Propionibacterium spp. (e.g. *P. acnes*, *P. propionicus*) are obligately anaerobic bacteria that are found in dental plaque; *P. propionicus* has been isolated from cases of actinomycosis and lacrimal canaliculitis (infection of the tear duct). *Corynebacterium* (formerly *Bacterionema*) *matruchotii*, *Rothia dentocariosa*, and *Bifidobacterium dentium* are also regularly isolated from dental plaque. Two species of bifidobacteria have been reclassified as *Scardovia inopinata* (formerly *B. inopinatum*) and as *Parascardovia denticolens* (formerly *B. denticolens*), but their role in the mouth is yet to be determined. *Alloscardovia omnicolens* has been isolated from saliva. *C. matruchotii* has an unusual cellular morphology having a long filament growing out of a short, fat rod-like cell, thus earning its description of 'whip-handle' cell. *Rothia* is isolated on very rare occasions from cases of infective endocarditis. *Rothia mucilaginosa* (formerly *Stomatococcus mucilaginosus*) produces an extracellular slime, and is isolated almost exclusively from the tongue. Some bacteria previously classified as *Actinomyces* have been placed in new genera; *Actinomyces bernardiae* has been reclassified as *Arcanobacterium bernardiae* while other species have been placed in the genus, *Actinobaculum*. Bacteria originally described as 'anaerobic lactobacilli' have been placed in new genera such as *Olsenella*, e.g. *O. uli* (formerly *Lactobacillus uli*), which has been isolated from periodontal pockets, and *Atopobium* spp. (e.g. *A. rimae* and *A. parvulum*). *Filifactor* (e.g. *F. alocis*) is found in endodontic infections.

SUMMARY

Gram positive bacteria are commonly distributed on most surfaces of the mouth. The predominant genera are *Streptococcus* and *Actinomyces*; representative species are found at healthy sites, although many can also act as opportunistic pathogens. For example, mutans streptococci are implicated in dental caries while the intermedius- and the mitis-groups of streptococci are recovered commonly from abscesses and infective endocarditis, respectively; *Actinomyces israelii* is implicated in actinomycosis.

GRAM NEGATIVE COCCI

Neisseria are aerobic or facultatively anaerobic Gram negative cocci that are isolated in low numbers from most sites in the oral cavity. They are among the earliest colonizers of teeth, and make an important contribution to plaque formation by consuming oxygen and creating conditions that permit obligate anaerobes to grow. Some *Neisseria* spp. can produce extracellular polysaccharides and some streptococcal strains can metabolize these polymers, effectively using them as external carbohydrate reserves. The taxonomy of this group remains confused, but common species include *N. subflava*, *N. mucosa*, *N. flavescens* and *N. pharyngis*. *Moraxella catharrhalis* is a commensal of the upper respiratory tract, but it is also a well-established opportunistic pathogen; many strains produce a β-lactamase that can lead to complications during antibiotic treatment.

Veillonella are strictly anaerobic Gram negative cocci; several species are recognised: *V. parvula*, *V. dispar*, *V. atypica*, *V. denticariosi* (more common in carious dentine) and *V. rogosae* (more common in caries-free individuals). *Veillonella* spp have been isolated from most surfaces of the oral cavity although they occur in highest numbers in dental plaque. *Veillonella* spp. lack glucokinase and fructokinase and, therefore, are unable to metabolize carbohydrates. Instead, they utilize several intermediary metabolites, in particular lactate, as energy sources and, consequently, play an important role in the ecology of dental plaque and in the aetiology of dental caries. Lactic acid is the strongest acid produced in quantity by oral bacteria and is implicated in the dissolution of enamel (dental caries; Ch. 6). *Veillonella* can reduce the potentially harmful effect of lactic acid by converting it to weaker acids (predominantly propionic acid). Some bacteria originally thought to belong within the family *Veillonellaceae* have been classified as *Anaeroglobus geminatus*. *Megasphaera* are also Gram negative anaerobic cocci that have been isolated occasionally from dental plaque.

GRAM NEGATIVE RODS

Facultatively anaerobic and capnophilic genera

The majority of facultatively anaerobic Gram negative rods in the mouth were originally assigned to the genus *Haemophilus*. These organisms were not detected in early studies until appropriate isolation media were used that contained essential growth factors required by members of this genus – haemin (X-factor) and nicotinamide adenine dinucleotide, NAD (V-factor). This group of bacteria have been reclassified, and the only species of *Haemophilus* found commonly in the mouth is *H. parainfluenzae* (V-factor requiring); *H. parahaemolyticus* is isolated from soft tissue infections of the oral cavity, but is probably not a regular member of the oral microflora. Organisms previously classified as haemophili have been placed in the new genus, *Aggregatibacter*, e.g. *A. aphrophilus* (can cause brain abscesses and infective endocarditis) and *A. segnis* (only occasionally isolated from infections). In addition, an important periodontal pathogen, *Actinobacillus actinomycetemcomitans*, implicated in a particularly aggressive form of periodontal disease in adolescents, has also been reclassified as *Aggregatibacter actinomycetemcomitans* (Fig. 3.6A). Strains are capnophilic often requiring 5–10% CO_2 for growth. Cells have surface layers containing molecules that stimulate bone resorption, as well as serotype-determining polysaccharides. Freshly isolated strains possess fimbriae, although these can be lost on sub-culture. *A. actinomycetemcomitans* produces a range of virulence factors including a powerful leukotoxin, collagenase, immunosuppressive factors and proteases capable of cleaving IgG; in addition, strains can be invasive for epithelial cells. *A. actinomycetemcomitans* is also an opportunistic pathogen, being isolated from cases of endocarditis, brain and subcutaneous abscesses, osteomyelitis, and periodontal disease (Ch. 6). Recently, a highly virulent clone of strains of *A. actinomycetemcomitans* has been recognised, whose distribution is restricted to only certain adolescents with a high risk of aggressive periodontitis, all of which generally have a North West African origin.

Other facultatively anaerobic Gram negative rods include *Eikenella corrodens*. Colonies of this species characteristically pit the surface of agar plates. Strains of *E. corrodens* have been isolated from a range of oral infections including endocarditis and abscesses, and have been implicated in periodontal disease. *Capnocytophaga* are CO_2-dependent Gram negative rods, with a gliding motility, and are found in subgingival plaque, and increase in proportions in gingivitis. A number of species have been recognised (including *C. gingivalis*, *C. ochracea*, *C. sputigena*, *C. granulosa*, *C. haemolytica* and *C. leadbetteri*). *Capnocytophaga* are opportunistic pathogens and have been isolated from a number of infections in immunocompromised patients; some strains produce an IgA1 protease.

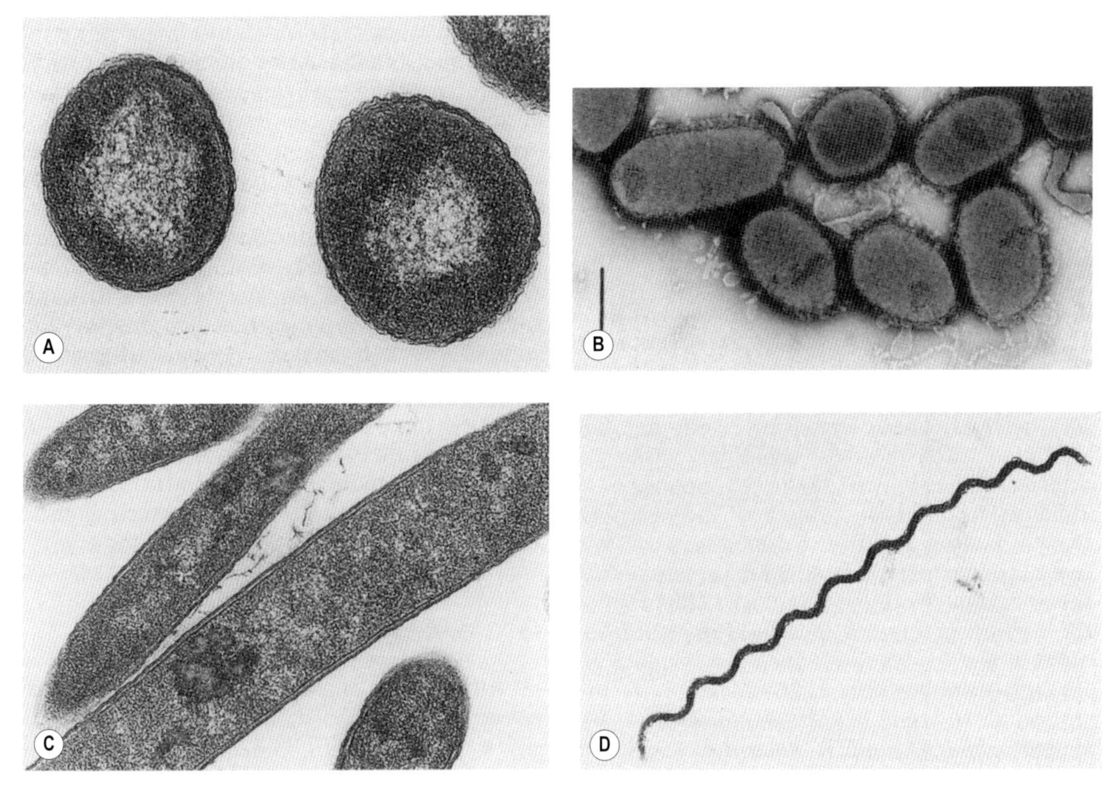

Fig. 3.6 Electron micrographs of: (A) *Aggregatibacter actinomycetemcomitans*, (B) *Porphyromonas gingivalis*, (C) *Fusobacterium nucleatum* and (D) an oral spirochaete.

Kingella (e.g. *K. oralis*) is a coccobacillus that has been isolated from several oral sites. The gliding bacterium *Simonsiella* has been isolated from epithelial surfaces of the oral cavity of man and a variety of animals. These organisms have a unique cellular morphology being composed of unusually large, multi-cellular filaments in groups, or multiples of eight cells.

Obligately anaerobic genera

Obligately anaerobic Gram negative rods comprise a large proportion of the microflora of dental plaque and the tongue. The classification of many of these organisms has proved difficult; many strains grow poorly so that clear results in fermentation tests are not obtained, and the concentration of metabolites is too low to be analyzed satisfactorily. The development and application of new types of test such as lipid analyses and enzyme mobilities has enabled the speciation of isolates that appeared non-reactive by conventional methods. New species that are at present unculturable in the laboratory have been identified in clinical samples using molecular approaches, such as amplification of 16S rRNA genes followed by cloning and sequence analysis (Figs 3.2 and 3.3).

Most of the cultivable oral obligate anaerobes belong to the genera *Prevotella* and *Porphyromonas*. Some organisms from these genera produce colonies with a characteristic brown or black pigment when grown on blood agar (Fig. 3.7). This pigment may act as a defence mechanism helping to protect the cells from the toxic effects of oxygen. These organisms are referred to collectively as black-pigmented anaerobes. Haemin is an essential growth factor and is obtained in the host from the catabolism of haeme-containing molecules such as haemoglobin.

Prevotella spp. are moderately saccharolytic (i.e. able to ferment carbohydrates), producing acetic, succinic and other acids from glucose. Species with pigmented strains include *Prevotella intermedia*, *P. nigrescens*, *P. melaninogenica*, *P. loescheii*, *P. pallens* and some strains of *P. denticola*. *Prevotella intermedia* and *P. nigrescens* are difficult to distinguish using simple physiological tests, but *P. intermedia* is associated with periodontal disease while *P. nigrescens* is isolated more often, and in higher numbers, from

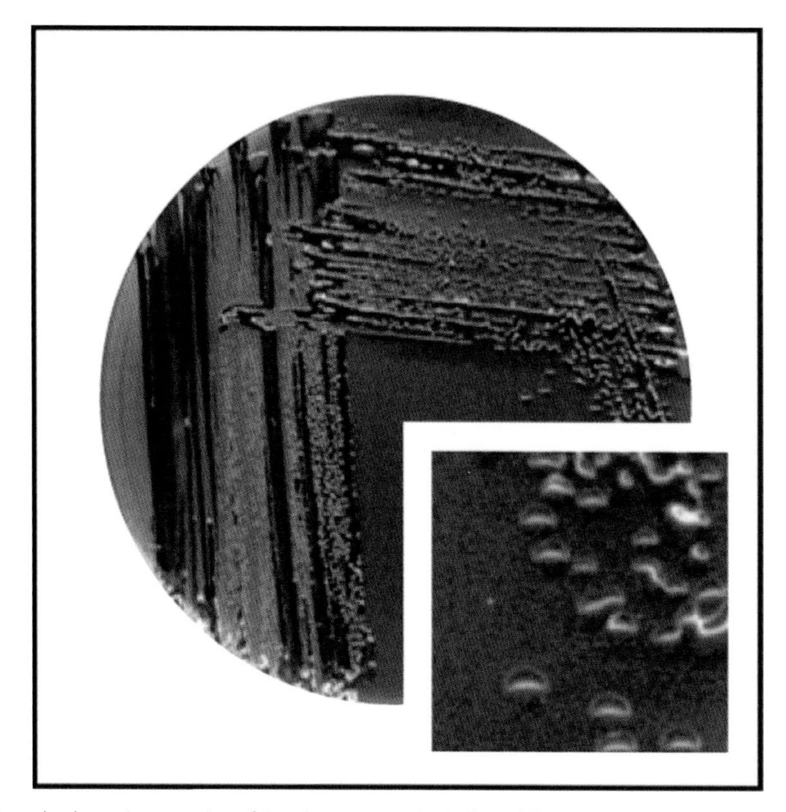

Fig. 3.7 Haemolysis and colony pigmentation of *Porphyromonas gingivalis* on blood agar after 10 days of anaerobic incubation. Courtesy of Professor M Curtis and the American Society for Microbiology (see Curtis et al Infect Immun 2002 70:6968-6975).

healthy sites. There are a large number of oral non-pigmented species including *Prevotella buccae, P. buccalis, P. oralis, P. oris, P. oulora, P. veroralis, P. dentalis, P. tannerae, P. enoeca, P. bergensis, P. multisaccharivorax, P. marshii, P. baroniae, P. shahii, P. multiformis, P. salivae, P. maculosa* and *P. zoogleoformans*. The majority of these species can be isolated on occasions from dental plaque, particularly from subgingival sites. Some species are associated with disease and increase in numbers and proportions during periodontal disease, and have also been recovered from abscesses (Chs 6 and 7).

Porphyromonas spp. are mainly asaccharolytic, and use proteins and peptides for growth. *Porphyromonas gingivalis* (Figs 3.6B and 3.7) is isolated mainly from subgingival sites, especially in advanced periodontal lesions, although it has also been recovered from the tongue and tonsils. Six serotypes have been recognised based on capsular polysaccharides (K antigens). *P. gingivalis* is highly virulent in experimental infection studies in animals, and produces a range of putative virulence factors associated with tissue destruction and subversion of the host defences. These include highly active proteases, with specificity for arginine-x bonds and lysine-x bonds (arg- and lys-gingipains, respectively), that can degrade host molecules such as immunoglobulins, complement, and iron- and haeme-sequestering proteins and glycoproteins, as well as molecules that the host produces to regulate the host inflammatory response. *P. gingivalis* also produces a haemolysin, collagen-degrading enzymes, cytotoxic metabolites, and a capsule (Ch. 6). *P. gingivalis* has fimbriae on its cell surface that mediate adherence to oral epithelial cells and to saliva-coated tooth surfaces. *Porphyromonas endodontalis* has been mainly recovered from infected root canals. In contrast, *Porphyromonas catoniae* is found mainly at healthy sites or in shallow pockets.

Another major group of obligately anaerobic Gram negative bacteria belong to the genus *Fusobacterium*. Cells are characteristically in the form of long filaments (5–25 μm in length; Fig. 3.6C) or pleomorphic rods, and cells characteristically produce butyric acid as the major end product of metabolism. The most common species is *F. nucleatum*, and several subspecies have been recognised: subspecies *nucleatum*, subsp.

polymorphum and subsp. *vincentii*. These subspecies may have different associations with health and disease; *F. nucleatum* subsp. *polymorphum* is commonly isolated from the normal gingival crevice whereas subspecies *nucleatum* is recovered mainly from periodontal pockets. Other oral fusobacteria include *F. periodonticum* which is isolated from sites with periodontal disease. Fusobacteria are often described as being asaccharolytic, although they can take up carbohydrates for the synthesis of intracellular storage compounds composed of polyglucose. Fusobacteria catabolise amino acids such as aspartate, glutamate, histidine and lysine to provide energy; these can be obtained from the metabolism of peptides if free amino acids are not available. *F. nucleatum* is able to remove sulphur from cysteine and methionine to produce ammonia, butyrate, hydrogen sulphide and methyl mercaptan, and these compounds contribute to the odour associated with halitosis. Fusobacteria are able to aggregate with most other oral bacteria and, consequently, are believed to be an important bridging organism between early and late colonizers during plaque formation (coadhesion and coaggregation, Ch. 5).

Other oral Gram negative anaerobic and microaerophilic bacteria include *Leptotrichia buccalis* (cells also have a filamentous morphology with a pointed end but produce lactate as their major fermentation product). Species include *L. buccalis, L. hofstadii, L. shahii* and *L. wadei. Wolinella succinogenes* is an asaccharolytic and formate/fumarate-requiring strain. A number of campylobacter species have been recognised (cells have a spiral morphology) including *Campylobacter concisus, C. gracilis* (formerly *Bacteroides gracilis*), *C. showae, C. sputorum, C. curvus* and *C. rectus* (the latter two species were previously classified as *Wolinella curva* and *W. recta*, respectively). *C. concisus* was isolated in higher proportions from relatively shallow pockets and healthy subgingival sites whereas *C. rectus* is found more commonly at sites with active periodontal disease, especially in immunocompromised patients. Some strains of *C. rectus* produce a cytotoxin which shares some sequence homology with the leukotoxin of *A. actinomycetemcomitans. Selenomonas sputigena, S. noxia, S. flueggei, S. infelix, S. dianae* and *S. artemidis* have been found in plaque from the human gingival crevice.

Some of the species described above have flagella and are motile. The *Wolinella* and *Campylobacter* species have a single flagellum, while *Selenomonas* spp. are curved to helical bacilli with a tuft of flagella. Another helical or curved Gram negative oral anaerobe is *Centipeda periodontii* which has numerous flagella which spiral around the cell. There have been reports of *Helicobacter pylori* in dental plaque; this species is usually isolated from the stomach where it is associated with gastritis, peptic ulcers and gastric cancer. It may be present in the mouth transiently following reflux from the stomach. Some newly described genera include: *Johnsonii* (*J. ignava*) and *Cantonella* (*C. morbi*), which are associated with gingivitis and periodontitis, respectively; *Dialister* (*D. pneumosintes* and *D. invisus*) which can be found in endodontic infections and periodontitis; *Flavobacterium*; and *Tannerella forsythia* (formerly *Bacteroides forsythus* or *T. forsythensis*) which is commonly isolated from advanced periodontal disease.

Organisms such as sulphate-reducing bacteria (e.g. *Desulfobacter, Desulfobulbus, Desulfomicrobium* and *Desulfovibrio*) and methanogens (e.g. *Methanobrevibacter* spp.), which use terminal end products of metabolism, such as hydrogen, CO_2, and organic acids, have been detected in dental plaque. Sulphate-reducing bacteria produce hydrogen sulphide, which can contribute to mouth odour. These bacteria are extremely difficult to grow in the laboratory because of their sensitivity to even trace amounts of oxygen, and their requirement for a very low redox potential for growth (Ch. 2).

Spirochaetes are numerous in subgingival plaque and can readily be detected using dark-field or electron microscopy (Fig. 3.6D). Several morphological types can be distinguished according to cell size and the arrangement of periplasmic flagella (endoflagella). Spirochaetes possess an outer membrane and an inner membrane (which encloses the protoplasmic cylinder); the periplasmic flagella lie in the periplasmic space between these two membranes. The periplasmic flagella attach at either pole of the cell by means of a basal hook, and wrap themselves around the helical protoplasmic cylinder. Some of the oral spirochaetes adhere to surfaces in a polar orientation; this type of adhesion results in gross alterations to host cell morphology facilitating penetration into underlying tissues. The numbers of spirochaetes are raised in advanced periodontal diseases, and are diagnostic for necrotizing ulcerative periodontitis (Ch. 6), but whether they cause disease or merely increase following infection is still to be resolved.

Oral spirochaetes fall within the genus *Treponema* and a large number of species have been proposed, including *T. denticola*, *T. socranskii* (subspecies *socranskii*; subspecies *buccale*; subspecies *paredis*), *T. maltophilum*, *T. amylovorum*, *T. parvum*, *T. pectinovorum*, *T. putidum*, *T. lecithinolyticum*, *T. medium* and *T. vincentii*. In addition to their detection from periodontally-inflamed sites, some of these species have also been detected in primary endodontic infection. Little is known about the physiology of these organisms because of difficulties associated with their laboratory cultivation. However, *T. denticola* has been grown using appropriate methods, and has been shown to have potent degradative enzyme activity, including an arginine-specific ('trypsin-like') protease. *T. denticola* can also degrade collagen and gelatin, and appears to be more proteolytic than other oral spirochaetes. The use of culture-independent molecular approaches, in which 16S rRNA gene sequences have been compared from clinical samples, is emphasizing the diversity that exists within oral spirochaetes; for example, 47 as yet uncultivated *Treponema* species were identified in one study of subgingival sites in health and disease (Fig. 3.3A).

As stated earlier in this chapter, only about 50% of the microorganisms that can be visualized in the mouth by microscopy are at present able to be cultivated. This is due not only to ignorance of the growth requirements of these organisms but also because some bacteria have evolved to grow in partnership (physically and nutritionally) with other microbes. New families of unculturable bacteria are being identified by molecular ecological approaches, e.g. *Bacteroidales* and *Lachnospiraceae*, while some of the unculturable bacteria show sufficient genetic similarity to known cultivable species that they can be placed within a genus, for example, the unculturable spirochaetes are assigned to the genus, *Treponema* (Fig. 3.3A). Others represent novel evolutionary lineages, which are found in a number of habitats, and are designated simply by the phyla in which they are grouped. Most oral examples belong to the TM7 phylum, and have been described as a sheathed filament. They can be numerous in subgingival plaque, and can be visualized by fluorescent *in situ* hybridization (FISH) by combining oligonucleotide probes (coupled to a fluorescent tag) with specialized microscopy techniques (epifluorescence or confocal laser scanning microscopy) (Fig. 3.3B). Some organisms detected by molecular approaches in samples from subgingival plaque, and from periodontal lesions and endodontic infections, belong to a new candidate phylum 'Synergistetes', and one example has been identified as *Jonquetella anthropi*. Increasing our understanding of the role of these unculturable bacteria in health and disease is now an important goal for oral microbiologists.

SUMMARY

Oral Gram negative bacteria are diverse, and include species that are facultatively and obligately anaerobic, as well as species that are microaerophilic and capnophilic. *Veillonella* are anaerobic Gram negative cocci that play an important role in dental plaque by converting lactate to weaker acids. Most of the anaerobic Gram negative bacilli are found in dental plaque, and have an asaccharolytic metabolism, and depend on proteins and glycoproteins for their nutrition; some common genera include *Prevotella* and *Fusobacterium*. The diversity of species increases in periodontal disease, and many of these are 'unculturable' at present. The taxonomy of Gram negative bacteria has been transformed by molecular techniques such as 16S rRNA gene sequencing.

FUNGI

Fungi generally constitute a relatively small proportion of the oral microflora. The 'perfect fungi' (fungi that divide by sexual reproduction) are rarely isolated from the oral cavity but are occasionally found infecting patients with advanced acquired immunodeficiency syndrome (AIDS). The main 'perfect fungi' causing oral infection are *Aspergillus*, *Geotrichium* and *Mucor* spp.. The perfect yeast species seen in healthy individuals may be transient rather than resident members of the oral microflora. In contrast, the 'imperfect yeasts', e.g. *Candida* spp. (which divide by asexual reproduction) are commonly found in the mouth (Ch. 9).

The largest proportion of the fungal microflora in the human mouth is made up of *Candida* spp. *Candida albicans* is by far the most common species, but a large number of other yeasts have been isolated, including *C. glabrata*, *C.tropicalis*, *C. krusei*, *C. parapsilosis*, and *C. guilliermondii*, as well as *Rhodotorula* and *Saccharomyces* spp.. Estimations of carriage rates of *Candida* species in the mouth vary markedly because of the different isolation techniques used and the population groups investigated (Ch. 9). Carriage rates range from 2 to 71% in asymptomatic adults, but this increases, and approaches 100%, in medically-compromised patients or those on broad spectrum antibacterial agents.

Candida are distributed evenly throughout the mouth but the most common site of isolation is the dorsum of the tongue. The isolation of *Candida* increases with the presence of intra-oral devices such as dentures or orthodontic appliances, particularly in the upper jaw on the fitting surface; indeed, *Candida* spp. can attach tenaciously to acrylic. Plaque can also harbour *Candida* spp., but the exact proportion and significance of these yeasts in health and disease is unclear. The mouth may be the source of yeast colonization of the gut, and saliva is the vehicle for the transmission of *Candida* spp. to other areas of the body. Colonization of the mouth by yeasts occurs either at birth or soon afterwards. The carriage rate falls in early childhood and increases during middle and later life for reasons that are as yet unclear.

MYCOPLASMA

Bacteria belonging to the genus *Mycoplasma* are primarily characterized through the absence of a cell wall. This feature makes these bacteria appear Gram negative upon Gram staining, although due to their small size (<1 µm; they are the smallest of all free-growing cells) they are difficult to visualize by normal light microscopy.

Analysis of *Mycoplasma* genome sequences (16S rDNA) suggests that these organisms are most closely related to *Bacillus–Lactobacillus* and *Streptococcus* subgroups of Gram positive bacteria. Mycoplasma are notoriously slow growing bacteria and require specialized microbiological culture media enriched in proteins and with an elevated carbon dioxide atmosphere for growth. Mycoplasmas are pleomorphic, and several cell shapes can occur depending on the environment.

Mycoplasmas are most prevalent on mucosal surfaces, and infections of the respiratory tract and urinary tract are associated with these organisms. Oral carriage rates of between 6 and 32% have been reported in humans with a number of species recovered from saliva (*M. salivarium, M. pneumoniae, M. hominis*), the oral mucosa (*M. buccale, M. orale, M. pneumoniae*) and dental plaque (*M. pneumoniae, M. buccale, M. orale*). *Mycoplasma orale* and *M. salivarium* have also been isolated from salivary glands where it has been postulated that they play a role in salivary gland hypofunction. Periodontal disease has also been associated with the presence of members of this genus.

VIRUSES

The presence of viruses in the mouth has been studied extensively over recent years (Ch. 10), especially since the advent of polymerase chain reaction (PCR) techniques. It is now no longer necessary to use time-consuming and often unreliable methods of detection of viruses, such as tissue culture or electron microscopy. Indeed, some viruses have only been detected by the use of molecular approaches and have never been grown (e.g. hepatitis C and hepatitis G).

The virus most frequently encountered in saliva and the orofacial area is Herpes simplex type 1 (HSV-1). The vast majority (80–90%) of adults in the Western World have suffered from infection with HSV-1, which is the cause of cold sores. Molecular techniques have revealed that HSV is persistent within the oral tissues and can also be detected occasionally by culture in saliva in the absence of cold sores, which indicates periodic shedding. The virus also remains latent, in the trigeminal nerve ganglion, where it may be reactivated by UV light or stress. Once reactivated, the genome passes back down the peripheral nerve to cause the characteristic cold sores, which rupture to release further virus particles.

Cytomegalovirus is present in most individuals. It has been detected in the saliva of symptomless adults, but its portal of entry into the oral cavity is not clear. Coxsackie virus A2, 4, 5, 6, 8, 9, 10, and 16 have all been detected in saliva and in the oral epithelium. The detection of these viruses has usually been associated with hand, foot and mouth disease or herpangina. There are more than 100 types of human papilloma virus (HPV), a number of which have been isolated from the oral cavity, usually within the tissue of localized hyperplastic warty like lesions (verruca vulgaris). HPV types 2, 4, 6, 11 and 16 have been detected relatively frequently in oral lesions of patients with AIDS. Extensive studies have been undertaken to explore the possible role of HPV in oral cancer, but no link has been identified as yet.

Hepatitis viruses and human immunodeficiency virus (HIV) can be found in the oral cavity, especially in saliva, where their presence poses a significant cross-infection threat. One of the most important aspects of infection control relates to the presence of hepatitis B virus in the saliva of asymptomatic individuals who may carry the virus for many years. Both groups of viruses are discussed in detail in Chapters 10 and 12. Other viruses found in the oral cavity are measles and mumps, but usually in association with oral lesions.

Bacteriophage (viruses for which bacteria are the natural hosts) have been observed in samples of saliva and dental plaque, but few have been isolated. Bacteriophage specific for *S. mutans*, *Lactobacillus*, *Actinomyces*, *Veillonella* and *Aggregatibacter* spp. have been described. Some phage with activity against non-oral bacteria (e.g. *Proteus mirabilis*) have been detected, and this might contribute to the ability of the resident oral microflora to exclude exogenous species (colonization resistance; Ch. 4).

PROTOZOA

Protozoa are defined as unicellular eukaryotic microorganisms that lack a cell wall. Several species are known to cause human diseases and examples of these include members of the genus *Plasmodium* (malaria), *Entamoeba histolytica* (amoebiasis) and *Cryptosporidium* spp. (diarrhoeal infection in susceptible individuals following ingestion of protozoan cysts).

Two protozoan species are frequently recovered from the mouth, namely *Trichomonas tenax* (previously referred to a *T. buccalis* and *T. elongate*) and *Entamoeba gingivalis*. Their oral prevalence is variable but estimates report carriage rates of between 4 and 52% in the healthy population. The reason for this variation in incidence is unclear, but probably reflects difficulties in conventional detection approaches either by culture or microscopic visualization. In recent years, molecular analytical techniques have allowed researchers to use PCR techniques to detect oral protozoa through amplification of small ribosomal RNA gene sequences. Such investigations have indicated a 2% incidence of *T. tenax* in healthy oral cavities, increasing to 21% in patients with periodontal disease.

Both of the oral protozoan species are motile, and in the case of *T. tenax*, its characteristic 'tumbling' motility is mediated through the presence of four anterior flagella and a fifth recurrent flagellum, attached to an undulating membrane along the length of the cell. *Trichomonas tenax* and *E. gingivalis* are heterotrophic, acquiring their carbon requirements through ingestion of other microorganisms, host leukocytes and dead organic matter within the mouth and, in this sense, they are truly parasitic. Both species are strictly anaerobic and, while generally considered to be harmless commensals, there are reports associating their presence with periodontal disease. *Trichomonas tenax* does exhibit proteolytic activity through the production of cysteine proteinases and metalloproteinases and these enzymes could conceivably induce damage to host connective tissues. However, whether these organisms play an active role in periodontal disease still remains unclear, although it is apparent that their incidence does increase in individuals with poor oral hygiene.

CHAPTER SUMMARY

The healthy mouth supports the growth of a wide range of microorganisms including bacteria, yeasts, mycoplasmas, viruses, and even protozoa. Bacteria are the predominant components of the resident oral microflora; a list of the major genera is given in Table 3.4. Many of these bacteria are fastidious in their nutritional requirements, while others are obligate anaerobic and highly sensitive to oxygen, and some have evolved to grow in mixed culture. Some organisms are slow growing and relatively unreactive in tests used in conventional identification schemes, and novel approaches have been devised to differentiate them, such as analysis of cell wall components or whole cell protein profiles. At present, only about 50% of the organisms in plaque can be isolated in pure culture in the laboratory. Molecular approaches, based on comparisons of 16S rRNA gene sequences, have revolutionized our understanding of the complexity of the resident oral microflora, and resolved many long-standing problems with the classification of several groups of oral bacteria (for an example, see Fig. 3.5). These approaches have identified many new genera and species, including currently unculturable phyla such as TM7 (Fig. 3.3B). The use of specific oligonucleotide probes is leading to rapid (and relatively simple) techniques to detect, visualize and identify even the most fastidious of oral microbe in clini-

Table 3.4 The principal bacterial genera found in the oral cavity

Gram positive		Gram negative	
Cocci	Rods	Cocci	Rods
Abiotrophia	*Actinobaculum*	*Anaeroglobus*	*Aggregatibacter*
Enterococcus	*Actinomyces*	*Mega sphaera*	*Campylobacter*
Finegoldia	*Alloscardovia*	*Moraxella*	*Cantonella*
Gemella	*Arcanobacterium*	*Neisseria*	
Granulicatella	*Atopobium*	*Veillonella*	*Capnocytophaga*
Peptostreptococcus	*Bifidobacterium*		*Centipeda*
Streptococcus	*Corynebacterium*		*Desulfomicrobium*
	Cryptobacterium		*Desulfovibrio*
	Eubacterium		*Dialister*
	Filifactor		*Eikenella*
	Lactobacillus		*Flavobacterium*
	Mogibacterium		*Fusobacterium*
	Olsenella		*Haemophilus*
	Parascardovia		*Johnsonii*
	Propionibacterium		*Kingella*
	Pseudoramibacter		*Leptotrichia*
	Rothia		*Methanobrevibacter*
	Scardovia		*Porphyromonas*
	Shuttleworthia		*Prevotella*
	Slackia		*Selenomonas*
	Solobacterium		*Simonsiella*
			Tannerella
			Treponema
			Wolinella

- Mycoplasma are also isolated from the mouth
- There are also unculturable bacteria that have yet to be placed in a genus; some belong to the phylum, TM7.

cal samples. The resultant benefits in classification and detection will increase the likelihood of finding closer associations between particular species or taxa with sites in health and disease.

The high diversity of the oral microflora reflects the wide range of nutrients available endogenously in the mouth, the varied types of habitat for colonization, and the opportunity provided by biofilms such as plaque for survival on surfaces. Despite this diversity, many microorganisms commonly isolated from neighbouring ecosystems, such as the skin and the gut, are not found in the mouth, emphasising the unique and selective properties of the mouth for microbial colonization.

FURTHER READING

Comprehensive sources on the properties of microorganisms include recent editions of reference works such as Topley & Wilson's Principles of Bacteriology, Virology and Immunity, Bergey's Manual of Determinative Bacteriology, and The Prokaryotes (Editor in Chief: M Dworkin).

Some specific references are listed below:

Aas JA, Paster BJ, Stokes LN, Olsen I, Dewhirst FE 2005 Defining the normal bacterial flora of the oral cavity. J Clin Microbiol 43: 5721-5732.

Citron DM 2002 Update of the taxonomy and clinical aspects of the genus *Fusobacterium*. Clin Infect Dis 35:S22-S27.

Downes J, Munson MA, Spratt DA et al 2001 Characterisation of *Eubacterium*-like strains isolated from oral infections. J Med Microbiol 50:947-951.

Ellen RP, Galimanas VB 2005 Spirochetes at the forefront of periodontal infections. Periodontology 2000 38:13-32.

Fine DH, Kaplan JB, Kachlany SC, Schreiner HC 2006 How we got attached to *Actinobacillus actinomycetemcomitans*: a model for infectious diseases. Periodontology 2000 42:114-157.

Hitch G, Pratten J, Taylor PW 2004 Isolation of bacteriophages from the oral cavity. Lett Appl Microbiol 39:215-219.

Holt SC, Ebersole JL 2005 *Porphyromonas gingivalis, Treponema denticola*, and *Tannerella forsythia*: the 'red complex', a prototype polybacterial pathogenic consortium in periodontitis. Periodontol 2000 38:72-122.

Li L, Redding S, Dongari-Bagtzoglou A 2007 *Candida glabrata*: an emerging oral opportunistic pathogen. J Dent Res 86:204-215.

Macuch PJ, Tanner AC 2000 Campylobacter species in health, gingivitis and periodontitis. J Dent Res 79:785-792.

Sakamoto M, Umeda M, Benno Y 2005 Molecular analysis of human oral microbiota. J Periodont Res 40: 277-285.

Tanner ACR, Izard J 2006 *Tannerella forsythia*, a periodontal pathogen entering the genomic era. Periodontology 2000 42:88-113.

Wade W 2004 Non-culturable bacteria in complex commensal populations. Adv Appl Microbiol 54:93-106.

Williams DW, Lewis MA 2000 Isolation and identification of *Candida* from the oral cavity. Oral Dis 6:3-11.

The Human Oral Microbiome Database (HOMD) provides comprehensive information on the microorganisms found in the human oral cavity. This is an on-going project and the database will be continuously updated. The database can be accessed at: www.homd.org

Chapter 4

Acquisition, adherence, distribution and metabolism of the oral microflora

The foetus in the womb is normally sterile. Despite the widespread possibility of contamination, the mouth of the newborn baby is usually sterile. However, from the first feeding onwards, the mouth is regularly inoculated with microorganisms and the process of acquisition of the resident oral microflora begins.

ACQUISITION OF THE RESIDENT ORAL MICROFLORA

Acquisition depends on the transmission of microorganisms to the site of potential colonization. Initially, in the mouth, this is by passive inoculation from the mother, from other individuals in close proximity to the baby, and from ingested milk and water. Acquisition of microorganisms such as yeasts and lactobacilli from the birth canal itself may be only transient, but the role of saliva in the process of acquisition has been confirmed conclusively.

The ability to type strains (Fig. 3.1) has confirmed the transfer of *Streptococcus salivarius*, mutans streptococci and some other species from mother to child via saliva. Similarly, comparisons of the DNA fingerprints (genotyping) of a variety of oral bacterial species have shown that the same digest pattern (and hence presumably the same **clonal type**) is commonly found within family groups, and that different patterns are usually observed between such groups. Nevertheless, strains of some bacteria can be acquired occasionally by young children from other family members, while some strains seem to be distinct from any found in close relatives. The genotypes of mutans streptococci found in children were identical to those of their mothers in 71% of 34 infant-mother pairs examined (**vertical transmission**). Little evidence of father-infant (or father–mother) transmission of mutans streptococci was observed, although **horizontal transmission** between spouses, and vertical transmission within family units, can occur with some periodontal pathogens, such as *Porphyromonas gingivalis* and *Aggregatibacter actinomycetemcomitans*.

Pioneer community and microbial succession

The mouth is highly selective for microorganisms even during the first few days of life. Very few of the species common to the oral cavity of adults, and even fewer of the large number of bacteria found in the environment, are able to colonize the mouth of the newborn. The first microorganisms to colonize are termed **pioneer species**, and collectively they make up the **pioneer microbial community**. These pioneer species continue to grow and colonize until environmental resistance (physical and chemical) is encountered. In the mouth, physical factors include the shedding of epithelial cells (desquamation), and the shear forces from chewing and saliva flow. Nutritional restrictions and unfavourable conditions of Eh or pH, and the antibacterial properties of saliva, are chemical barriers that can limit growth.

One genus or species is usually predominant during the development of the pioneer community. In the mouth, the predominant cultivable organisms are streptococci, and in particular *S. salivarius*, *S. mitis* and *S. oralis*. Many of the pioneer species possess IgA_1 protease activity, which may enable producer organisms to evade the effects of this key host defence factor. Over time, the metabolic activity of the pioneer community modifies the environment providing conditions suitable for colonization by a succession of other populations. This may be by:

- modifying or exposing new receptors for attachment ('cryptitopes' – Ch. 5),
- changing the local pH or reducing oxygen levels and lowering the redox potential, Eh, or
- generating additional nutrients, for example, as end products of metabolism (lactate, succinate) or as breakdown products (peptides, haemin) which can be used by other organisms as part of a food chain.

As outlined above, the pioneer community influences the pattern of **microbial succession**. This involves the progressive development of a pioneer community (containing few species) through several stages in which the number of microbial groups increases, until an equilibrium is reached; this is termed the **climax community**, and generally has a high species diversity (Fig. 4.1). Succession is associated with a change from a site possessing few niches (roles – Ch. 1) to one with a multitude of potential niches. A climax community reflects a highly dynamic situation between the host, the environment and the microflora, and must not be regarded as a static state.

The oral cavity of the newborn contains only epithelial surfaces for colonization. The pioneer populations consist of mainly aerobic and facultatively anaerobic species. In full-term babies, a range of streptococcal species have been recovered during the first few days of life, and *S. oralis*, *S. mitis* biovar 1 and *S. salivarius* were numerically dominant (Table 4.1). The diversity of the streptococcal microflora increases with time; after one month, all babies were colonized by at least two species of *Streptococcus*, with *S. salivarius*

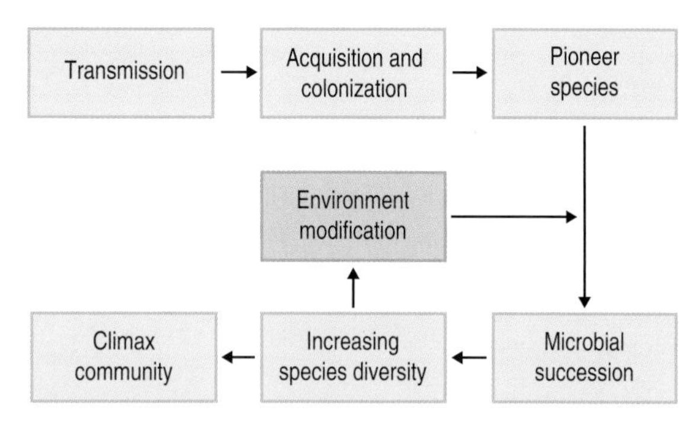

Fig. 4.1 Ecological stages in the establishment of a microbial community. As microbial diversity increases, the metabolism of the pioneer species modifies the local environment making conditions suitable for secondary colonizers.

Table 4.1 Streptococcal species isolated from the mucosal surfaces of babies.

Streptococcus	**Percentage viable count**		
	Age		
	1–3 days	**2 weeks**	**1 month**
S. oralis	41	24	20
S. mitis biovar 1	30	28	30
S. mitis biovar 2	4	1	1
S. salivarius	10	30	28
S. sanguinis	4	3	2
S. anginosus	3	5	5
S. gordonii	1	2	4

and *S. mitis* biovar 1 being isolated most commonly (Table 4.1). In contrast, the prevalence of *S. sanguinis* increased only after 12 months. *Actinomyces odontolyticus* was isolated from oral mucosal surfaces in infants as young as two months; *A naeslundii* was generally only present in older babies (ca. 12 months old) once teeth had erupted.

The diversity of the pioneer oral community increases during the first few months of life, with some Gram negative obligate anaerobes appearing. *Prevotella melaninogenica* was the most frequently isolated anaerobe, being recovered from 76% of edentulous infants (mean age = 3 months; range: 1–7 months) (Table 4.2). Other commonly isolated bacteria were *Fusobacterium nucleatum* (present in 67% of infants), *Veillonella* spp. (63%), and non-pigmented *Prevotella* spp. (62%), while *Eikenella corrodens* and *Wolinella succinogenes* were found only in a single mouth (Table 4.2). The number of different anaerobes in the same mouth varied from 0–7 species.

The same infants were followed longitudinally during the eruption of the primary dentition. Gram negative obligately anaerobic bacteria were isolated more commonly, and a greater diversity of species were recovered from around the gingival margin of the newly erupted teeth (mean age of the infants = 32 months) (Table 4.2). These findings confirm that the eruption of teeth has a significant ecological impact on the oral environment and its resident microflora.

During the first year of life, members of the genera *Neisseria, Veillonella, Actinomyces, Lactobacillus,* and *Rothia* are commonly isolated, particularly after tooth eruption. Studies using molecular detection assays have shown that some of the obligately anaerobic species implicated in periodontal diseases can be detected on occasions from tooth and tongue samples from young children (aged 18–36 months). *Porphyromonas gingivalis, Tannerella forsythia* and *Aggregatibacter actinomycetemcomitans* were detected in approximately 10–30% of 18-month-old infants. When present, these bacteria are at very low levels and are not of any clinical relevance. However, these bacteria can be carried, and at some point exploit either a change in local environmental conditions or a suppression of the host defences, to outcompete species associated with oral health, thereby predisposing such sites to disease. **An appreciation of this dynamic relationship between the host and the oral microflora is central to understanding the aetiology of most dental diseases.**

Allogenic and autogenic microbial succession

The establishment of a climax community at any oral site involves a series of phases of development during which the complexity of the microflora increases (**microbial succession**; Fig. 4.1). Two distinct types of succession have been identified (Fig. 4.2). In **allogenic succession**, factors of non-microbial origin are responsible for an altered pattern of community development. For example, the frequency of detection of mutans streptococci and *S. sanguinis* in the mouth increases markedly once hard, non-shedding

Table 4.2 The effect of tooth eruption on the composition of the cultivatable oral microflora in 21 young children.

Bacterium	**Percentage isolation frequency**	
	Mean age	
	3 months	**32 months**
Prevotella melaninogenica	76	100
non-pigmented *Prevotella*	62	100
Prevotella loescheii	14	90
Prevotella intermedia	10	67
Prevotella denticola	ND*	71
Fusobacterium nucleatum	67	100
Fusobacterium spp.	ND	71
Selenomonas spp.	ND	43
Capnocytophaga spp.	19	100
Leptotrichia spp.	24	71
Campylobacter spp.	5	43
Eikenella corrodens	5	57
Veillonella spp.	63	63

*ND = not detected.

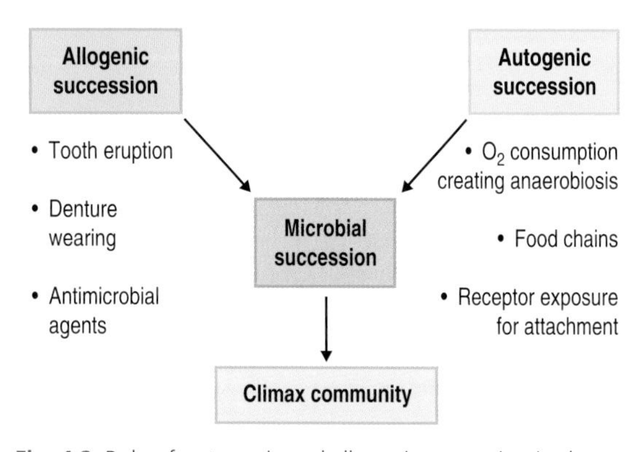

Fig. 4.2 Role of autogenic and allogenic succession in the development of oral microbial communities.

surfaces are present. This is usually following tooth eruption, but it can also occur after the insertion of dentures or removable orthodontic appliances, and acrylic obturators in children with cleft palate.

The increase in number and diversity of obligate anaerobes once teeth are present is an example of **autogenic succession** in which community development is influenced by microbial factors (Fig. 4.2). The metabolism of the aerobic and facultatively anaerobic pioneer species lowers the redox potential in plaque and creates conditions suitable for colonization by strict anaerobes (Ch. 5). Other examples of autogenic succession are the development of food chains and food webs, whereby the metabolic end product of one organism becomes a primary nutrient source for another:

complex substrate —(primary feeder)→ product —(secondary feeder)→ simpler product

A further example of autogenic succession is the exposure of new receptors for bacterial adhesion ('cryptitopes'; Ch. 5) following microbial modification of host macromolecules.

The gross composition of the oral microflora can remain relatively stable over time at individual sites, especially when analyzed at the genus or species level. Ribotyping (Ch. 3) can discriminate among strains within a species on the basis of genetic variation, thereby allowing specific **clonal types** to be recognised. Relatively few clones are found within species of pathogenic bacteria, and a limited number of these may be responsible for the majority of infections. In contrast, species that comprise the resident human microflora generally display large numbers of clones, and this may be a strategy to help such species evade the host defences. Clones of some species appear to persist for long periods at a site whereas others appear to be transient, and undergo replacement by fresh clones. For example, clonal replacement appears to maintain *S. mitis* biovar 1 in the mouth of neonates; 93 clonal types were detected among 101 strains of *S. mitis* colonizing 40 infants over a one month period. The clonal types that could be isolated were found to vary at different sampling times, suggesting that individual clones did not persist and were replaced by new clones. In a further study of the clonal diversity of *S. mitis* biovar 1, limited sharing of genotypes was found among three members of a particular family, and each individual carried between 6 and 13 types. Differences were also found between isolates recovered from the pharyngeal and buccal mucosa of the same individual. The reasons for, and the mechanisms involved in, the persistence of certain clones of some species but the continual turnover of clones of other species is not yet understood. It may be that the niche (function) occupied by these clonal types is similar, but that turnover may represent a longer-term survival strategy. Wide variations in the expression of carbohydrate and protein antigens have been found among the different genotypes of *S. mitis* biovar 1 from the family group, suggesting that this 'turnover' might play a role as an 'immune-evasion' mechanism for this species.

In contrast to the situation for *S. mitis*, a particular clone of *Aggregatibacter actinomycetemcomitans* has been implicated in an aggressive form of periodontitis in young adults (Ch. 6). The JP2 clone has a 530 base pair deletion in the promoter region of the leukotoxin gene operon, resulting in increased production of the leukotoxin. Adolescents harbouring this clone are more likely to suffer loss of attachment between the tooth and the periodontium than those who have non-JP2 types. In the future, the ability to recognise virulent clones of an organism may result in the better diagnosis and prediction of sites/individuals at risk of disease.

SUMMARY

The mouth is usually sterile at birth. The acquisition of the normal oral microflora follows a specific ecological progression from a small number of pioneer species, especially *S. salivarius, S. mitis* and *S. oralis*, to a diverse climax community containing many obligately anaerobic and nutritionally-fastidious bacteria. This development involves both allogenic and autogenic succession; in allogenic succession, community development is influenced by non-microbial factors while microbial factors are responsible for autogenic succession. There is a dynamic relationship between the host, the environment and the resident microflora.

AGEING AND THE ORAL MICROFLORA

The acquisition of the oral microflora continues with age. Following tooth eruption, the isolation frequency of spirochaetes and black-pigmented anaerobes increases. In one study, the latter group of organisms was recovered from 18 to 40% of children aged 5 years but were found in over 90% of teenagers aged 13–16 years. The increased prevalence of spirochaetes and black-pigmented anaerobes during puberty might be due to hormones entering the gingival crevice and acting as a novel nutrient source. The rise in *Prevotella intermedia* in plaque during the second trimester of pregnancy has also been ascribed to the elevated serum levels of oestradiol and progesterone which can satisfy the naphthaquinone requirement for growth of this organism. Increases in the numbers of black-pigmented anaerobes have also been observed in women taking oral contraceptives. Other studies have failed to show similar associations between black-pigmented anaerobes and pregnancy, while the recent application of more sensitive molecular techniques have detected these organisms in prepubertal children, implying that hormonal changes cannot be the only factor affecting the prevalence of these fastidious bacteria.

In adults, the composition and proportions of the resident oral microflora remain reasonably stable over time and this microflora coexists in relative harmony with the host. This stability (termed **microbial homeostasis**; Ch. 5, Fig. 5.18) is not a passive response to the environment, but is due to a dynamic balance being achieved from numerous inter-bacterial and host- bacterial interactions. The diversity of the oral microflora in a healthy individual is typically between 50-100 species.

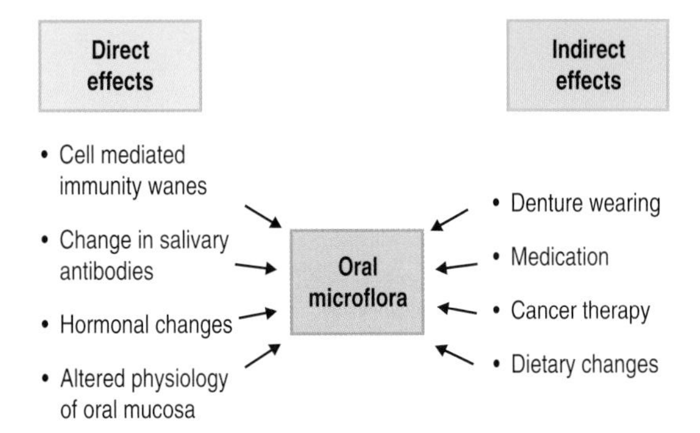

Fig. 4.3 Direct and indirect effects of ageing on the oral microflora.

Some variations in the oral microflora have been discerned in later life and can be attributed to both direct and indirect effects of ageing (Fig. 4.3). In the case of the latter, variations can occur if the habitat or environment is severely perturbed. For example, the risk of cancer rises with age, and cytotoxic therapy or myelosuppression combined with the disease itself is associated with the increased carriage of *Candida albicans* and non-oral opportunistic pathogens such as enterobacteria (e.g. *Klebsiella* spp., *Escherichia coli, Pseudomonas aeruginosa*) and *Staphylococcus aureus*. The wearing of dentures also increases with age and this also promotes colonization by *C. albicans*. Many elderly subjects take a variety of medications, the side-effects of which can reduce the flow of saliva and thereby perturb the normal balance of the resident oral microflora.

Information is now emerging on direct age-related changes to the oral microflora. Significantly higher proportions and isolation frequencies of lactobacilli and staphylococci (mainly *S. aureus*) in saliva were found in healthy subjects aged 70 years or over while yeasts were isolated more often and in higher numbers from saliva in those aged 80 years or more. Cell-mediated immunity declines with age, but the precise effect of old age on the innate and adaptive host defences of the mouth has yet to be established definitively. Serum IgM antibody titres to selected oral and gut commensal bacteria are lower in elderly subjects. These antibodies represent the initial response by the host to infection, and such a decrease in titre may be one explanation for the increased susceptibility to disease seen in older subjects. Age-related changes in salivary antibodies have also been reported. In general, activities of specific salivary IgG and IgM antibodies decreased in the elderly, whereas specific sIgA antibodies increased with age.

The incidence of oral candidosis is more common in the elderly and this has been attributed not only to the increased likelihood of denture wearing but also to physiological changes in the oral mucosa, malnutrition, and to trace element deficiencies. There have been reports of increased isolations of enterobacteria from the oropharynx of the elderly, but this seems to be related in many cases to the health of the individual rather than to their age *per se*, with the highest incidences being in the most debilitated individuals. One of the fundamental problems in determining whether the oral microflora changes in old age is that the chronological age of a person does not always equate to their physiological age!

Social habits can perturb the balance of the oral microflora. The regular intake of dietary carbohydrates can lead to the enrichment of aciduric (acid-tolerant) and cariogenic species such as mutans streptococci and lactobacilli. Furthermore, mutans streptococci and *S. sanguinis* are not detected in the mouths of individuals who have full dentures when these surfaces are not worn, although both groups of bacteria can reappear when these 'hard surfaces' are inserted again. Smoking has been shown to affect bacterial counts, and is a significant risk factor for periodontal diseases.

METHODS OF DETERMINING THE COMPOSITION OF THE RESIDENT ORAL MICROFLORA

There are a number of challenges when attempting to determine the composition of the microbial communities at sites in the mouth. These range from the basic problem of removing the majority of the microorganisms from their habitat (many of which are by necessity bound tenaciously to a surface or to each other, and the site may be difficult to access) to their eventual identification (Table 4.3; Ch. 3). The main approaches to determining the microbial composition of the oral microflora are illustrated in Fig. 4.4, while the main differences between culture-dependent and -independent approaches were highlighted in Figure 3.2. Some of the issues are discussed in more detail below:

Sample taking

The microflora can vary in composition over relatively small distances. Therefore, large plaque samples

Table 4.3 Some properties of the oral microflora that contribute to the difficulty in determining its composition.

Property	Comment
High species diversity	The oral microflora, and especially dental plaque, consists of a diverse number of microbial species, some of which are present only in low numbers.
Surface attachment/coaggregation (coadhesion)	Oral microorganisms attach firmly to surfaces and to each other and, therefore, have to be dispersed without loss of viability.
Obligate anaerobes	Many oral bacteria lose their viability if exposed to air for prolonged periods.
Fastidious nutrition/unculturable	Some bacteria are difficult to grow in pure culture and may require specific cofactors etc. for growth. Some groups (e.g. certain spirochaetes; TM7 group) cannot as yet be cultured in the laboratory.
Slow growth	The slow growth of some organisms makes enumeration time consuming, (e.g. they may require14–21 days incubation).
Identification	The classification of many oral microorganisms still remains unresolved or confused; simple criteria for identification are not always available (particularly for some obligate anaerobes).

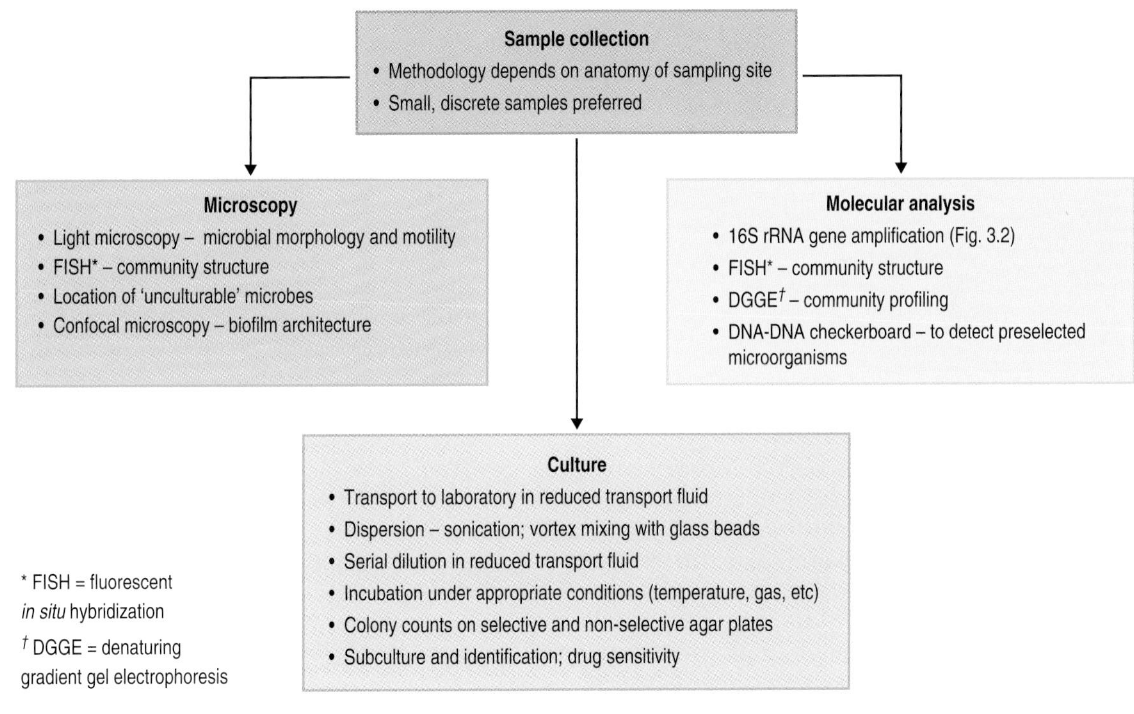

Fig. 4.4 Stages in the microbiological analysis of the oral microflora. Culture, microscopy and molecular approaches can be used to characterize the oral microflora.

or a number of smaller pooled samples from different sites can be of little value because important site-specific differences will be obscured. Consequently, small samples from discrete sites are preferable, but the method of sampling will depend on the anatomy and properties of the site to be studied.

The oral mucosa can be sampled by swabbing, direct impression techniques, or by removing epithelial cells by scraping or scrubbing with a blunt instrument into a container. Microbial counts can then be related to a fixed area or to an individual epithelial cell. Saliva can be collected by expectoration into a sterile container; the saliva flow can be at a normal resting rate (unstimulated) or it can be stimulated by chemical means or by chewing. Although a greater volume is collected by stimulation, such samples will also contain many more organisms that have been dislodged from oral surfaces.

There is no universally accepted way of sampling dental plaque. The accessible smooth surfaces of enamel pose few problems and a range of dental instruments have been used. Dental probes, scalers, dental floss and abrasive strips have been used to remove plaque from approximal surfaces between teeth. Fine probes, pieces of wire, blunt hypodermic needles, and toothpicks have been used to sample plaque from fissures, although the amount of biofilm removed can depend on the anatomy of the site. Subgingival plaque is difficult to sample because of the inaccessibility and anaerobic nature of the site. High numbers of obligately anaerobic bacteria are found in the gingival crevice and periodontal pocket, most of which will lose their viability if exposed to air. In disease, the anatomy of the site means that those organisms at the base of the pocket, near the advancing front of the lesion, are likely to be of most interest (Ch. 6). Again, it is important to avoid removing plaque from other areas within the pocket so as not to obscure significant relationships between particular bacteria and disease. A common approach is to insert paper points into pockets but the number of firmly adherent organisms removed from the root of the tooth will be small. Samples have also been taken by irrigation of the site and retrieval of the material through syringe needles; however, this method will obviously remove plaque from the whole depth of the pocket. A particularly sophisticated method employed a broach kept withdrawn in a cannula that was flushed constantly with oxygen-free nitrogen. The broach was used to sample plaque only when the cannula was in position near the base of the pocket. After sampling, the broach was retracted into the cannula and withdrawn. Another approach has been to use a curette or scaler after the supragingival area has been cleared. The scaler tips can be detached and placed immediately in gas-flushed tubes containing reduced (anaerobic) transport fluid for delivery to the laboratory. Alternatively, when periodontal surgery is needed, plaque has been removed from extracted teeth or from surfaces exposed when 'gingival flaps' are reflected. It is important to appreciate, particularly when comparing studies in which different sampling procedures have been used, that the results will, to a certain extent, reflect the method adopted.

Transport and dispersion

Cultural studies require that samples should be transported to the laboratory for processing as quickly as possible. Specially designed transport fluids containing reducing agents to maintain a low redox potential will help reduce the loss of viability of anaerobic organisms during delivery to the laboratory.

Clumps and aggregates of bacteria must be dispersed efficiently (ideally to single cells) prior to dilution and plating of the specimen. Plaque poses a particular problem in this respect because, by definition, it is a mixture of a diverse range of microorganisms bound tenaciously to one another. One of the most efficient methods, particularly for subgingival plaque, is to vortex samples with small, sterile glass beads, ideally in a tube filled with inert gas. Mild sonication produces the maximum number of particles from a specimen but it exerts a selective effect by specifically damaging spirochaetes and some other Gram negative bacteria, particularly *Fusobacterium* species.

Cultivation

Once dispersed, samples are usually serially diluted in a suitable fluid (usually a transport fluid) and aliquots are spread on to a number of freshly prepared, pre-reduced agar plates, and incubated to allow cells to form microbial colonies. These media are designed to grow either (a) the maximum number of bacteria (e.g. blood agar) or, (b) only a limited number of species (**selective media**) in order to recover minor components of the microflora. For example, the addition of vancomycin to blood agar plates will inhibit most Gram positive bacteria, while a high sucrose concentration encourages the growth of oral streptococci, and plates with a low pH favour lactobacilli. It should be emphasised that these media are selective and not specific for any type of microbe. The identity of the colonies on these plates must be confirmed; colonial appearance or mere growth on a particular medium is not diagnostic. Media need to be incubated for different times and under different atmospheric conditions depending on the bacteria being cultivated. For example, 7–14 days incubation at 37 °C in an anaerobic jar or cabinet filled with a gas mix containing

$CO_2/H_2/N_2$ will be needed to grow some obligate anaerobes; in contrast, *Neisseria* require only 2 days incubation in air. Some organisms are capnophilic (CO_2-loving) and grow optimally in 10% CO_2 in air. Other media require supplementation with growth factors in order to enable certain fastidious organisms to grow (Ch. 3). As mentioned previously, at present only about 50% of the resident oral microflora can be cultured in the laboratory.

Enumeration and Identification

Colonies are counted and their concentration in the original sample is determined by compensating for the dilution steps, and expressed as colony forming units (CFU). Representative colonies are subcultured to check for purity and for subsequent identification; isolates can also be tested for antimicrobial susceptibility. Colony counting assumes that:

(a) cells of the same microorganism produce colonies with an identical morphology,

(b) cells of different species produce distinct morphologies, and

(c) one colony arises from a single cell.

Generally, these assumptions hold true except for (c), as most colonies inevitably arise from small aggregates of cells; this emphasizes the need for efficient dispersion of samples. It is also advisable to take several examples of a particular colony type to ensure that some species are not overlooked due to their appearance being similar to a numerically dominant organism. One strategy to determine the predominant microflora involves identifying 30–50 random colonies, irrespective of their morphology, rather than selecting only those colony types that appear different.

The first level of discrimination involves the Gram staining of subcultured colonies; bacteria are then grouped according to whether their cells are Gram positive or Gram negative, and are rod- or coccal-shaped. This dictates which tests will be necessary to achieve speciation. Some bacteria can be identified using simple criteria, for example, sugar fermentation tests or the detection of preformed enzymes using commercial kits. Other bacteria require a more sophisticated approach such as the application of gas–liquid chromatography to determine their acid end-products of metabolism (Table 3.2). The use of probes (antibody or oligonucleotide) on isolates can speed up identification and distinguish between strains of the same species (for example, by ribotyping); this level of discrimination is essential for studies of bacterial transmission. Other issues relating to bacterial identification are discussed in Chapter 3.

Microscopy

As an alternative to many of the lengthy steps associated with conventional culture techniques, the principal morphological groups of bacteria can be determined using light microscopy (Fig. 4.4). Dark-field illumination or phase contrast techniques have been used to quantify the numbers of motile bacteria (including spirochaetes) directly in dental plaque (particularly from subgingival sites). Such organisms are related to the severity of some periodontal diseases, and this approach has been used in the clinic to monitor sites undergoing treatment. However, most of the putative pathogens cannot be recognized by morphology alone. To overcome this problem, cells can be identified by reaction with antisera (monoclonal or specific polyclonal), oligonucleotide probes or tagged with a fluorescent label (Fig. 3.3).

Scanning and transmission electron microscopy have proved useful in studying plaque formation, and have also been used to show that bacteria invade gingival tissues in aggressive forms of periodontal disease. Electron dense markers (ferritin, peroxidase, gold granules) conjugated with antibodies can label specific surface antigens on bacteria and facilitate their identification within plaque. Electron microscopy requires samples to be processed before viewing which can distort the structure of plaque. Non-invasive techniques such as confocal laser scanning microscopy are now being used, with and without the use of specific probes (antibody or oligonucleotide), to determine the true architecture of plaque and the location of selected bacteria within the biofilm (Ch. 5). Confocal microscopy involves the generation of numerous focussed images throughout the depth of an untreated specimen (optical sections); image analysis software is then used to combine these sections and reconstruct the three-dimensional structure of the original specimen (for an example, see Fig. 4.6). Confocal microscopy has shown that plaque may have a more open architecture than previously thought from studies involving electron microscopy.

In situ models

As a result of some of the methodological problems outlined above, various devices have been developed that can be worn in the mouth by volunteers, containing model surfaces for microbial colonization. These devices can be removed from the mouth to facilitate sampling. The microbiology of fissure plaque has been studied using artificial or natural fissures mounted in a crown or in an occlusal filling. Removable pieces of enamel or denture acrylic have been placed on natural teeth or dentures in a desired position and have been used for studies of the structural development of dental plaque. Removable appliances have the additional advantages that experiments can be performed on the surfaces when out of the mouth that would not be permitted on natural teeth, such as the effect of regular sugar applications, or the evaluation of novel antimicrobial agents.

Molecular approaches

The limitations and bias of culture approaches can be avoided by applying molecular approaches to microbial detection and identification. 16S rRNA gene sequences can be amplified with universal oligonucleotide primers, cloned, and compared to existing sequences in databases; these approaches were discussed in Chapter 3 and have enabled the recognition in clinical specimens of species that are as yet unculturable in the laboratory (Fig. 3.2). The location of these organisms can be determined in biofilms such as dental plaque by *in situ* hybridization, usually with a fluorescent label (Fig. 3.3). A molecular approach such as denaturing gradient gel electrophoresis (DGGE) can be used to compare the diversity of oral microbial communities from different sites in health and disease. Likewise, checkerboard DNA–DNA hybridization techniques can be used to simultaneously screen multiple clinical samples for around 40 different preselected microbial species (Ch. 3).

DISTRIBUTION OF THE RESIDENT ORAL MICROFLORA

The populations making up the resident microbial community of the oral cavity are not found with equal frequency throughout the mouth. The composition of these communities varies on distinct surfaces due to differences in the biological and physical properties of each site. In the following sections the predominant microflora from several different sites in the oral cavity will be compared (Fig. 4.5, Table 4.5).

Lips and palate

The lips form the border between the skin microflora (which consists predominantly of staphylococci, micrococci and Gram positive rods such as

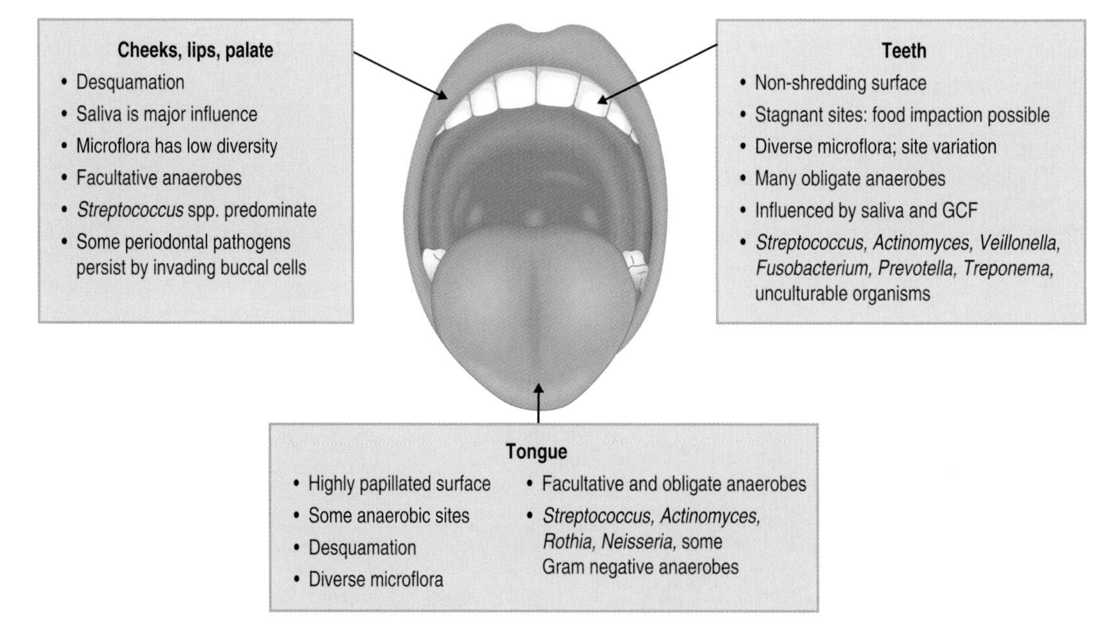

Fig. 4.5 Distribution of the microflora at distinct sites in the mouth.

Corynebacterium and *Propionibacterium* spp.), and that of the mouth (which contains many Gram negative species and few of the organisms commonly found on the skin surface). Facultatively anaerobic streptococci comprise a large part of the microflora on the lips. *Veillonella* and *Neisseria* have also been found, but only in very low numbers (<1.0% of the total cultivable microflora). *Streptococcus vestibularis* is recovered most commonly from the 'gutter' between the lower lip and the gums, and occasionally black-pigmented anaerobes and fusobacteria have been detected; between 3-9 species are usually present in this region. *Candida albicans* can colonize damaged lip mucosal surfaces in the corners of the mouth ('angular cheilitis'; Ch. 9). Molecular techniques have confirmed the presence of a range of streptococci on the lips, especially *S. mitis, S. oralis* and *S. constellatus;* some obligate anaerobes are also detected occasionally, including *P. melaninogenica.*

The microflora of the normal palate can show large variations between subjects, not only in the total colony forming units removed (which may reflect differences in the area sampled or the success in removing organisms) but also in the proportions of the individual species. The majority of the bacteria are streptococci and actinomyces; veillonellae, haemophili and Gram negative anaerobes are also regularly recovered but at lower levels (Table 4.4). *Candida* are not regularly isolated from the normal palate except when dentures are worn; in this situation, the mucosa of the palate can become infected with *C. albicans* (denture stomatitis; Ch. 9).

Table 4.4 Predominant cultivable microflora of the healthy human palatal mucosa.

Microorganism	Percentage of the total cultivable microflora	Percentage isolation frequency
Streptococcus	52	100
Actinomyces	15	100
Lactobacillus	1	87
Neisseria	2	93
Veillonella	1	100
Prevotella	4	100
Candida	+*	7

*present, but in numbers too low to count.

Studies using culture independent molecular approaches have detected a more diverse microflora including a range of streptococci (*S. mitis, S. oralis,* and *S. infantis*), as well as *Gemella* spp., *Neisseria* spp., *Veillonella* spp., *Capnocytophaga gingivalis* and *Prevotella melaninogenica* (and other *Prevotella* spp.) in samples from the palate from healthy adults. The number of species present ranged from 4 to 21 per person in a survey of 5 people.

Cheek

Streptococci are the predominant bacteria from the cheek (buccal mucosa), especially members of the mitis-group, and *H. parainfluenzae* is also commonly isolated (Table 4.5). *Simonsiella* spp. are isolated primarily from the cheek cells of humans and animals. Obligate anaerobes are not present in high numbers, although spirochaetes and other motile organisms have been observed by microscopy to be attached to the buccal mucosa. Molecular techniques have confirmed the presence of a range of streptococcal species on buccal cells, as well as *Granulicatella* and *Gemella* spp.; obligate anaerobes were less commonly detected, although *Veillonella* and *Prevotella* spp. were present. Between 4 and 20 species can be detected in a sample from the buccal mucosa.

Recent studies, in which fluorescent *in situ* hybridization (FISH) was combined with confocal microscopy, have shown that some of the species implicated in periodontal disease (*A. actinomycetemcomitans, P. gingivalis, F. nucleatum, P. intermedia, T. forsythia*) can gain refuge inside buccal epithelial cells in healthy people, where they persist as intracellular polymicrobial communities (Fig. 4.6). Furthermore, *F. nucleatum* can transport non-invasive species, such as *S. cristatus,* into human oral epithelial cells via inter-bacterial coaggregation. Streptococci were the most common organisms found intracellularly in about 30% of buccal epithelial cells, followed by *Granulicatella adiacens* and *Gemella haemolysans.* These studies imply that oral mucosal cells could serve as a reservoir for periodontal pathogens.

Tongue

The dorsum of the tongue with its highly papillated surface has a large surface area and supports a higher bacterial density and a more diverse microflora than other oral mucosal surfaces (Table 4.5), with around 20 species being present in a typical sample. Streptococci are the most numerous group

Table 4.5 Proportions of some cultivable bacterial populations at different sites in the normal oral cavity.

Bacterium	Saliva	Buccal mucosa	Tongue dorsum	Supragingival plaque
Streptococcus sanguinis	1	6	1	7
S. salivarius	3	3	6	2
S. oralis / S. mitis	21	29	33	23
mutans streptococci	4	3	3	5
Actinomyces naeslundii	2	1	5	5
A. odontolyticus	2	1	7	13
Haemophilus spp	4	7	15	7
Capnocytophaga spp	<1	<1	1	<1
Fusobacterium spp	1	<1	<1	<1
Black-pigmented anaerobes	<1	<1	1	+*

*detected on occasions.

of bacteria (approximately 40% of the total cultivable microflora) with salivarius- and mitis-group organisms predominating. Anaerobic streptococci have also been isolated while *Rothia mucilagenosa* is found almost exclusively on the tongue. Other major groups of bacteria (and their proportions) include *Veillonella* spp. (16%), Gram positive rods (16%) of which *Actinomyces naeslundii* and *A. odontolyticus* are common, and haemophili (15%). Both pigmenting (*Prevotella intermedia, P. melaninogenica*) and non-pigmenting anaerobes can be recovered from the tongue and this site is regarded as a potential reservoir (along with the tonsils) for some of the organisms implicated in periodontal diseases. Other organisms, including lactobacilli, yeasts, fusobacteria, spirochaetes and other motile bacteria, have been found in low numbers (<1% of the total microflora) on the tongue.

Similar findings have been obtained from a comprehensive study of the anterior dorsal surface of the tongue in infants (aged 8–13 months). Streptococci accounted for 52% of the microflora, and *S. salivarius* and *S. mitis* were the predominant species (Table 4.6). *Rothia mucilaginosa* was recovered from almost half of the samples. High proportions of *Neisseria* (20%) were also found, together with lower levels of *Actinomyces* (5%) and occasional Gram negative species including haemophili, fusobacteria, *Prevotella, Capnocytophaga* and *Aggregatibacter*.

Molecular studies, in which 16S rRNA gene sequences (Ch. 3) were determined on DNA from scrapings of the tongue dorsum, have been carried out to more fully characterize the microflora of the tongue. The microflora was shown to be even more diverse than predicted from culture studies, and about 30% of the bacterial populations detected were found only on the tongue, suggesting that the properties of this habitat are distinct from those of other oral surfaces. 16–22 species were detected in each tongue sample, and the most common isolates were *Rothia mucilagenosa, S. salivarius* and a *Eubacterium* spp.. Studies using DNA–DNA checkerboard techniques found a number of Gram negative bacteria on the tongue, including *P. melaninogenica, V. parvula* and *C. gingivalis*, while other studies commonly detected *Granulicatella* and *Gemella* spp..

Oral malodour is associated with the microflora of the tongue. A higher bacterial load, especially of Gram negative anaerobes (including *Porphyromonas, Prevotella* and *Fusobacterium* spp.), was isolated from the tongue of subjects with high odour. An even more diverse microflora was found when culture independent molecular methods were applied; species associated with halitosis included *Atopobium parvulum, Dialister* spp., *Eubacterium sulci, Solobacterium moorei*, an uncharacterized *Streptococcus*, and members of the uncultivable group, TM7 (Ch. 3; Fig. 3.3B). The chemical basis of odour is not fully understood, but

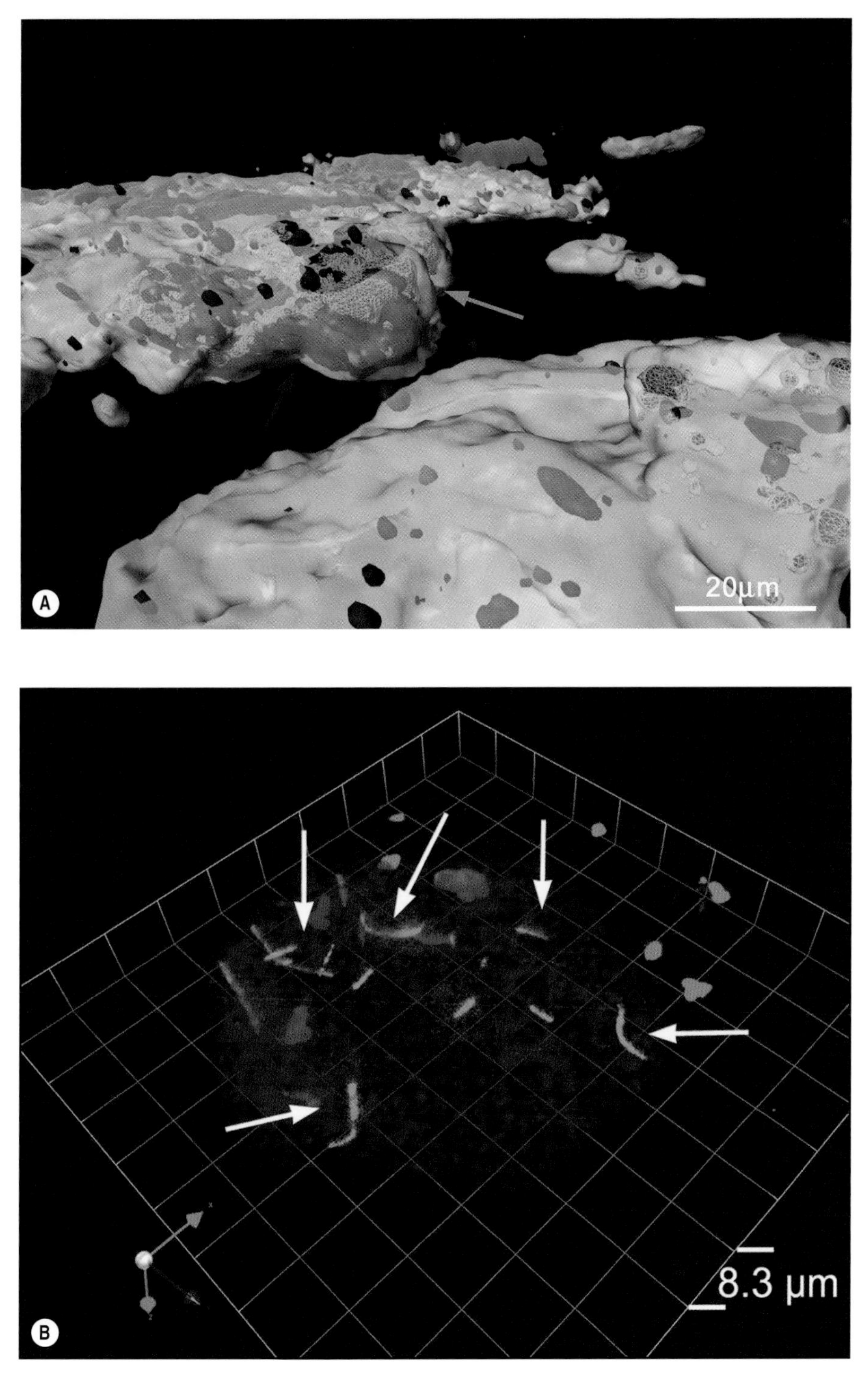

Fig. 4.6 Intracellular colonization of buccal epithelial cells. (A) Three-dimensional reconstruction of a buccal epithelial cell (BEC). Bacteria recognized only by a universal bacterial probe are shown in solid red, while co-localization of the *Aggregatibacter actinomycetemcomitans* and universal probes is depicted by a green wireframe over a red interior. Reconstructed BEC surfaces are presented in blue. The red and green colours are muted when bacterial masses are intracellular, and brighter when bacteria appear to project out of the surface. The large mass indicated by red and green arrows is a cohesive unit containing *A. actinomycetemcomitans* in direct proximity to other species. Published with permission: Rudney et al, J Dent Res 2005 84:59–63. (B) Buccal cell dominated by presumed streptococci that were labelled by a universal bacterial probe (red). The sample also was treated with a *Fusobacterium nucleatum*-specific probe, and the buccal cell shown contained several yellow *F. nucleatum* cells (arrows) in close association with cocci. Published with permission: Rudney et al, J Dent Res 2005 84:1165–1171.

Table 4.6 The predominant cultivable microflora of the tongue from pre-school children.

Bacterium	Mean proportion (%)	Isolation frequency (%)
Streptococcus anginosus	4.7	42
Streptococcus oralis	3.8	30
Streptococcus mitis	11.8	75
Streptococcus mutans	1.0	8
Streptococcus sobrinus	0.5	2
Streptococcus salivarius	22.3	94
Streptococcus sanguinis	7.6	58
Total streptococci	**51.7**	
Actinomyces naeslundii	4.2	46
Actinomyces odontolyticus	1.1	17
Rothia dentocariosa	0.9	21
Rothia mucilaginosa	5.5	46
Corynebacterium matruchotii	0.1	4
Lactobacillus spp.	0.3	6
Total Gram positive rods	**12.1**	
Neisseria spp.	20.2	>90
Veillonella spp.	6.3	73
Total Gram negative cocci	**26.5**	
Prevotella spp.	0.4	15
Fusobacterium spp.	0.6	25
Leptotrichia spp.	0.2	13
Haemophilus spp.	0.6	19
Aggregatibacter spp.	0.1	4
Capnocytophaga spp.	0.1	6
Aerobic Gram negative rods	2.3	40
Anaerobic Gram negative rods	1.8	40
Yeasts	1.0	4

Data are from 9 children, aged 8 –13 months.

includes the production of volatile sulphur compounds by the resident microflora; some implicated compounds are described later in this Chapter.

Saliva

Although saliva contains up to 10^8 microorganisms ml^{-1} it is not considered to have its own resident microflora. The normal rate of swallowing ensures that bacteria cannot be maintained in the mouth by multiplication in saliva. The organisms found are derived from other surfaces, especially the tongue (Table 4.5), as a result of oral removal forces (saliva and GCF flow, chewing, oral hygiene). The microbial profile of saliva (in particular, the level of mutans streptococci and/or lactobacilli) has been used as an indicator of the caries susceptibility of an individual, and commercially-available kits for their culture are available. People with high counts of these potentially cariogenic bacteria are considered to be 'at-risk', and can be targeted for intense oral hygiene, antimicrobial therapy and dietary counselling (Ch. 6).

Teeth

The microbial community associated with teeth is referred to as dental plaque. Its composition varies at each tooth surface due to the local environmental conditions (Ch. 2). For these reasons, plaque is described on the basis of the sampling site by terms such as smooth surface, approximal, fissure, or gingival crevice plaque, while the terms supragingival and subgingival plaque are used to describe samples taken above or below the gum margin, respectively (Fig. 2.2). The detailed composition of dental plaque from these sites will be given in Chapter 5. As teeth are non-shedding surfaces, the highest numbers of microorganisms are found in stagnant sites which afford protection from removal forces; a typical sample of plaque might contain around 20 species. Dental plaque is an example of a biofilm; bacteria growing in biofilms can display novel properties, including an enhanced tolerance of antimicrobial agents. The properties of plaque as a biofilm are discussed in Chapter 5.

Gram positive rods and filaments (mainly *Actinomyces* species) are among the major groups of bacteria cultured from plaque (Table 4.5). Mutans streptococci and members of the mitis- and anginosus-groups of streptococci are found in highest numbers on teeth whereas, in contrast to mucosal surfaces, *S. salivarius* is only a minor component of dental plaque. Obligate anaerobes are found in high numbers particularly in the gingival crevice, and oral spirochaetes are almost uniquely associated with this region. There are high proportions of bacteria belonging to groups that cannot, as yet, be cultured in the laboratory. Molecular (culture-independent) studies of early colonization of removable enamel chips confirmed streptococci as the predominant colonizers of early plaque (at 4 and 8 hours), but also found representatives of the genera *Actinomyces, Gemella, Granulicatella, Neisseria, Prevotella, Rothia* and *Veillonella*. FISH-studies showed streptococci and *Prevotella* spp. existing as small multi-generic clusters of cells, which may aid their co-survival during early biofilm development. Thus, the composition of dental plaque differs both qualitatively and quantitatively from the communities of other oral surfaces.

SUMMARY

Oral populations are not distributed evenly in the mouth. Large differences occur in the prevalence of individual species at particular oral sites (Table 4.5), resulting in each habitat having a characteristic microflora. Desquamation ensures that the microbial load on most mucosal surfaces is low, although the papillated surfaces of the tongue promote the accumulation of complex microbial communities, including obligate anaerobes. Dental plaque, especially at stagnant sites on teeth, harbours the most diverse microflora.

FACTORS INFLUENCING THE DISTRIBUTION OF ORAL MICROORGANISMS

For successful colonization, microorganisms must first adhere to a surface and then be able to multiply. In order to overcome the oral removal forces, microbes either seek out habitats that offer protection (refuge) from the environment, or they deploy specific adherence mechanisms. The distribution of many oral populations is related to their ability to adhere to specific surfaces, and this property is referred to as a **tissue tropism**. However, the final proportions of attached microorganisms are determined by their subsequent ability to grow and compete successfully with neighbouring species. As discussed in Chapter 2, the degree of anaerobiosis (redox potential; Eh) and nutrient availability will determine whether the attached cells can grow at a site. The sites with the lowest Eh (and the highest number of obligate anaerobes) are those associated with stagnant areas on the teeth. Also, in a biofilm such as dental plaque, oxygen consumption by aerobic and facultatively anaerobic organisms can create anoxic (oxygen-depleted) and reduced conditions over relatively short distances, which will also facilitate the growth of obligate anaerobes. The increased proportions of many asaccharolytic but proteolytic bacteria in subgingival plaque during various periodontal diseases is due, in part, to the provision of additional nutrients (proteins, glycoproteins) by GCF (Ch. 6).

The presence of some other species can be attributed to the provision of nutrients by other oral bacteria in food chains.

SUMMARY

The distribution of microorganisms in the mouth is related to the redox potential (Eh) and nutrient availability at individual sites, and also to the strength of adherence between an organism and a surface.

HOST AND BACTERIAL FACTORS INVOLVED IN ADHERENCE

Oral microorganisms do not encounter naked host surfaces. Molecules are absorbed from saliva on to the tooth and mucosal surfaces to form a conditioning film (the acquired pellicle). The first stage of adherence involves the initial interaction between the external surfaces of both the microbe and the substrate, and adhesion will be influenced by the properties of the suspending medium (saliva). The initial process can be described in terms of precise physicochemical interactions of attraction and repulsion (Ch. 5). Subsequently, attachment involves specific molecular interactions between complementary molecules on the microbial and host surface. In general, the term 'adhesin' is used to describe the microbial components which function in adherence while the host-derived factors are termed 'receptors'. A microbial cell surface can express multiple types of adhesin while the host surface can contain several classes of receptor. Bacteria can also contain receptors that react with adhesins on other microbial types during cell-cell attachment (coaggregation or coadhesion; Ch. 5). Some polymers of host and bacterial origin that are involved in adherence are discussed below.

Host receptors

Epithelial cells, especially the buccal epithelium, have sialic acid exposed on their surfaces which can interact with adhesins on bacteria such as *S. mitis*. If the sialic acid residue is removed, for example, by bacterial neuraminidases, then another receptor (a galactosyl residue) can be exposed which is recognised by *Actinomyces* spp., and Gram negative bacteria including *Fusobacterium nucleatum*, *Prevotella intermedia* and *Eikenella corrodens*. Collagen fibres, which are major structural components of connective tissue, can also act as receptors for certain mutans streptococci (*S. cricetis*, *S. ratti*) and *Porphyromonas gingivalis*, while specific domains for the attachment of streptococci or spirochaetes can be found on fibronectin.

Pellicles form on all oral surfaces (hard and soft) and are not identical; the components that adsorb to cementum are not the same as enamel, and both will differ from those that form on the oral mucosa. These differences are sometimes acknowledged by the use of different terminologies, such as the acquired enamel pellicle or the acquired cementum pellicle, while the pellicle that forms on epithelial surfaces is referred to as the mucus coat. Pellicle forms as soon as a clean surface is exposed to saliva; it takes around 90–120 minutes for the adsorption of molecules to reach a plateau and cease (Fig. 5.3). Pellicles contain proteins, lipids and glycolipids; once formed, the composition and structure of pellicles will change and be modified.

Within the enamel pellicle, acidic proline-rich proteins and statherin promote the adherence of *Actinomyces naeslundii*, some *S. mutans* strains and black-pigmented anaerobes. Amylase, lysozyme, albumin and immunoglobulins, as well as some bacterial components, including glucosyltransferases (GTFs) and glucans, have also been detected in the acquired pellicle. The adsorbed enzymes in the pellicle are still able to function and the glucans produced can bind to molecules (glucan-binding proteins) on mutans streptococci, thereby increasing their ability to colonize. The polymer synthesised by adsorbed GTF on the tooth surface has a different chemical structure to that produced by free-living bacteria.

Bacterial adhesins

Many bacterial adhesins are lectins (carbohydrate-binding proteins) that bind to carbohydrate receptors on a surface. Often these adhesins are associated with surface structures termed fibrils or fimbriae. Fibrils are short and narrow while fimbriae have a measurable width (3–14 nm) and a variable length up to 20 µm. Some cells possess both fibrils and fimbriae, and strains can have different functional types of each structure. For example, *S. salivarius* has a complex fibrillar mosaic comprising four different classes of fibril, each with a specific length. The 91 nm fibrils are responsible for coaggregation with *Veillonella parvula* while the 73 nm fibrils are involved with adhesion to buccal epithelial cells. The longest (178 nm) and shortest (63 nm) fibrils have yet to be assigned a function. Similarly, *A. naeslundii* possesses two types of fimbriae. Type 1 fimbriae mediate the binding of cells to adsorbed proline-rich proteins and to statherin in salivary pellicle on enamel whereas type 2 fimbriae are associated with a galactosyl-binding lectin which mediates attachment to host cells and to other bacteria (coadhesion or coaggregation). The presence of fibrils is not limited to Gram positive oral bacteria. Strains of *Prevotella* spp. (Fig. 4.7) carry peritrichous fibrils, the morphology, cellular density and length of which can vary markedly.

A significant adhesin is the antigen I/II family of cell surface-anchored polypeptides found in most oral streptococci. These linear polypeptides are structurally complex, multi-functional adhesins, with multiple receptor binding sites. Discrete regions within these peptides bind to human salivary glycoproteins (agglutinins), other microbial cells (coaggregation; Ch. 5), and calcium. Sequences within the N-terminal region preferentially bind salivary glycoproteins in solution, while the C-terminal half of the polypeptide contains species-specific adhesion-mediating sequences that bind only to surface-associated glycoproteins.

Other bacterial adhesins include glucosyltransferases (GTFs) which are found on the surface of several oral streptococci. Some species produce more than one GTF (see later this Chapter). These GTFs can interact with receptors in pellicle such as blood group reactive proteins or adsorbed dextrans and glucans. The latter can also react with glucan-binding proteins expressed by other streptococci. The polysaccharides synthesized by GTFs help consolidate bacterial attachment to hard surfaces in the mouth and contribute to the plaque biofilm matrix (Ch. 5). GTFs are secreted and have been found both in pellicle and on the surface of unrelated bacteria where they retain biological function. Thus, some species may produce extracellular polysaccharides (EPS) in plaque using a surrogate enzyme from another organism. Many oral Gram positive bacteria are negatively charged due to the penetration of the cell wall by lipoteichoic acid (LTA). These anionic polymers are composed of sugar phosphates, usually glycerol and ribitol phosphate, and interact with blood group reactive substances in pellicle. The surface of oral bacteria is a complex mosaic of multi-functional molecules, many of which can play a role in attachment. The cell surface of a Gram positive bacterium is shown schematically in Fig. 4.8. The production of molecules such as peptidoglycan, LTA, polysaccharide, proteins and lipoproteins can be influenced by the growth environment. Oral bacteria may be able to detect that they are on a surface, and therefore modify their pattern of gene expression to suit the new environmental conditions.

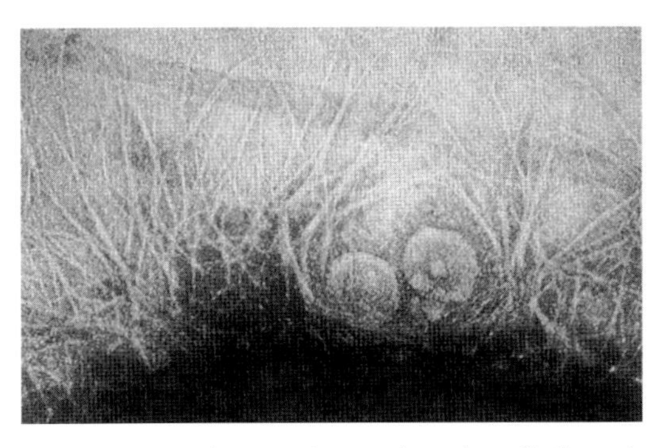

Fig. 4.7 Scanning electron micrograph to show fibrils on the cell surface of *Prevotella nigrescens*.

SUMMARY

The acquisition of the resident oral microflora involves the interaction between adhesins on the microbial cell surface and receptors on the host surface. Desquamation ensures that the microbial load is light on mucosal surfaces. A wide range of potential receptors are adsorbed onto teeth and form the acquired pellicle, increasing the potential for diversity in terms of microbial colonization. Furthermore, the fact that teeth are non-shedding surfaces means that large accumulations of microorganisms can develop. These accumulations, or biofilms, are termed dental plaque; the properties and composition of dental plaque are discussed in Chapter 5.

FUNCTIONS OF THE CLIMAX COMMUNITY: COLONIZATION RESISTANCE

One of the main beneficial functions of the resident microflora at any site is its ability to prevent colonization by exogenous (and often pathogenic) organisms (**colonization resistance**; Table 4.7). A strain of *S. salivarius* (strain TOVE)

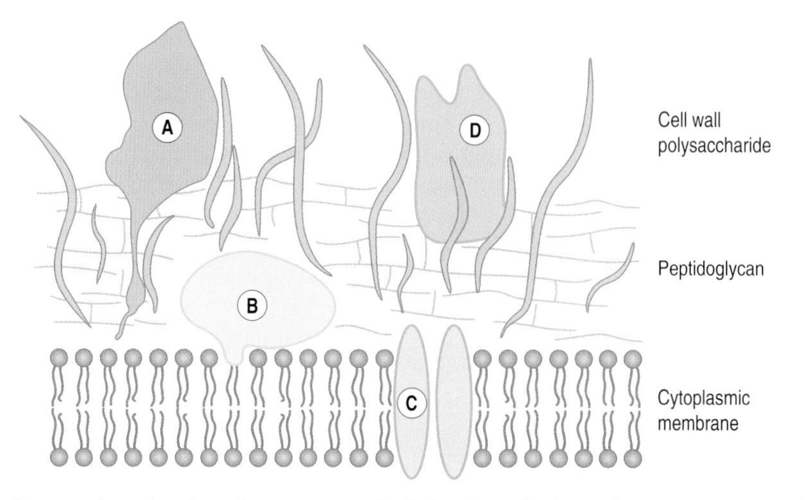

Fig. 4.8 Diagram to illustrate the cell surface of a streptococcal cell showing adhesins and receptors associated with adherence, and solute transport. (A) cell wall anchored polypeptide; (B) membrane anchored polypeptide; (C) transmembrane polypeptide (e.g. in transport of solutes); (D) extracellular polypeptide (e.g. GTF).

Table 4.7 Functions of the resident oral microflora that contribute to colonization resistance.

Function
Competition for receptors for adhesion
Competition for essential endogenous nutrients and cofactors
Creation of microenvironments that discourage the growth of exogenous species
Production of inhibitory substances (bacteriocins, H_2O_2, bacteriophage, etc.)

has been shown to displace virulent strains of *S. mutans* from teeth in experimental animal studies. Other strains of *S. salivarius* produce an inhibitor (termed enocin or salivaricin) that can prevent or reduce colonization by pathogenic Lancefield Group A streptococci (*S. pyogenes*) on mucosal surfaces. In some countries, children are being deliberately colonized by bacteriocin-producing strains of *S. salivarius* in order to reduce the incidence of streptococcal sore throats, and the use of oral probiotics is being considered to boost the benefits of the resident oral microflora in an analogous manner to that used to improve gastric health. The properties of some of these probiotic streptococcal strains (e.g. S. *salivarius* K12) may also include the down-regulation of proinflammatory responses to resident bacteria by the host.

Attempts have been made to enhance the colonization resistance of the resident oral microflora. As the mother is the major source of bacteria (including cariogenic species) in the infant, levels of mutans streptococci have been suppressed in expectant mothers by professional oral hygiene, dietary counselling with, if necessary, treatment with chlorhexidine or fluoride (Ch. 6). The result is that the natural microflora of the infant increases in diversity in the absence of mutans streptococci. The subsequent colonization by these cariogenic streptococci is delayed, as is the average time for the first caries lesion to form. Other approaches include the preemptive colonization of teeth with either low virulence mutants of *S. mutans* or with harmless plaque organisms that are more competitive than wild-type *S. mutans* strains (**replacement therapy**). A strain of *S. mutans* has been genetically engineered by replacing lactate dehydrogenase with an alcohol dehydrogenase gene from an unrelated organism; such mutants grow well but produce no detectable lactic acid. This strain has also been engineered to produce a bacteriocin that will inhibit the growth of wild-type mutans streptococci. The use of probiotic bacteria to inhibit oral bacteria implicated in dental disease is also being considered.

Colonization resistance can be impaired by factors that compromise the integrity of the host defences or perturb the resident microflora. These include the side effects of cytotoxic therapy or the long-term use of broad spectrum antibiotics, but more subtle mechanisms can apply. Fibronectin has been shown to prevent adherence of *Pseudomonas aeruginosa* to buccal epithelial cells. Levels of fibronectin in seriously ill adults and in infants are lower that those in healthy adults and may account for the higher rates of colonization by Gram negative bacilli in these subjects.

METABOLISM OF ORAL BACTERIA

The persistence of the resident oral microflora is dependent on their ability to obtain nutrients and grow in the mouth. Nutrients are derived mainly from the metabolism of endogenous substrates present in saliva and GCF, and these often require the concerted action of consortia of microorganisms (Ch. 5; Figs 5.13 and 5.16). Superimposed on these components are the exogenous nutrients that are supplied intermittently via the diet; the most significant of these for the oral microflora are fermentable dietary carbohydrates, starches and casein. The concentration of nutrients will affect the growth rate and physiology of the microflora, as will any changes in pH resulting from their metabolism. Microbial gene expression will vary with changes in environmental conditions; bacteria are able to sense their environment via membrane-bound two component signal transduction pathways consisting of a sensor histidine kinase and a response regulator. These systems enable bacteria to detect signals and respond to environment changes through specific gene activation or repression. The fluctuating conditions of nutrient supply (feast–famine) and environmental change require the oral microflora to possess biochemical flexibility. Indeed, the pattern of metabolism is closely related to whether the resident microflora enjoys a pathogenic or commensal relationship with the host.

Carbohydrate metabolism

Most attention has been paid to the metabolism of carbohydrates because of the relationship between dietary sugars, acid production and dental caries (Chs 2 and 6). The metabolic fate of dietary carbohydrates is illustrated in simplified form in Fig. 4.9.

Sucrose (a disaccharide of glucose and fructose) is the most widely used sweetening agent, and can be:

- broken down by extracellular bacterial invertases (α-glucosidases) and the resultant glucose and fructose molecules taken up directly by bacteria,

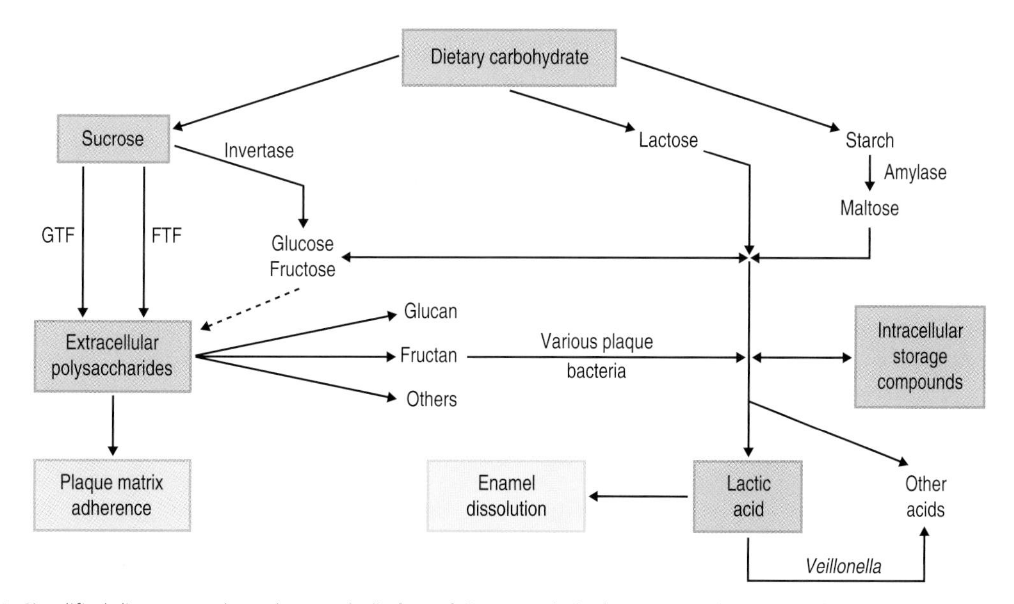

Fig. 4.9 Simplified diagram to show the metabolic fate of dietary carbohydrates. GTF, glucosyltransferase; FTF, fructosyltransferase.

- transported intact as the disaccharide or disaccharide phosphate, and cleaved inside the cell by an intracellular invertase or a sucrose phosphate hydrolase,
- utilized extracellularly by glycosyltransferases. Glucosyltransferases (GTF) produce both soluble and insoluble glucans (with a release of fructose) which are important in plaque formation and in the consolidation of bacterial attachment to teeth. Fructosyltransferases (FTF) produce fructans (and liberate glucose), some of which can be metabolized by other plaque organisms.

Starches, which contain mixtures of amylose and amylopectin, can be broken into their constituent sugars by amylases of salivary and bacterial origin. Some streptococci (*S. gordonii, S. mitis*) are able to bind amylase, which provides them with an additional metabolic capability. *S. mutans* possesses a spectrum of enzymes with the potential to catabolize dietary starches including an extracellular pullanase, which degrades pullulan and debranches amylopectin, as well as an amylase; there is also an extracellular endo-dextranase and an intracellular exo-dextranase.

Some aspects of the metabolism of carbohydrates will be considered in more detail in the following sections.

Sugar transport and acid production

All substrates have to be transported across the cytoplasmic membrane and into the bacterial cell if they are to be of value for biomass production or as an energy source. Oral bacteria can transport carbohydrates by three known processes:

- the phosphoenolpyruvate-mediated phosphotransferase (PEP-PTS) transport system,
- the multiple sugar metabolism system (Msm), and
- a glucose permease.

The most significant system is the PEP-PTS, which is the high-affinity sugar transport system for mono- and disaccharides in acidogenic oral bacteria (*Streptococcus, Actinomyces, Lactobacillus*). The PEP-PTS is a carrier-mediated, group translocation system involving phosphoryl-transfer from PEP via two non-sugar-specific, general cytoplasmic proteins, HPr and enzyme I (E1), to a sugar-specific, membrane-bound enzyme II complex (EII), that catalyzes the transport and phosphorylation of the incoming sugar (Fig. 4.10). The phosphate group of E1~P, generated from PEP, is transferred to HPr, forming HPr~P, and then to the EII complex.

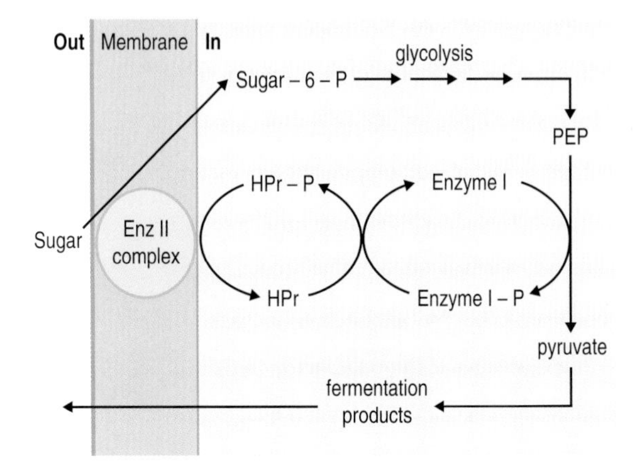

Fig. 4.10 Diagrammatic representation of a phosphoenolpyruvate (PEP)-mediated sugar phosphotransferase (PTS) system. Enz I and HPr are cytoplasmic proteins; EII is a membrane-associated sugar specific protein that may exist on its own, or as a complex with sugar-specific, cytoplasmic-associated proteins IIA, IIB and IIC.

The PEP-PTS is constitutive for some sugars, such as glucose, mannose and sucrose, but must be induced for the transport of lactose and sugar alcohols such as mannitol and sorbitol. The components induced are those in the EII complex as well as additional enzymes required to convert the substrate to a component of the glycolytic pathway. For example, when *S. mutans* is grown on lactose there is co-induction of the lactose-PTS and phospho-β-galactosidase, which cleaves intracellular lactose-phosphate to galactose-6-phosphate and glucose. The activity of the PEP-PTS in oral streptococci is modulated by environmental conditions. It is optimal under conditions of carbohydrate-limitation, neutral pH and slow rates of bacterial growth. In contrast, it is repressed under conditions of excess sugar, low pH and high growth rates. This is significant because oral streptococci in dental plaque are continually exposed to transitory conditions of low pH and high sugar concentration.

Many strains of *S. mutans* possess a second system to transport sugars into the cell (the multiple sugar metabolism, Msm, transport system). The existence of this system was inferred entirely from the finding of sequence homology of genes cloned from *S. mutans* with known gene products from Gram negative bacteria. The Msm system is analogous to the binding-protein-dependent system that is normally found in Gram negative bacteria, and is capable of transporting various common sugars including sucrose, as well as melibiose, raffinose and maltose (a derivative of starch). The exact role of this system in plaque ecology is unknown, but it might be involved in transporting the breakdown products of extracellular polysaccharide degradation during periods between meals when the supply of the more refined dietary mono- and di-saccharides is negligible.

At high sugar concentrations, PEP-PTS activity is repressed and sugar transport is augmented by an ATP-dependent glucose permease; this system also functions at high growth rates and at low pH. The sugar is transported into the cell where it is phosphorylated on the inner surface of the membrane. Some bacteria can form glycogen under conditions of carbohydrate-excess in order to reduce the toxic intracellular levels of glycolytic intermediates. Organisms with this ability, therefore, are able to cope better than most other oral bacteria with the fluctuating 'feast-and-famine' conditions in the mouth in terms of the availability of dietary sugars.

The resident oral microflora can also obtain carbohydrates for biomass and energy from the catabolism of host glycoproteins present in saliva (such as mucins) and in GCF (e.g. transferrin). Bacteria produce a range of glycosidases that can remove sugars sequentially from the oligosaccharide side chains of these glycoproteins, and these can be transported by systems such as the PEP-PTS. Generally, bacteria interact synergistically to fully degrade these molecules (Ch. 5), as no single organism can optimally produce all the enzymes required. Acid production from these glycoproteins is slow compared to that from exogenous sugars, and would not cause significant enamel demineralization.

Streptococcus oralis is highly prevalent being found on most oral surfaces; it can also act as an opportunistic pathogen and is commonly isolated from cases of infective endocarditis. Sialidase (neuraminidase) and *N*-acetylglucosaminidase activities are induced when *S. oralis* grows in the presence of glycoproteins, which cleave sialic acid and *N*-acetylglucosamine, respectively, from the oligosaccharide side chains. These sugars are then transported inside the cell, and key intracellular enzymes associated with the catabolism of *N*-acetyl sugars are also induced. These include *N*-acetylneuraminate pyruvate lyase, *N*-acetylglucosamine-6-phosphate deacetylase and glucosamine-6-phosphate deiminase. Significant concentrations of lactate are not produced from sialic acid metabolism; the main fermentation products are formate and ethanol.

Once sugars have been transported into the bacterial cell, they can be used either in anabolic pathways to generate biomass, or they can be broken down to organic acids (which are subsequently excreted) to generate energy. Acid production has been studied intensively because of its role in the demineralization of enamel. Bacteria catabolise sugars by glycolysis to pyruvate; the fate of pyruvate will depend on the particular organism and the availability of oxygen. Most oral bacteria metabolize pyruvate anaerobically to organic acids, the pattern of which can sometimes be used to identify particular genera. Oral streptococci, convert pyruvate to lactate by lactate dehydrogenase when sugars are in excess, while formate, acetate and ethanol are the products of metabolism by mutans streptococci and *S. sanguinis* (but not *S. salivarius*) under carbohydrate limitation (Fig. 4.11). Other bacterial genera produce acetate, butyrate, propionate, and formate as primary products of metabolism.

The mechanism of excretion of lactic acid has been determined in *S. mutans*. Lactate and protons are translocated across the cell membrane as lactic acid in a carrier-mediated, electroneutral process. After the addition of a fermentable substrate to cells, lactate begins to accumulate, and protons are pumped out of the cell by an ATP synthase (an F_1F_0-ATPase). This generates a transmembrane pH gradient, which can then be used as the driving force to transport lactate as lactic acid out of the cell. Once this process is energized, the ATP synthase is only needed to maintain the pH gradient if protons enter the cell by leakage or in symport with substrates such as amino acids. Thus, once the process is initiated no metabolic energy is needed for lactate efflux, thereby maximizing the energy (ATP) return from carbohydrate catabolism.

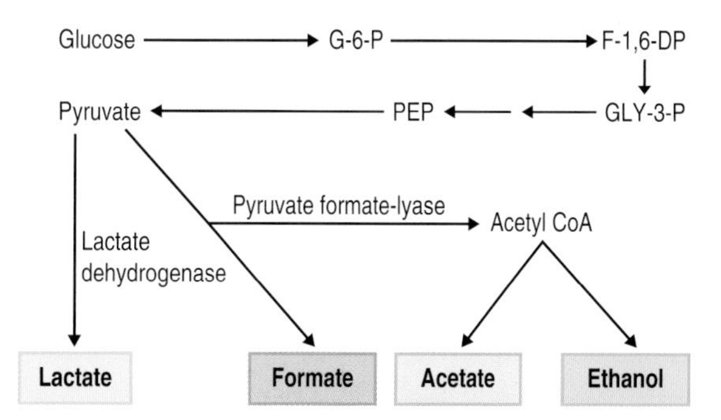

Fig. 4.11 Formation of end products of sugar metabolism by mutans streptococci. G-6-P, glucose-6-phosphate; F-1,6-DP, fructose-1,6-diphosphate; GLY-3-P, glyceraldehyde-3-phosphate; PEP, phosphoenolpyruvate.

Different species produce acid at different rates, and vary in the terminal pH reached, and in their ability to survive under such conditions. Generally, mutans streptococci produce acid at the fastest rates while lactobacilli generate the lowest environmental pH; both groups are also aciduric and can tolerate conditions of acidity that most other oral bacteria would find inhibitory or even lethal (Fig. 2.4); the biochemical mechanisms behind this tolerance are described below.

Variations are found in the profiles of acids found in plaque at different times of the day. Acetic, succinic, propionic, valeric, caproic and butyric acids are found in human plaque sampled after overnight fasting. These profiles reflect hetero-fermentation and amino acid catabolism. Following exposure to sucrose, the concentration of volatile acids falls while lactic acid becomes the predominant fermentation product. Such a switch in metabolism would encourage demineralization.

Acid tolerance

Although many of the saccharolytic bacteria found in dental plaque can generate a low terminal pH from sugar metabolism, few species can survive such conditions for prolonged periods. One of the prime distinguishing features of cariogenic bacteria such as mutans streptococci and lactobacilli is their ability to tolerate a low pH stress.

Microbial survival in acidic environments depends on the ability of a cell to maintain intracellular pH homeostasis. The mechanisms by which *S. mutans* achieves this include:

- proton extrusion via membrane-associated, proton-translocating ATP synthase (H^+/ATPase), and
- acid end-product efflux (see previous section).

These mechanisms ensure that the intracellular pH remains higher (i.e. more alkaline) than that of the external environment during acid production. Acid tolerant organisms such as mutans streptococci and lactobacilli have higher levels of ATP synthase activity, and the pH optimum for their activity is lower than for less tolerant species such as *S. sanguinis* or *A. naeslundii*.

Streptococcus mutans undergoes a specific alteration in its physiology in order to survive in an acidic environment (Table 4.8), providing cells with a competitive advantage at low pH over organisms associated with enamel health that lack this response, such as *S. sanguinis*. Other species cope with the stress of a low environmental pH by up-regulating genes involved in base production. For example, urease (urea is converted to two molecules of ammonia) gene expression by *S. salivarius* is enhanced significantly at low pH, while the arginine deiminase system (which degrades arginine to ornithine, CO_2 and ammonia) of *S. sanguinis* is active at pH values lower (pH 4.0) than it can grow (pH 5.2) or carry out glycolysis. A number of proteins are up-regulated when streptococci are exposed to low pH, but the function of some of these still remains to be determined, and they may form part of a co-ordinated acid stress response.

Table 4.8 Metabolic strategies adopted by *Streptococcus mutans* to cope with low pH stress.

Metabolic strategy
• increase in glycolytic activity
• shift to lower pH optimum for glucose transport, glycolysis and proton impermeability.
• decrease in activity of specific components of the PEP-PTS sugar transport system
• increased activity of the H^+/ATP synthase
• increased capacity to maintain transmembrane pH gradients at lower pH values
• shift to homo-fermentative metabolism.
• synthesis of stress response proteins

Polysaccharide production

Bacteria in the mouth are subjected to continual cycles of 'feast and famine' with respect to dietary carbohydrates. As a consequence, the resident microflora has developed strategies to store these carbohydrates during their brief exposure to these energy sources. These strategies help to avoid the lethal effects of the build up of intracellular glycolytic intermediates, and provide a source of carbon and energy for the subsequent periods of 'famine'. The most common strategy is to store these carbohydrates as intracellular polysaccharides (IPS) (Fig. 4.9), and many species of oral streptococci can synthesise polymers that resemble glycogen (1,4-α-glucan), although other polymers might also be formed. IPS metabolism is a virulence factor for *S. mutans* since mutants defective in this property cause less caries in animal models.

Many species of oral bacteria are also able to synthesize extracellular polysaccharides (EPS) from carbohydrates, especially from sucrose (Table 4.9). The polysaccharides can be soluble or insoluble; the former are more labile and can be metabolized by other bacteria, while the latter make a major contribution to the structural integrity of dental plaque (plaque matrix; Ch. 5) and can consolidate the attachment of bacteria in plaque. Sucrose has a unique property as a substrate in that the bond between the glucose and fructose moieties has sufficient energy on cleavage to support the synthesis of polysaccharide. The polysaccharides formed are either glucans or fructans, and are synthesized by glucosyltransferases (GTFs), and fructosyltransferases (FTFs), respectively:

$$n\text{-sucrose} \xrightarrow{\text{glucosyltransferase}} (\text{glucan})_n + n\text{-fructose}$$

$$n\text{-sucrose} \xrightarrow{\text{fructosyltransferase}} (\text{fructan})_n + n\text{-glucose}$$

GTFs can be divided into four groups depending on whether they produce a soluble dextran (GTF-S enzymes synthesize predominantly α,1-6 linked glucan) or an insoluble glucan (GTF-I enzymes synthesize predominantly α,1-3 polymers), and whether or not they require a dextran primer for activity. *S. mutans* possesses three GTFs (encoded for by *gtfB*, *gtfC* and *gtfD* genes) which synthesize α,1-3- and α,1-6-linked glucan polymers (Table 4.9). In *S. mutans*, the *gtfB* and *gtfC* genes encode for enzymes that produce water insoluble glucans, consisting primarily of α,1-3 linkages. These gene products contribute to cell adhesion, and plaque formation and structure, and are also essential for the initiation of caries on smooth surfaces of teeth in animal models. In contrast, the *gtfD* gene encodes a primer-dependent enzyme responsible for the formation of glucan, predominantly with α,1-6 linked glucose units, that is much more water soluble. The basic structure of some glucans is shown in Fig. 4.12.

Streptococcus mutans has a single FTF (produced by the *ftf* gene) which catalyzes the incorporation of the fructose component of the sucrose molecule into a fructan polymer with an inulin-type structure, composed mainly of β,2-1 linked fructose units. Fructans are not involved in adhesion, and do not appear to last for long periods in plaque. These molecules are believed to act more as extracellular carbohydrate storage compounds in plaque biofilms, being broken down to fructose (which can be transported by the PEP-PTS for glycolysis) by fructan hydrolases produced by a range of oral bacteria.

Table 4.9 Extracellular polysaccharide-producing bacterial populations found in the oral cavity.

Population	Carbohydrate substrate	Type of polymer (with predominant linkages[1])
Streptococcus mutans	Sucrose	Water-insoluble and soluble glucans α,1-3-; α,1-3- + 1-6- ; α,1-6-.
	Sucrose	Fructan 2, 1-*β*-
Streptococcus sanguinis[3]	Sucrose	Water-insoluble glucan α,1-3- + α,1-6-
	Sucrose	Water soluble glucan (dextran) α,1-6-
Streptococcus salivarius[4]	Sucrose	Fructan (levan) β, 2-6-
Actinomyces naeslundii	Sucrose	Fructan (levan) β, 2-6-
	-[2]	Heteropolysaccharide (60% N-acetyl glucosamine)
Lactobacillus sp.	-[2]	Glucan
		Heteropolysaccharide
Eubacterium spp.	-[2]	Heteropolysaccharide (predominantly acetate)
		Homopolysaccharide (D-glycero-D-galacto-heptose)
Rothia dentocariosa	Glucose	Heteropolysaccharide
	Sucrose	Levan
Rothia mucilaginosa	-[2]	Heteropolysaccharide (hexoses, hexosamines, amino acids)
Neisseria sp.	Sucrose	Glycogen-like

1. Where known.
2. No specific substrate required.
3. Some strains produce a fructan.
4. Some strains produce a glucan.

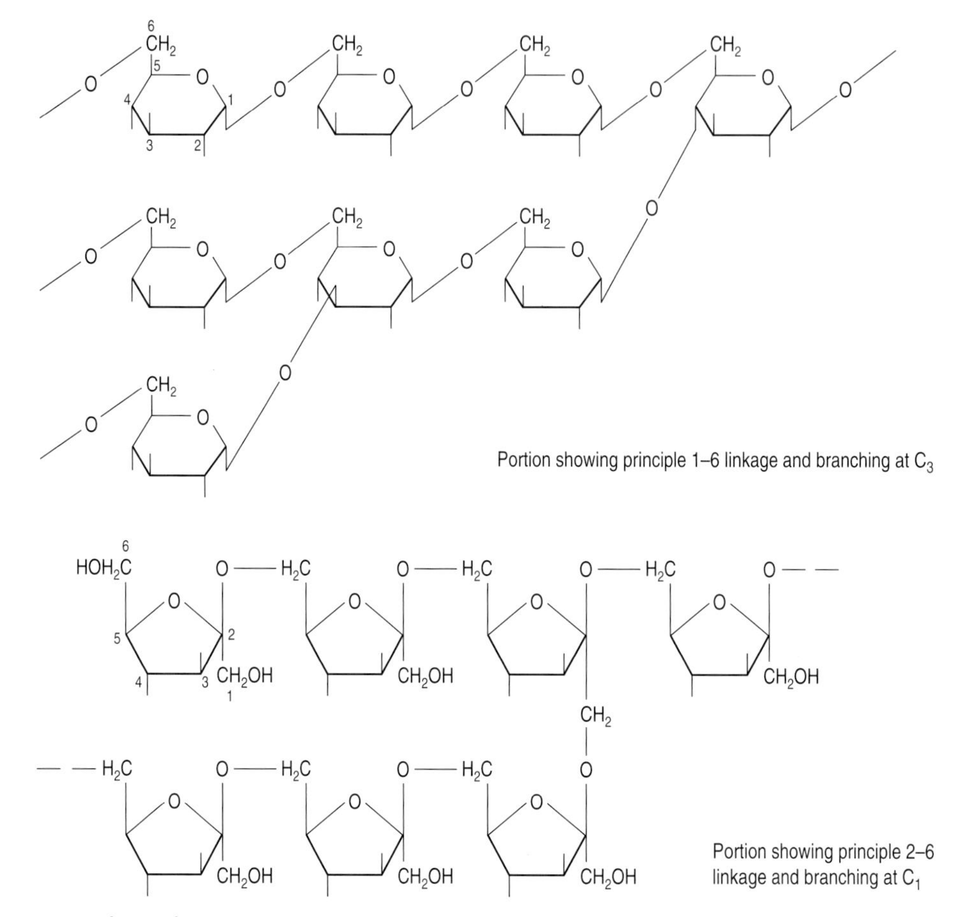

Fig. 4.12 Structure of part of a glucan chain, showing α,1-6,- and α,1-3,- linkages, and a fructan, showing an α,2-6,- linkage.

Other streptococci possess different numbers of GTF genes. Four GTF activities have been detected in *S. sobrinus* including a primer-dependent GTF-I which synthesizes a glucan with predominantly α,1-3 linked glucose residues. There are two gene products which produce polymers with mixed α,1-3 and α,1-6 linked glucose molecules, and a primer-independent GTF-S producing a linear glucan composed predominantly of α,1-6 residues. *S. salivarius* also produces four GTFs, although their properties differ from those described for *S. sobrinus*. In contrast, *S. gordonii* possesses only a single GTF, although this can form both soluble and insoluble glucan depending on the prevailing environmental conditions. Less is known about the products of *S. sanguinis* or *S. oralis*, although they probably only synthesize one enzyme. *Streptococcus salivarius* also produces a fructan, but in contrast to that of *S. mutans*, it is a levan with a characteristic β,2-6 linkage (Table 4.9). The FTF of *S. salivarius* is cell associated, whereas those of most other organisms are secreted.

Other species that produce EPS are listed in Table 4.9. The hetero-polysaccharides are generally complex in composition; for example, the polymer produced by a strain of *Actinomyces naeslundii* contains *N*-acetyl glucosamine (62%), galactose (7%), glucose (4%), uronic acids (3%), and small amounts of glycerol, rhamnose, arabinose, and xylose. *Actinomyces naeslundii* also has FTF activity, and synthesizes a fructan with a levan-type structure containing mainly β,2-6 linkages. Different strains of *A. naeslundii* produce fructanases with distinct specificities; some break down (a) only levans, (b) only inulins, sucrose or raffinose, but not levans, or (c) levans, inulins, sucrose or raffinose, indicating the importance of these polymers to these oral bacteria. Some of the homo- and heteropolysaccharides can be metabolized by other oral bacteria; this aspect will be discussed in Chapter 5.

Nitrogen metabolism

Apart from casein, there is little evidence that dietary proteins are utilized to any great extent. Casein can be incorporated into dental plaque and degraded. *Streptococcus sanguinis* has been shown to have both endo- and exopeptidase (amino- and carboxy-terminal) activity that can cleave proteins such as casein into a range of peptide fragments. Exopeptidase activity is mainly cell-associated and up-regulated at high pH, whereas endopeptidase activity is extracellular and optimal at neutral pH. *Streptococcus sanguinis* can rapidly release arginine from C-terminal peptides, converting the released arginine to energy (and carbamyl phosphate) via the arginine deiminase pathway. Urea is present in relatively high concentrations (200 mg/litre) in saliva. Some oral species (e.g. *A. naeslundii* and *S. salivarius*) possess urease activity and can convert urea to carbon dioxide and ammonia. At acidic pH, decarboxylation of amino acids yields carbon dioxide and amines, while at high pH, deamination produces ammonia and keto acids, which can be converted to acetic, propionic, and possibly *iso*- and *n*-butyric acids. For example, some periodontal pathogens can convert histidine, glutamine or arginine to acetate and butyrate. In this way, amino acid metabolism might be an important mechanism by which oral microorganisms counter the extremes of pH caused by the catabolism of carbohydrates and urea.

Essential amino acids can be obtained from the environment or synthesized by the cell. Ammonia can be converted into a number of amino acids, for example:

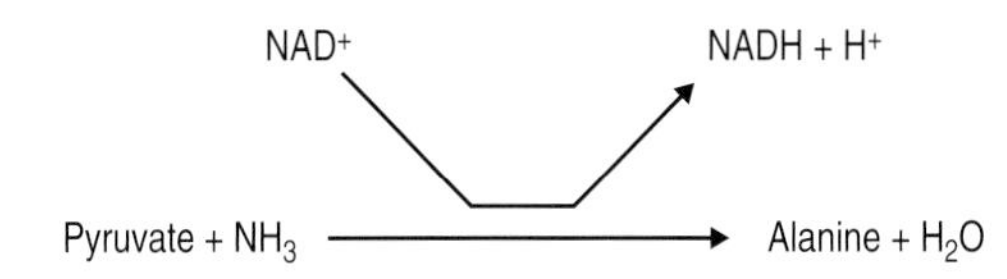

Further transamination reactions can provide other essential amino acids. The Stickland reaction can occur in dental plaque; this involves the coupled oxidation-reduction of suitable pairs of amino acids, and is a mechanism whereby various biochemical processes can be balanced in plaque.

The transport of amino acids such as glutamate and aspartate in *S. mutans* is by a primary transport system driven by ATP hydrolysis, whereas branched-chain amino acids (such as leucine) are taken up by an energized membrane- (proton motive force) driven carrier system. Essential amino acids can also be derived from the metabolism of peptides either inside or outside of the cell. Both *S. mutans* and *S. sanguinis* can transport tri-peptides (with an X-proline-Y structure) that are degraded intracellularly by cytoplasmic dipeptidyl peptidases, and then by an enzyme that breaks down X-proline dipeptides. This process is energetically very favourable for the cells because all of the amino acids present in the peptide are obtained for the same energy cost as the transport of a single amino acid.

Many of the microorganisms from the periodontal pocket are asaccharolytic (i.e. do not gain energy from the conversion of sugars to acidic fermentation products) but proteolytic, and depend for their growth on their ability to utilize the nutrients provided by GCF. During inflammation, many novel nutrients (e.g. haemoglobin, transferrin, haemopexin, haptoglobin) are provided by the host, and this can lead to the enrichment of highly proteolytic periodontal pathogens such as *Porphyromonas gingivalis*. These host molecules can be degraded to provide peptides and amino acids, as well as haeme, which is an essential cofactor for black-pigmented anaerobes. Although *P. gingivalis* can directly transport and utilize some amino acids, it prefers to take up short peptides for bioenergetic reasons; such peptides are then broken down within the cell by intracellular peptidases. The main proteases produced by *P. gingivalis* belong to the cysteine proteinase family, with specificity for arginine and lysine residues, and are termed Arg-gingipain (RgpA and RgpB) and Lys-gingipain (Kgp), respectively. RgpA and Kgp have C-terminal adhesin domains, and these can bind to host molecules. For example, *P. gingivalis* preferentially utilizes haemoglobin-derived haeme, and this is acquired through the ability of the RgpA-Kgp proteinase-adhesin extracellular complexes to bind and hydrolyze haemoglobin, releasing haeme at the cell surface. Indeed, Kgp has been shown to be essential for the formation of the black pigment associated with *P. gingivalis* colonies on blood agar (Fig. 3.7); the pigmentation is due to the deposition of haeme, as a μ-oxo dimer on the cell surface.

In addition to obtaining essential nutrients from GCF, many subgingival organisms are also able to degrade structural proteins and glycoproteins associated with the pocket epithelium. The production of enzymes such as chondroitin sulphatase, hyaluronidase, and collagenase contributes to tissue damage and pocket formation. Arg-gingipain is also important in virulence, and can deregulate and subvert the host inflammatory response by degrading host molecules designed to control inflammation, and this leads to 'by-stander' damage to the periodontal tissues (Ch. 6). The pH optimum of some of these enzymes is at neutral or slightly alkaline pH, which corresponds to that of the inflamed periodontal pocket.

Synergistic interactions occur in the breakdown of host molecules, and mutually beneficial associations occur between organisms with complementary patterns of enzyme activity (Ch. 5). The endopeptidase activity of *P. gingivalis* can provide appropriate peptides from the catabolism of host molecules for the growth of *F. nucleatum*. Similarly, *F. nucleatum* can support the growth of *P. gingivalis* in oxygenated environments. This might explain why these two species are frequently found together in periodontal pockets. The concept of plaque behaving as a microbial community in terms of the breakdown of complex host molecules and environment modification is developed further in Chapter 5.

Collectively, these findings emphasise the significance of nitrogen metabolism in oral microbial ecology. Host and bacterial proteases are associated directly and indirectly with tissue destruction in periodontal disease, while it has been argued that caries results not so much from an over-production of acid but more from a deficiency in base production by plaque bacteria.

Oxygen metabolism

The mouth is an overtly aerobic environment and yet the majority of bacteria are either facultatively anaerobic or obligately anaerobic, especially in dental plaque. Early colonizers tend to be more tolerant of the toxic effects of oxygen metabolism, especially with respect to hydrogen peroxide and hypothiocyanite, than later colonizers, which may depend on inter-species metabolic interactions within the biofilm structure of plaque in order to cope with oxygen and toxic radicals.

All plaque bacteria, including obligate anaerobes, are able to metabolize oxygen, albeit at different rates. Aerobic bacteria (such as *Neisseria* spp.) may use cytochrome-containing electron transport chains for oxygen reduction and coupled ATP synthesis. In contrast, facultatively anaerobic lactic acid producing species have a flavin-containing NADH oxidase and NADH peroxidase; similarly, even *Treponema denticola* (which is highly anaerobic), possesses NADH oxidases and NADH peroxidases, enabling it to scavenge low levels of oxygen in the subgingival environment. Some of these reactions are illustrated below:

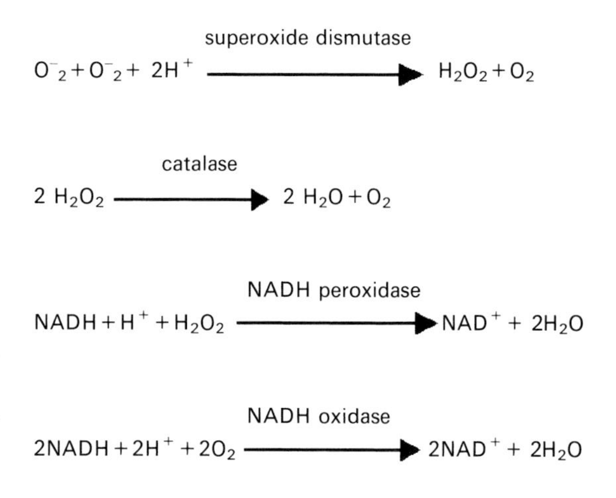

Although oxygen itself is not toxic, the production of oxygen metabolites can be, and so oral bacteria possess molecular defence mechanisms to prevent or reduce oxidative damage. These mechanisms involve the production of catalase, peroxidases and superoxide dismutase. Thus, oral organisms as metabolically diverse as mutans streptococci and *Porphyromonas gingivalis* produce protective enzymes: mutans streptococci produce superoxide dismutase, NADH peroxidase and glutathione reductase, while *P. gingivalis* has a superoxide dismutase, NADH oxidase and NADH peroxidase. The activities of these enzymes increase when cells of *P. gingivalis* are exposed to oxygen. The characteristic black pigmentation of colonies of *P. gingivalis* growing on blood agar can also provide protection against oxidative damage. When haeme is released from haemoglobin it can react with oxygen to form dimers that accumulate on the cell surface of *P. gingivalis*. These aggregated dimers can provide antioxidant protection, serving as a physical barrier to environmental oxygen, as well as acting as a buffer system to hydrogen peroxide, due to a catalase-like activity inherent to the layer.

Oral malodour (halitosis)

Oral malodour is a relatively common condition in the adult population, and is associated with the metabolism of bacteria located on the tongue. High odour subjects generally have a higher total bacterial load on the tongue, and higher numbers of Gram negative anaerobes, including *Porphyromonas, Prevotella, Fusobacterium* and *Treponema* spp..

Malodour production is strongly associated with high proteolytic activity and the production of volatile sulphur compounds. The predominant sulphur compounds are hydrogen sulphide [H_2S], and methyl mercaptan [CH_3SH], with smaller concentrations of dimethyl sulphide [$(CH_3)_2S$] and dimethyl disulphide [$(CH_3S)_2$]. Hydrogen sulphide is generated principally by the action of L-cysteine dehydrosulphatase on L-cysteine, while methyl mercaptan (methanethiol) is produced by the oxidation of L-methionine. *Fusobacterium* spp. and *Parvimonas micra* (formerly *Peptostreptococcus micros*) are able to form high concentrations of hydrogen sulphide from glutathione (a tripeptide: L-δ-glutamyl-L-cysteinylglycine), which is present in most tissue cells and would be available in the periodontal pocket. Treatment of periodontal disease usually results in the resolution of halitosis; tongue scraping to reduce the microbial load at this site can also be effective.

Metabolism and Inhibitors

Antimicrobial agents are used extensively in toothpastes and mouthrinses to help maintain dental plaque at levels compatible with oral health. Although they are often selected on the basis of a broad spectrum of antimicrobial activity, they frequently function in the mouth at sub-lethal concentrations and can interfere with carbohydrate and nitrogen metabolism (Fig. 6.19). For example, chlorhexidine can abolish the activity of sugar transport by the PEP-PTS, and thereby severely reduce glycolysis, and also inhibit the ATP-synthase and affect the maintenance of ion gradients in streptococci. Chlorhexidine can also interfere with nitrogen metabolism by inhibiting the arg-gingipain of *P. gingivalis* and arginine uptake by *S. sanguinis* (see Chapter 6).

SUMMARY

The oral microflora exhibits considerable biochemical flexibility in order to cope with the oscillating feast-famine conditions in the mouth. Dietary sugars are rapidly transported into cells (e.g. via the PEP-PTS) by cariogenic bacteria and converted to acidic fermentation products or to extracellular and intracellular polysaccharides. Mutans streptococci have specific strategies to cope with the resultant acid stress conditions. Subgingival bacteria rely on metabolizing proteins and glycoproteins supplied by GCF, often generating base, and raising the local pH to alkaline levels. Many of these proteolytic bacteria are obligately anaerobic, and they have specific mechanisms to cope with oxidative stress. Some of these important enzyme systems can be regarded as virulence factors, and are susceptible to inhibitors used in oral care products.

CHAPTER SUMMARY

Although the mouth is sterile at birth, the acquisition of the resident oral microflora begins within the first few hours of life. The biological properties of the mouth make it highly selective in terms of the types of microorganisms able to colonize. Few of the species found in the mouths of adults and even fewer of the organisms of the general environment are able to establish successfully. Acquisition of the resident microflora follows a pattern of ecological succession: relatively few organisms (pioneer species) are able to colonize, but their presence enables other species to establish; this process eventually leads to a climax community with a high species diversity. Many species are acquired from the mother by transmission via saliva, although studies of the clonal diversity of strains suggest that some organisms may be derived from more general sources. The development of a climax community in the mouth can involve both allogenic (non-microbial influenced) and autogenic (microbial influenced) succession.

The composition of the resident microflora varies at different sites around the mouth, with each site having a relatively characteristic microbial community. Mutans streptococci and *S. sanguinis* have preferences for hard surfaces for colonization, whereas species such as *S. salivarius* are recovered predominantly from the oral mucosa. The tongue has the highest number of microorganisms per area of oral mucosal surface, and can act as a reservoir for some Gram negative anaerobes that are implicated in periodontal diseases and halitosis.

The distribution of microorganisms is related to their ability to adhere at a site, as well as to their nutritional and environmental requirements (pH and redox potential) being satisfied. Many species of bacteria adhere by specific molecular interactions between adhesins located on their cell surface and receptors on the host; these receptors are found in the acquired pellicle and mucus coat on enamel and mucosal surfaces, respectively. The bacterial adhesins can be structurally complex, with multiple binding sites.

In order to cope with the fluctuating nutritional conditions in the mouth, the resident oral microflora is biochemically flexible. The primary source of nutrients is the endogenous supply of host proteins and glycoproteins from saliva and GCF. Superimposed on these are carbohydrates (and some proteins) provided by the diet. Carbohydrates can be transported into the bacterial cell by, for example, a high affinity PEP-PTS system, and either converted to organic acids or used to synthesize IPS. Potentially cariogenic bacteria deploy specific molecular strategies that enable them to tolerate low pH conditions that would be inhibitory to other species. Some disaccharides can be metabolized extracellularly into constituent sugars (for transport) or into EPS; these polysaccharides can function to consolidate attachment or used as extracellular storage compounds. The extracellular glucans and fructans are synthesized by glucosyl- and fructosyltransferases, respectively.

The metabolism of nitrogen compounds involves a wide range of exo- and endopeptidases; nitrogen metabolism can lead to base production which will help regulate environmental pH. The catabolism of complex host molecules requires bacteria with complementary patterns of enzyme activity to interact in order to ensure their complete breakdown. Obligate anaerobes are found commonly at many sites in the mouth. These bacteria survive oxygen exposure by interacting with oxygen-consuming species, and by the possession of a number of specific enzyme systems to scavenge oxygen and toxic radicals.

Halitosis involves the production of increased levels of malodorous compounds (such as hydrogen sulphide and methyl mercaptan) by proteolytic anaerobic bacteria; many of these organisms are located on the tongue. The metabolism of oral microorganisms is sensitive to many of the inhibitors used in preventive dentistry.

FURTHER READING

Aas JA, Paster BJ, Stokes LN, Olsen I, Dewhirst FE 2005 Defining the normal bacterial flora of the oral cavity. J Clin Microbiol 43:5721-5732.

Carlsson J 2000 Growth and nutrition as ecological factors. In Kuramitsu HK, Ellen RP (eds) Oral bacterial ecology. The molecular basis. Horizon Scientific Press, Wymondham, p 67-130.

Dashper SG, Cross KJ, Slakeski N et al 2004 Hemoglobin hydrolysis and heme acquisition by *Porphyromonas gingivalis*. Oral Microbiol Immunol 19:50-56.

Diaz PI, Rogers AH 2004 The effect of oxygen on the growth and physiology of *Porphyromonas gingivalis*. Oral Microbiol Immunol 19:88-94.

Diaz PI, Chalmers NI, Rickard AH 2006 Molecular characterization of subject-specific oral microflora during initial colonization of enamel. Appl Environ Microbiol 72:2837-2848.

Greenman J 1999 The microbial aetiology of halitosis. In Newman HN, Wilson M (eds) Dental plaque revisited: oral biofilms in health and disease. Cardiff, BioLine, Cardiff, p 419-442.

Kazor CE, Mitchell PM, Lee AM et al 2003 Diversity of bacterial populations on the tongue dorsa of patients with halitosis and healthy patients. J Clin Microbiol 41:558-563.

Könönen E 2000 Development of oral bacterial flora in young children. Ann Med 32:107-112.

Könönen E, Jousimies-Somer H, Bryk A, Kilpi T, Kilian M 2002 Establishment of streptococci in the upper respiratory tract: longitudinal changes in the mouth and nasopharynx up to 2 years of age. J Med Microbiol 51:723-730.

Lamont RJ, Jenkinson HF 2000 Adhesion as an ecological determinant in the oral cavity. In Kuramitsu HK, Ellen RP(eds) Oral bacterial ecology. The molecular basis. Horizon Scientific Press, Wymondham, p 131-168.

Lemos JA, Abranches J, Burne RA 2005 Responses of cariogenic streptococci to environmental stresses. Curr Issues Mol Biol 7:95-107.

Lingstrom P, van Houte J, Kashket S 2000 Food starches and dental caries. Crit Rev Oral Biol Med 11:366-380.

Mager DL, Ximenez-Fyvie LA, Haffajee AD, Socransky SS 2003 Distribution of selected bacterial species on intraoral surfaces. J Clin Periodontol 30:644-654.

Marquis RE 1995 Oxygen metabolism, oxidative stress and acid-base physiology of dental plaque biofilms. J Indust Microbiol 15: 198-207.

Percival RS 2009 Changes in oral microflora and host defences with advanced age In: Percival S, Hart A (eds) Microbiology and aging: clinical manifestations. Springer, New York, 131-152.

Rudney JD, Chen R, Sedgewick GJ 2005 Streptococci dominate the diverse flora within buccal cells. J Dent Res 84:1165-1171.
Sachdeo A, Haffajee AD, Socransky SS 2008 Biofilms in the edentulous oral cavity. J Prosthodont 17: 348-356.
Tanner AC, Milgrom PM, Kent R et al 2002 The microbiota of young children from tooth and tongue samples. J Dent Res 81:53-57.
Van Winkelhoff AJ, Boutaga K 2005 Transmission of periodontal bacteria and models of infection. J Clin Periodontol 32(suppl) 6:16-27.

Chapter 5

Dental plaque

Dental plaque is a general term for the complex microbial community that develops on the tooth surface, embedded in a matrix of polymers of bacterial and salivary origin. Plaque that becomes calcified is referred to as calculus or tartar. The presence of plaque in the mouth can readily be demonstrated by rinsing with a disclosing solution such as erythrosin (Fig. 5.1). The majority of plaque is found associated with the protected and stagnant regions of the tooth surface such as fissures, approximal regions between teeth, and the gingival crevice (see Figs 2.2 and 5.1). Plaque is found naturally on the tooth surface, and forms part of the host defences by excluding exogenous (and often pathogenic) species (**colonization resistance**) (Table 4.7). On occasions, however, plaque can accumulate beyond levels compatible with oral health, and this can lead to shifts in the composition of the microflora and predispose sites to disease (Ch. 6). Dental plaque is an example of a biofilm and a microbial community, and the significance of this will be explained in the following sections.

MICROBIAL BIOFILMS

Numerous studies of a range of distinct ecosystems have shown that the vast majority of microorganisms exist in nature associated with a surface. The term

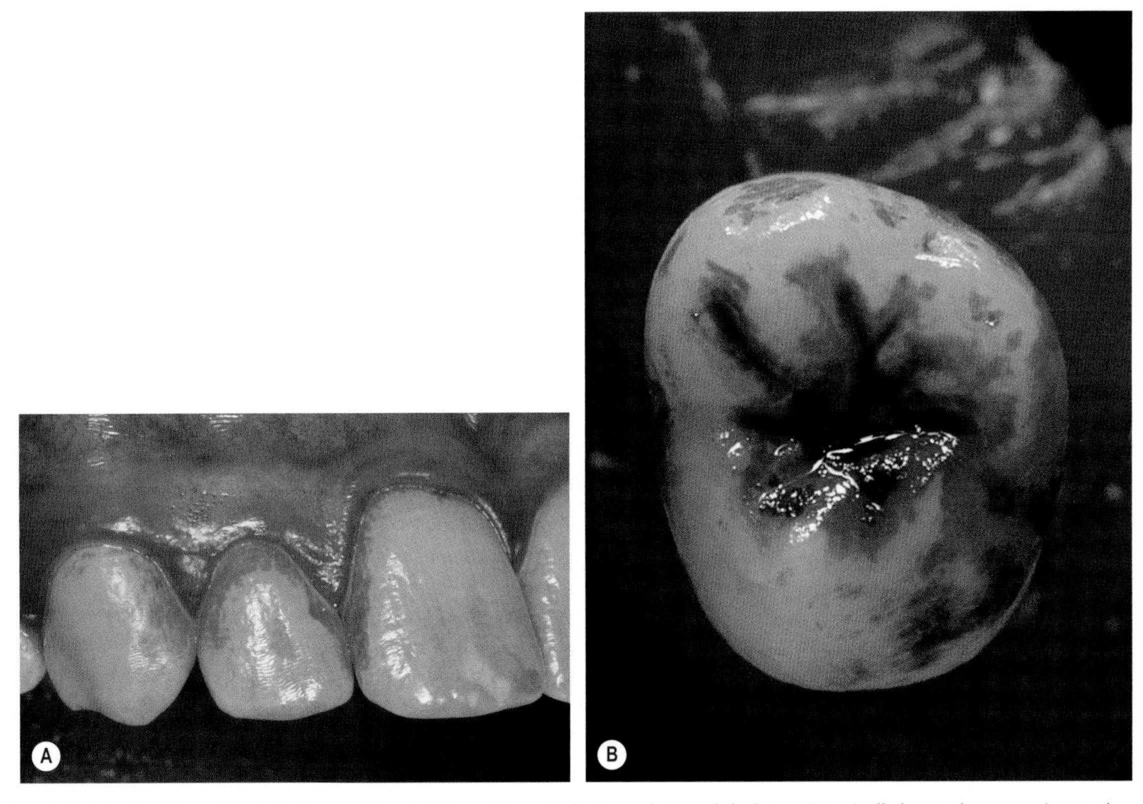

Fig. 5.1 Visualization of dental plaque after staining with a disclosing solution. (A) Plaque is typically located at retention and stagnation areas along the gingival margin and between teeth (approximal areas). (B) Heavy accumulation of plaque on the occlusal surface of an erupting third molar; plaque is preferentially located in the fissures. Taken from Marsh PD & Nyvad B, The oral microflora and biofilms on teeth, in dental caries. The disease and its clinical management, 2nd edn, Fejerskov O and Kidd EAM, Blackwell, Oxford, 2008; pp.163-187 – published with permission.

'biofilm' is used to describe communities of microorganisms attached to a surface; such microbes are usually spatially organized into a three-dimensional structure and are enclosed in a matrix of extracellular material (sometimes termed a 'glycocalyx') derived both from the cells themselves and from their environment. If (a) biofilm microbes were simply planktonic (liquid-phase) cells that had adhered to a surface, and (b) the properties of microbial communities were merely the sum of those of the constitutive populations, then scientific interest in such issues would be limited. However, research over recent years has revealed that cells growing as biofilms have unique properties, some of which are of clinical significance (Table 5.1), for example, biofilms can be up to 1000 times more tolerant of antimicrobial agents than the same cells growing in liquid culture, while communities of interacting species can be more pathogenic than pure cultures of the constituent microorganisms.

Originally, biofilms were considered to be dense, compressed accumulations of cells, and this compacted structure was believed to be responsible for many of the novel properties of biofilms. Recent advances in the study of biofilms have come from the application of novel techniques that enable biofilms to be studied *in situ* without any processing of samples that could distort their structure. A prime example has been the use of confocal laser scanning microscopy (CLSM) to study biofilm architecture without chemical fixation or embedding techniques. Optical thin sections can be generated throughout the depth of the biofilm, and these can be combined using imaging software to generate three-dimensional images. In addition, the location of specific organisms can be visualized with immunological or oligonucleotide probes, such as by fluorescent *in situ* hybridization, FISH, (Fig. 3.3), while other molecular probes can indicate the vitality and metabolic activity of cells. CLSM can also be used in

Table 5.1 General properties of biofilms and microbial communities.

General property	Dental plaque example
Open architecture	presence of channels and voids
Protection from host defences, desiccation, etc	production of extracellular polymers to form a functional matrix; physical protection from phagocytosis
Enhanced tolerance to antimicrobials*	reduced sensitivity to chlorhexidine and antibiotics; gene transfer
Neutralization of inhibitors	β-lactamase production by neighbouring cells to protect sensitive organisms
Novel gene expression*	synthesis of novel proteins on attachment; up-regulation of *gtfBC* in mature biofilms
Coordinated gene responses	production of cell-cell signalling molecules (e.g. CSP, AI-2)
Spatial & environmental heterogeneity	pH & O_2 gradients; coadhesion
Broader habitat range	obligate anaerobes in an overtly aerobic environment
More efficient metabolism	complete catabolism of complex host macromolecules (e.g. mucins) by microbial consortia
Enhanced virulence	pathogenic synergism in abscesses and periodontal diseases

*one consequence of altered gene expression can also be an increased tolerance of antimicrobial agents.

combination with 'reporter genes' to identify genes that are expressed only when cells form a biofilm. This technology involves the insertion of a marker into the bacterial chromosome downstream of a promoter so that a recognisable 'signal' (e.g. fluorescence) is produced when the gene is activated.

The application of these modern approaches to the general field of microbial ecology has shown that biofilms that develop in low-nutrient environments, especially those from aquatic habitats, have a more open structure than had been predicted previously from earlier studies employing electron microscopy. Channels have been observed in biofilms of environmental bacteria, enabling potentially growth-limiting factors such as nutrients and oxygen to penetrate more extensively than previously thought. In addition, the use of micro-electrodes and chemical probes have shown that considerable gradients in key factors (pH, redox potential, etc.) can occur over relatively short distances (a few microns, i.e. a few cell diameters) within biofilms. This produces spatial and temporal heterogeneity within the biofilm enabling fastidious bacteria to survive in apparently hostile or incompatible environments (Table 5.1).

A biofilm life-style may affect the properties of an organism in more than one way. Firstly, the attachment of cells to a surface may cause a **direct effect**, perhaps by triggering 'sensors' on the cell surface, and specifically inducing the expression of a subset of genes. Bacteria are able to sense their environment via membrane-bound two component signal transduction pathways consisting of a sensor histidine kinase and a response regulator. *Pseudomonas aeruginosa* is an environmental bacterium that can also act as an opportunistic pathogen, for example, in cystic fibrosis. Attachment leads to the up-regulation of genes (*algC* and *algG*) involved in exopolysaccharide (alginate) synthesis within 15 minutes of the initial contact of a cell with a surface. Secondly, the growth environment within the biofilm may differ significantly in respect to key factors (pH, oxygen and nutrient concentration) compared with planktonic culture. Again, this may result in altered gene expression, and hence an altered phenotype, but as an **indirect effect** of growing in a biofilm. Likewise, organisms in a biofilm will be growing more slowly, due to a particular nutrient limitation or an unfavourable pH, and this will also affect the properties of a cell. Often, it is difficult to resolve whether any observed phenotypic changes are due to the direct or indirect effects of being in a biofilm. For most practical purposes, the reasons for any change are less important than the biological significance of the change itself.

Biofilm bacteria are phenotypically distinct from planktonic cells, and one particularly important aspect of this is an increased tolerance of biofilm cells to antimicrobial agents. An extreme example was the finding that *P. aeruginosa* growing on urinary catheter material was between 500–1000 times more tolerant of the antibiotic, tobramycin, than the same cells in liquid (planktonic) culture. Conventionally, the sensitivity of bacteria to antimicrobial agents is determined on cells grown in liquid culture by the measurement of the minimum inhibitory concentration (MIC) or minimum bacteriocidal concentration (MBC) against relevant antimicrobial agents. Given the decreased sensitivity of an organism on a surface to antimicrobial agents, it has been argued that it would be more appropriate to determine the 'biofilm inhibitory concentration (BIC)' and 'biofilm killing concentration (BKC)' or 'biofilm eradicating concentration (BEC)'. As yet, these proposals have not been widely accepted, and there are no generally agreed methods by which these concentrations could be determined.

Microorganisms can become resistant to antibiotics due to mutations, the presence of drug efflux pumps and the production of neutralizing enzymes, but even innately sensitive organisms become apparently 'resistant' when growing on a surface in a biofilm. The mechanisms behind the increased tolerance of biofilms to antimicrobial agents are still not fully understood; a number of theories have been proposed, the relative significance or contribution of each may vary according to (a) the age, structure and location of the biofilm, and (b) the chemical properties of the agent. The structure of a biofilm may restrict the penetration of an antimicrobial agent; for example, positively-charged antibiotics such as aminoglycosides will bind to negatively-charged polymers that are present as part of the extracellular matrix (diffusion-reaction theory). Agents may also bind to and inhibit the organisms at the surface of the biofilm, leaving cells in the depths of the biofilm relatively unaffected, i.e. the agent is quenched at the surface. As stated earlier, microbes growing as a biofilm display a novel phenotype, and one possible consequence of this can be a reduced sensitivity to antimicrobial agents. The drug target may be modified or not expressed during growth on a surface, or the organism may use alternative biochemical strategies thereby diminishing the potential impact of the active agent. Cells also grow much slower in a mature biofilm and, as a consequence, are much less susceptible to antimicrobials than faster growing cells. The environment in the depths of a biofilm may also be unfavourable for the optimal action of some antimicrobial agents. In multi-species biofilms, a susceptible pathogen can be rendered resistant if neighbouring, non-pathogenic cells produce a neutralizing or drug-degrading enzyme – this is sometimes referred to as 'indirect pathogenicity'. In addition, biofilms provide ideal conditions for the transfer of resistance genes, e.g. via plasmids, among neighbouring cells in close proximity to one another (horizontal gene transfer).

BIOFILMS IN THE MOUTH

Dental plaque was probably the first biofilm to have been studied in terms of either its microbial composition or its sensitivity to antimicrobial agents. In the seventeenth century, Antonie van Leeuwenhoek pioneered the approach of studying biofilms by direct microscopic observation when he reported on the diversity and high numbers of 'animalcules' present in 'scrapings' taken from around human teeth. He also conducted early studies on the novel properties of surface-grown cells when he failed to kill plaque bacteria on his teeth by prolonged rinsing with wine-vinegar, while the organisms were 'killed' if they were first removed from his molars and mixed with vinegar *in vitro*.

Dental plaque is one of the best studied biofilms, and displays all of the characteristic features of a typical biofilm (Table 5.1). Compared to other habitats, dental plaque is relatively accessible for sampling, and can even be grown on relevant removable surfaces for subsequent investigation and experimentation in the laboratory (*in situ* models; Ch. 4). A large proportion of the key microorganisms can be identified, while the phenotype of such microbes (adhesins, metabolic potential, cell–cell interactions) is well-characterized. Extensive biofilms also develop on dentures, and the tongue. On other mucosal surfaces, bacteria attach to epithelial cells and may develop a surface-associated phenotype, but extensive 3-dimensional biofilms do not usually develop. Another dentally-relevant biofilm develops on the tubing used in dental unit water supply systems (DUWS); this will be discussed in Chapter 12 (see Fig. 12.6), but the principles governing the formation and properties of these biofilms will be similar to those described below for dental plaque.

MECHANISMS OF DENTAL PLAQUE FORMATION

The development of a biofilm such as dental plaque can be subdivided arbitrarily into several stages. As a bacterium approaches a surface a number of specific and non-specific interactions will occur between the substratum and the cell, and these will determine whether successful attachment and colonization will take place. Distinct stages in plaque formation are summarized below, and are shown schematically in Fig. 5.2.

However, it should be remembered that biofilm formation is a dynamic process and the phases distinguished above are only arbitrary and are for the benefit of discussion. The attachment, growth, removal and reattachment of bacteria are continuous processes, and a microbial biofilm such as plaque will undergo continuous reorganization.

1. Acquired pellicle formation

Bacteria rarely come into contact with clean enamel. As soon as a tooth surface is cleaned, salivary proteins and glycoproteins are adsorbed forming a surface conditioning film which is termed the acquired enamel pellicle. The major constituents of pellicle are salivary glycoproteins, phosphoproteins and lipids, including statherin, amylase, proline-rich peptides (PRPs) and host defence components (Chs 2 and 4). Bacterial components such as glucosyltransferases (GTFs) and glucan have also been detected in pellicle, and play a significant role in attachment. Depending on the site, pellicle can also contain components from gingival crevicular fluid (GCF).

Pellicle formation starts within seconds of a clean surface being exposed to the oral environment. An equilibrium between adsorption and desorption of salivary molecules occurs after 90–120 minutes. The thickness of the pellicle is influenced by the shear forces at the site of formation. After 2 hours, the pellicle on lingual surfaces is 20–80 nm thick whereas buccal pellicles can be 200–700 nm deep. Depending on the site, further increases in depth can occur over time. Pellicle has an electron dense basal layer covered by a more loosely arranged globular surface (Fig. 5.3). When salivary molecules bind to the tooth surface, they can undergo conformational changes. This can lead to exposure of new receptors for bacterial attachment (**cryptitopes**; see later) or,

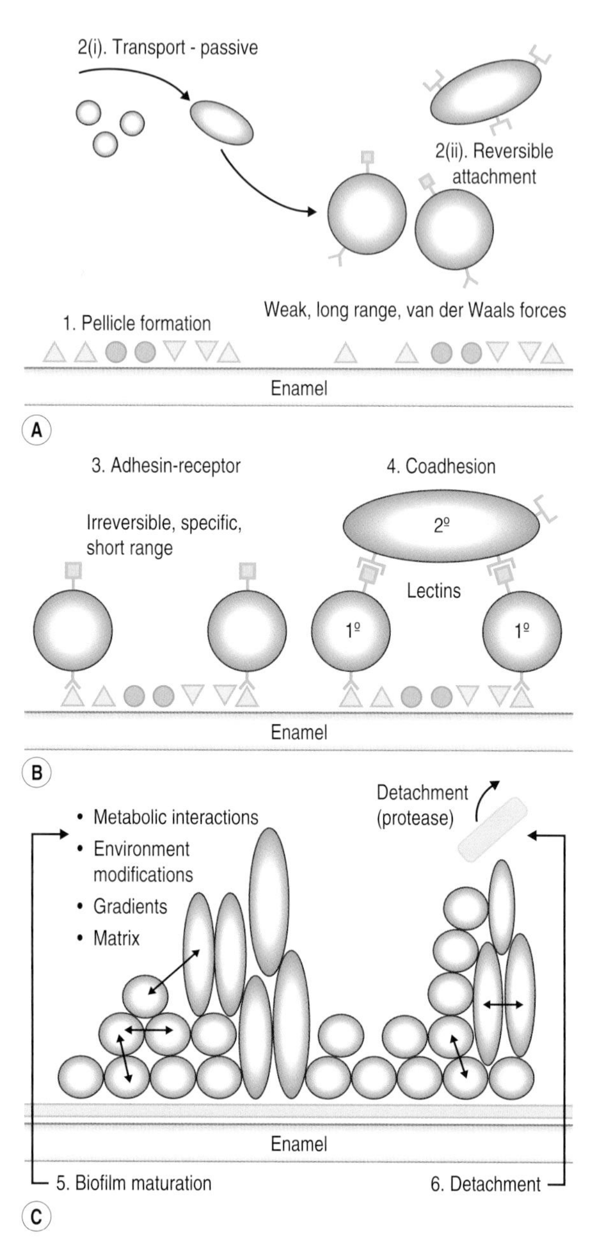

Fig. 5.2 Schematic representation of the different stages in the formation of dental plaque: (A) 1. Pellicle forms on a clean tooth surface. 2(i) Bacteria are transported passively to the tooth surface where they 2(ii) may be held reversibly by weak electrostatic forces of attraction. (B) 3. Attachment becomes irreversible by specific stereochemical molecular interactions between adhesins on the bacterium and receptors in the acquired pellicle, and 4. secondary colonizers attach to primary colonizers, often by lectin-like interactions (coadhesion). (C) 5. growth results in biofilm maturation, facilitating interbacterial interactions. 6. Eventually, detachment can occur, sometimes as a result of the degradation by bacteria of their adhesins.

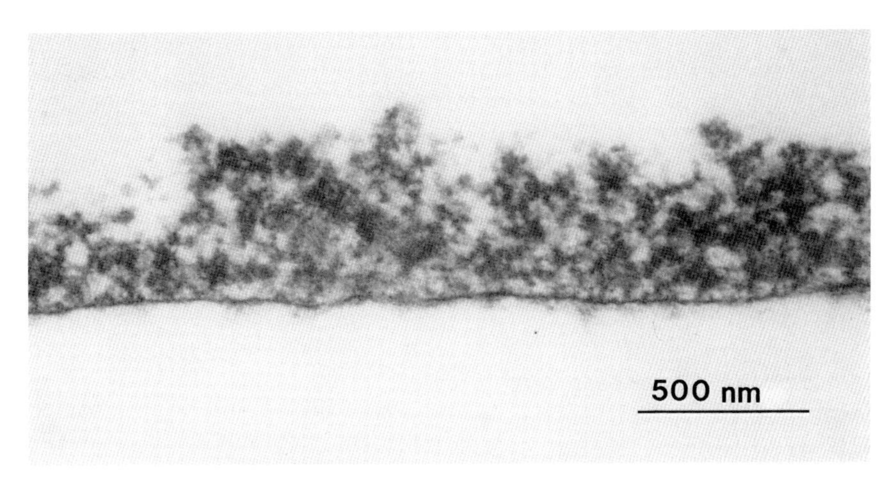

Fig. 5.3 Transmission electron micrograph (TEM) of the acquired pellicle on an enamel surface. Reproduced with permission of Prof M Hannig.

in the case of glucosyltransferases, an altered activity resulting in the synthesis of a glucan with a modified structure. The molecular composition and physicochemical properties of pellicle are critical in determining the pattern of microbial colonization.

2. Transport of microorganisms and reversible attachment

Microorganisms are generally transported passively to the tooth surface by the flow of saliva; few oral bacterial species are motile (e.g. possess flagella), and these are mainly located subgingivally.

As the cell approaches the pellicle-coated surface, long range but relatively weak physicochemical forces are generated. Microorganisms are negatively-charged due to the molecules on their cell surface, while many proteins present in the acquired pellicle also have a net negative charge. The Derjaguin and Landau and the Verwey and Overbeek (DLVO) theory has been used to describe the interaction between an inert particle (as a microorganism might be envisaged at large separation distances) and a substratum. This theory states that the total interactive energy, V_T, of two smooth particles is determined solely by the sum of the van der Waals attractive energy (V_A) and the usually repulsive, electrostatic energy (V_R). Particles in aqueous suspension and surfaces in contact with aqueous solutions can acquire a charge due to, for example, the preferential adsorption of ions from solution or the ionization of certain groups attached to the particle or surface. The charge on a surface in solution is always exactly balanced by an equivalent number of counter ions; the size of this electrical double layer is inversely proportional to the ionic strength of the environment. As a particle approaches a surface, therefore, it experiences a weak van der Waals attraction induced by the fluctuating dipoles within the molecules of the two approaching surfaces. This attraction increases as the particle moves closer to the substratum. A repulsive force is encountered if the surfaces continue to approach each other, due to the overlap of the electrical double layers. Curves can be plotted to show the variation of the total interactive energy, V_T, of a particle and a surface with the separation distance, h (Fig. 5.4).

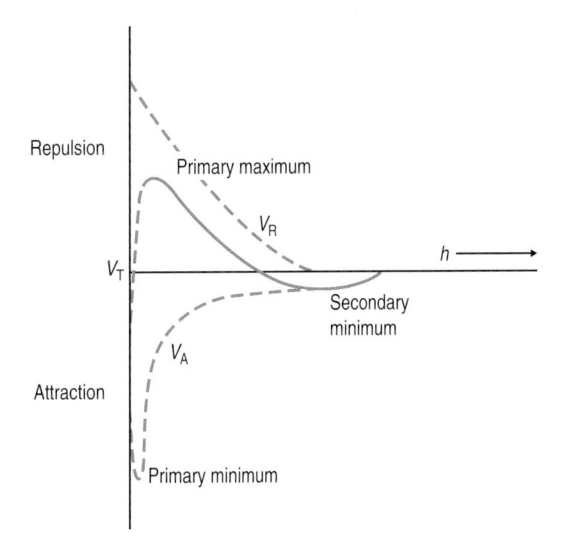

Fig. 5.4 Diagram illustrating the DLVO theory. The total interactive energy, V_T, between a particle and a surface is shown with respect to the separation distance, h. The total interaction curve is obtained by the summation of an attraction curve, V_A, and a repulsion curve, V_R.

A net attraction can occur at two values of h; these are referred to as the primary minimum (h very small) and the secondary minimum (h = 10–20 nm) and are separated by a repulsive maximum. The reversible nature of these initial interactions suggests that the primary minimum is not usually encountered while the high ionic strength of saliva increases the likelihood that oral bacteria could be retained near a surface by a secondary minimum area of attraction (e.g. about 10–20 nm from the surface).

3. Pioneer microbial colonizers and irreversible attachment (adhesin–receptor interactions)

Within a short time, these weak physicochemical interactions may become irreversible due to adhesins on the microbial cell surface becoming involved in specific, short-range interactions with complementary receptors in the acquired pellicle. For this to occur, water films must be removed from between the interacting surfaces. A major role of cell hydrophobicity and hydrophobic cell surface components is their dehydrating effect on this water film enabling the surfaces to get closer so that the short range interactions can occur. A direct relationship between the degree of cell surface hydrophobicity and the adhesion of oral bacteria to saliva-coated surfaces has often been demonstrated.

Irrespective of the type of tooth surface (enamel or cementum), the initial colonizers constitute a highly selected part of the oral microflora. Within minutes, coccal bacteria appear on the surface (Fig. 5.5A), and these pioneer organisms are mainly streptococci, especially members of the mitis-group of streptococci (e.g. *S. sanguinis, S. oralis* and *S. mitis* biovar 1) (Table 5.2). *Streptococcus sanguinis* and *S. oralis* produce an IgA_1 protease which may help them to survive and overcome a key element of the host defences during the early stages of plaque formation. *Actinomyces* spp. are also commonly isolated after 2 hours, as are *Haemophilus* spp. and *Neisseria* spp., while obligately anaerobic species are detected only rarely at this stage and are usually in low numbers. Some aggregates of mixtures of cells may also attach.

Once attached, these pioneer populations start to divide and form microcolonies; these early colonizers become embedded in bacterial extracellular slimes and polysaccharides together with additional layers of adsorbed salivary proteins and glycoproteins (Fig. 5.5, B and C). The early streptoccocal colonizers (mitis-group of streptococci) possess a range of glycosidase activities that enable them to interact and use salivary glycoproteins as substrates (Ch. 4; see Fig. 5.13 later). The fastest rates of multiplication occur during these early stages of plaque formation; the doubling times of pure cultures of *S. mutans* and *A. naeslundii* were 1.4 h and 2.7 hours, respectively, in studies using rodents.

Table 5.2 Proportions of bacteria in developing supragingival plaque.

Bacterium	Time of plaque development (h)		
	2	24	48
Streptococcus sanguinis	8	12	29
Streptococcus oralis	20	21	12
mutans streptococci	3	2	4
Streptococcus salivarius	<1	<1	<1
Actinomyces naeslundii	6	7	5
Actinomyces odontolyticus	2	3	6
Haemophilus spp.	11	18	21
Capnocytophaga spp.	<1	<1	<1
Fusobacterium spp.	<1	<1	<1
Black-pigmented anaerobes	0	<0.01	<0.01

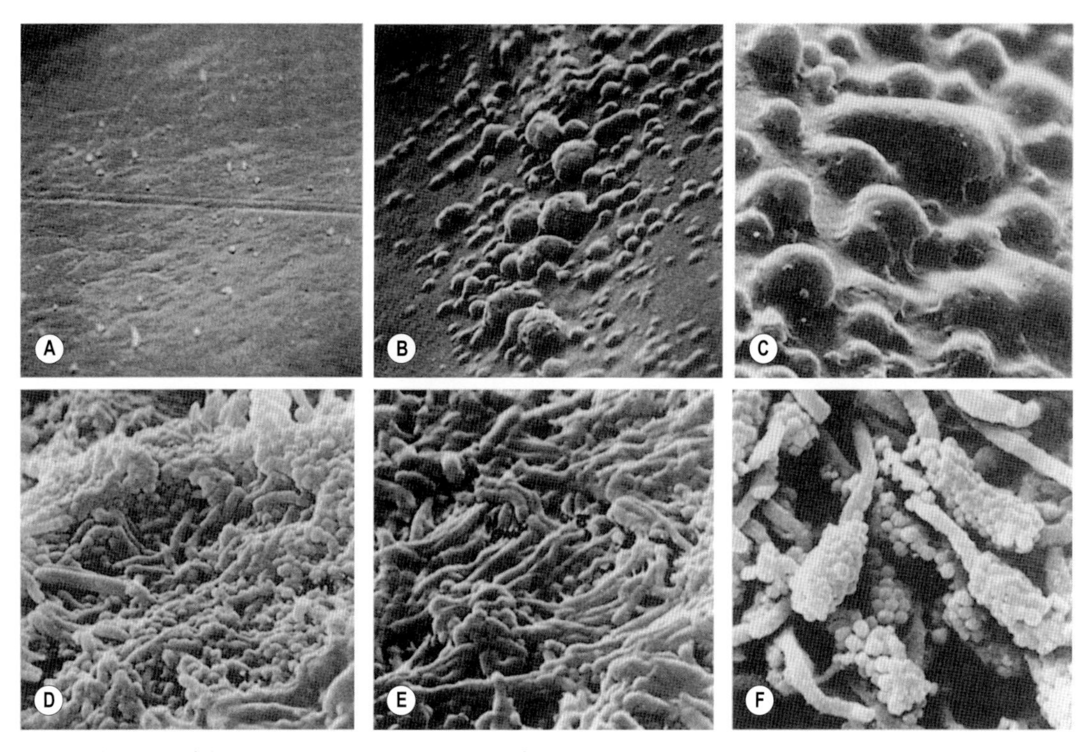

Fig. 5.5 Development of dental plaque on a clean enamel surface. Coccal bacteria attach to the enamel pellicle as pioneer species (A) and multiply to form microcolonies (B), eventually resulting in confluent growth (biofilm formation) embedded in a matrix of extracellular polymers of bacterial and salivary origin (C). With time, the diversity of the microflora increases, and rod and filament-shaped bacteria colonize (D and E). In the climax community, many unusual associations between different bacterial populations can be seen, including 'corn-cob' formations (F). (Magnification approx. × 1150) Published with permission of Dr A. Saxton.

The irreversible attachment of cells to the tooth involves specific, short range, stereochemical interactions between components on the microbial cell surface (**adhesins**) and complementary **receptors** in the acquired pellicle. These specific interactions contribute to the often observed associations (**tropisms**; Ch. 4) of certain organisms with a particular surface or habitat.

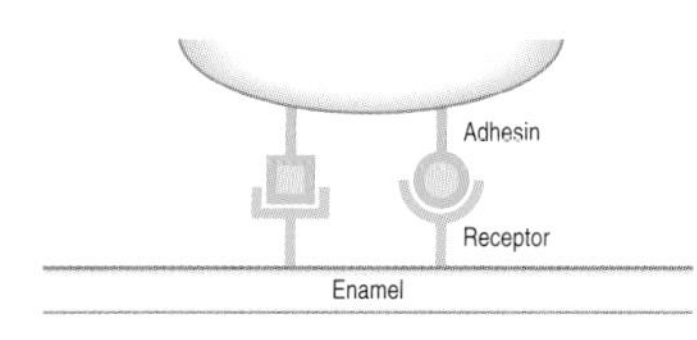

Several examples of these molecular interactions have been characterized, and some are listed in Table 5.3. Other examples of adhesins and their complementary receptors are described in Chapter 4. As examples, adhesins on *S. gordonii* can bind to α-amylase, while *A. naeslundii* and *F. nucleatum* interact with statherin. *Streptococcus mutans* (but not *S. sobrinus*), *P. gingivalis, P. loescheii* and *P. melaninogenica* adhere preferentially to hydroxyapatite coated with PRPs, although different regions of the molecule bind to particular organisms. Colonization by *S. sobrinus* is more dependent on sucrose-mediated mechanisms, including the interaction of glucans with receptors such as glucan binding proteins. Some adhesion mechanisms involve lectin-like bacterial proteins which interact with carbohydrates, or oligosaccharides, on glycoproteins adsorbed to the tooth surface. Thus, *S. sanguinis* can bind to terminal sialic acid residues in adsorbed salivary glycoproteins, while *S. oralis* expresses either a galactose-binding lectin or a lectin that interacts with a trisaccharide structure containing sialic acid, galactose and *N*-acetylgalactosamine.

Actinomyces spp. have two antigenically and functionally distinct types of fimbriae; type 1 fimbriae mediate bacterial adherence to PRPs and to statherin (a protein-protein interaction), whereas type 2 fimbriae are associated with a lactose-sensitive mechanism (a lectin-like activity) involving the adherence of cells to already attached bacteria (**coadhesion**; see later in this section) or to buccal epithelial cells.

Table 5.3 Some examples of host-bacterial interactions involved in adhesion.

Bacterium	Adhesin	Receptor
Streptococcus spp.	antigen 1/11	salivary agglutinin
Streptococcus spp.	LTA	blood group reactive glycoproteins
Mutans streptococci	glucan binding protein	glucan
Streptococcus parasanguinis	35 kDa lipoprotein	fibrin, pellicle
Actinomyces naeslundii	type 1 fimbriae	proline-rich proteins
Porphyromonas gingivalis	150 kDa protein	fibrinogen
Prevotella loescheii	70 kDa lectin	galactose
Fusobacterium nucleatum	42 kDa protein	coaggregation with *Porphyromonas gingivalis*

A number of proteins in the cell walls of streptococci have been identified as adhesins. A high molecular weight protein from *S. mutans*, (termed antigen I/II, B, P1 or Pac), interacts with salivary agglutinins. Antibody directed against this surface molecule can block the adhesion of *S. mutans* to saliva-coated surfaces. The large size of some of the bacterial cell wall proteins means that they may be involved in more than one function. For example, a protein of *S. gordonii* can interact both with salivary proteins and with *A. naeslundii* (coaggregation). Some of the other adhesins found on *S. sanguinis* and *S. gordonii* are now known to be lipoproteins (Ch. 4). Streptococci can use multiple adhesins to bind to saliva-coated surfaces; as an example, *S. sanguinis* can adhere via lectin-like, hydrophobic and/or specific protein (adhesin) interactions.

A critical factor in plaque formation concerns the site at which the specific interactions between bacterial adhesins and host receptors take place. The host-derived receptors reside on molecules that are not only adsorbed to the tooth surface but which are also freely accessible in solution in saliva. Some of these molecules are designed to aggregate bacteria in solution, thereby facilitating their removal from the mouth by swallowing (see Ch. 2). For plaque formation to proceed, however, it is implicit that not all bacteria are aggregated in saliva before they reach the tooth surface. A novel mechanism may function to overcome this problem. It was found that although *A. naeslundii* could bind to the acidic PRPs when the latter were bound to a surface, cells did not interact with these proteins in solution. It has been proposed that hidden molecular segments of PRPs become exposed only when the proteins are adsorbed to hydroxyapatite, as a result of conformational changes. Such hidden receptors for bacterial adhesins have been termed **'cryptitopes'**. In this way, a selective mechanism for facilitating natural plaque formation has evolved by which the host can promote the attachment of specific bacteria without compromising this process in the planktonic phase. Adhesins which recognise cryptitopes in surface-associated molecules would provide a strong selective advantage for any microorganism which colonizes a mucosal or tooth surface. Another example of a cryptitope involving conformational change is the binding of members of the mitis-group of streptococci to fibronectin when complexed to collagen but not to fibronectin in solution. This might also be a mechanism enabling certain oral streptococci to colonize damaged heart valves in infective endocarditis (Ch. 8). A different type of cryptitope involves the recognition of galactosyl-binding lectins by oral bacteria. Epithelial cells and the acquired enamel pellicle have mucins with oligosaccharide side chains with a terminal sialic acid. Bacteria such as *A. naeslundii* synthesize neuraminidase which cleaves the sialic acid exposing the penultimate galactosyl sugar residue. Many oral bacteria possess galactosyl-binding lectins including *A. naeslundii, L. buccalis, F. nucleatum, E. corrodens* and *P. intermedia*, and would benefit from the exposure of these cryptitopes. Similarly, the binding of *P. gingivalis* is greater to epithelial cells that have been mildly treated with trypsin. Some periodontal pathogens, including *P. gingivalis*, produce proteases with an arginine-x specificity (arg-gingipains) that may create appropriate cryptitopes for their colonization.

4. Coaggregation/coadhesion and microbial succession

Over time, the plaque microflora becomes more diverse; there is a shift away from the initial preponderance of streptococci to a biofilm with increasing proportions of *Actinomyces* and other Gram positive bacilli. Some organisms that were unable to colonize the pellicle-coated tooth surfaces are able to attach to already-adherent pioneer species by further adhesin–receptor interactions (coaggregation/co-adhesion). In addition, the metabolism of the pioneer communities alters the local environment and makes conditions more suited to the growth of some fastidious bacteria. Early colonizers are tolerant of a high redox potential; species such as *Neisseria* spp. can consume oxygen and produce carbon dioxide and more reduced end-products of metabolism. Gradually, conditions become more favourable for the growth of obligately anaerobic bacteria. Similarly, the metabolism of pioneer species generates nutrients (e.g. peptides) and fermentation products (lactate, butyrate, acetate) that can be used by other organisms as primary nutrient sources (i.e. food-chains develop; see later, Fig 5.15 and 5.16). Thus, the composition of the plaque microflora changes over time due to a series of complex interactions; these changes are termed **microbial succession** (Fig. 4.1).

Coaggregation or coadhesion (the term co-adhesion is used by some to distinguish between the adhesive interaction of cells on a surface rather than those in suspension) is the cell-to-cell recognition of genetically distinct partner cell types, and is a key process in microbial succession and biofilm formation. Coaggregation occurs among isolates representing most oral bacterial genera (Fig. 5.6). Early plaque accumulation is facilitated by intrageneric coaggregation among streptococcal spp. and among *Actinomyces* spp., as well as by intergeneric coaggregation between streptococci and *Actinomyces*. The subsequent development of dental plaque will involve further intergeneric coaggregation between other genera and the primary colonizers.

Coaggregation often involves lectins; these proteins bind to the complementary carbohydrate-containing receptor on another cell. Thus, the lectin-mediated interaction between streptococci and *Actinomyces* can be blocked by adding galactose or lactose, or by treating the receptor with a protease. Coaggregation can result in some unusual morphological formations, e.g. 'corn-cob' structures (Fig. 5.5F). 'Corn-cobs' can be formed between streptococci with certain types of fibrils (Chs 3 and 4) and *C. matruchotii*; similar associations occur between *Eubacterium* and *Veillonella* spp..

Fusobacteria have been found to coaggregate with the widest range of bacterial genera although, curiously, they do not coaggregate with each other. Early colonizers of plaque coaggregate extensively with *F. nucleatum*, while later colonizers such as *Selenomonas* spp. or *Eubacterium* spp. do not coaggregate with early colonizers but do coaggregate with *F. nucleatum*. It has been proposed that fusobacteria act as an important 'bridge' between early and late colonizing bacteria (Fig. 5.6).

Coaggregation may also be an important mechanism in the functional organization of microbial communities such as dental plaque. The persistence and survival of obligately anaerobic bacteria in an essentially aerobic habitat such as the mouth is enhanced if they are physically close to oxygen-consuming species such as *Neisseria* spp.; such interactions can be mediated by coaggregation, with fusobacteria facilitating the interaction of otherwise non-coaggregating species. The development of food-chains, including those between streptococci and *Veillonella* spp., might also be facilitated by coaggregation. Coaggregation could be a mechanism to increase the probability that species that need to interact and collaborate (in order to survive) will actually combine physically, especially during the earlier stages of plaque development. Cell-cell signalling can occur between bacteria, such as streptococci and *Veillonella* spp., to facilitate their involvement in a food chain (see later sections).

5. Mature biofilm formation

The microbial diversity of plaque will increase over time due to successive waves of microbial succession and subsequent growth. The growth rate of individual bacteria within plaque slows as the biofilm matures, and the mean doubling times of 1–2 hours observed during the early stages of plaque formation rise to between 12–15 hours after 1–3 days of biofilm development. Confluent growth on the tooth surface produces a biofilm with a 3-dimensional structure (Fig. 5.5, D, E). Some of the adherent bacteria synthesize extracellular polymers (soluble and insoluble glucans, fructans and heteropolymers) which will make a major contribution to the **plaque matrix**. Glucans are synthesized by glucosyltransferases; these enzymes can be secreted, and adsorb onto other bacteria or on to the tooth surface to form part of the acquired pellicle, where they can remain functional and contribute further to matrix formation. In contrast, the fructans produced by fructosyltransferases, FTFs, are short-lived in plaque,

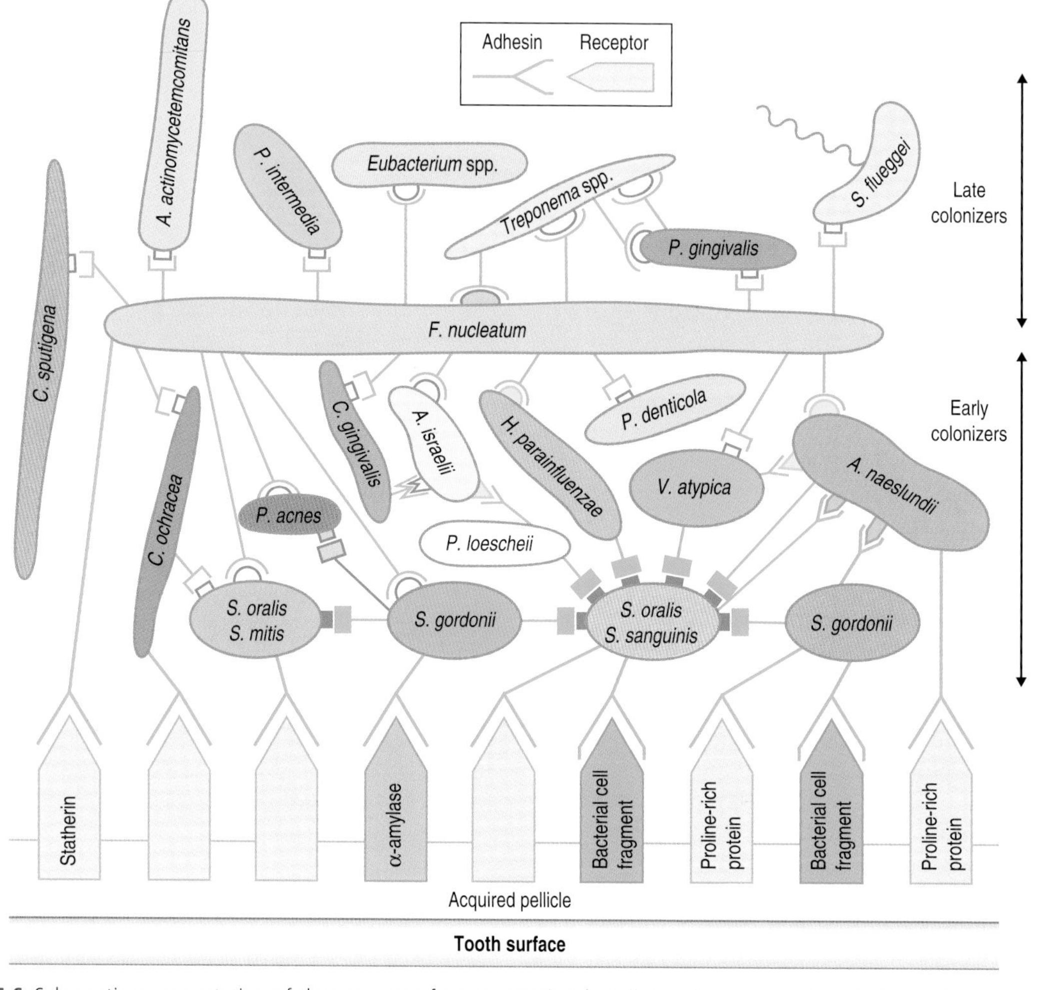

Fig. 5.6 Schematic representation of the patterns of coaggregation (coadhesion) in human dental plaque. Early colonizers bind to receptors in the acquired pellicle; subsequently, other early and later colonizers bind to receptors on the surface of these already attached cells (coadhesion). Adhesins (symbols with stems) are cell components that are heat or protease sensitive; the receptor (complementary symbol) is insensitive to either treatment. Identical symbols do not imply identical molecules. The symbols with rectangular shapes represent lactose-inhibitable coaggregations. Reproduced from Kolenbrander and London, J Bacteriol 1993 175:3247-3252; with permission from the American Society for Microbiology.

and act as extracellular nutrient storage compounds for use by other plaque bacteria (Ch. 4).

A matrix is a common feature of all biofilms, and is more than a chemical scaffold to maintain the shape of the biofilm. It makes a significant contribution to the structural integrity and general tolerance of biofilms to environmental factors (e.g. desiccation) and antimicrobial agents. The matrix can be biologically active and retain water, nutrients and enzymes within the biofilm. The chemistry of the matrix can also help exclude, or restrict the penetration of, other types of molecules including some charged antimicrobial agents.

In mature plaque, the microflora displays maximum diversity. A small sample of plaque may contain 12–27 distinct species, but the bacterial composition will vary at distinct anatomical sites due to the prevailing biological conditions. The distribution of the main groups of microorganism at distinct sites on the tooth will be described later

(Fig. 5.9). Gradients continue to develop in factors that are critical to microbial growth so that sites close together may be vastly different in the concentration of key nutrients and toxic products of metabolism, as well as in terms of pH and Eh, etc. These gradients are not necessarily linear; zones of quite different pH have been detected adjacent to each other in laboratory-generated plaque biofilms. Such **vertical and horizontal stratifications** will cause local environmental heterogeneity resulting in a **mosaic of microhabitats or microenvironments**. Such heterogeneity can explain how organisms with apparently contradictory growth requirements in terms of nutritional, atmospheric or pH requirements are able to coexist in plaque at the same site. Each microhabitat potentially could support the growth of different populations and hence a different microbial community. Similarly, organisms residing in apparently the same general environment might be growing under quite dissimilar conditions and, therefore, exhibiting a different phenotype. This is another reason why it is essential when studying plaque to take small samples from defined areas (Ch. 4).

Multi-species biofilms create opportunities for numerous interactions among the constitutive species that are physically close to one another. These include examples of the conventional antagonistic and synergistic interactions described later in this Chapter. Additional types of interaction have been recognised in oral biofilms including gene transfer via plasmids and cell–cell signalling mediated by small diffusible molecules that enable similar bacteria to communicate with each other and coordinate their activities. More details of these will be given in a subsequent section.

6. Detachment from surfaces

Shear forces can remove microorganisms from oral surfaces, but some bacteria can actively detach themselves from within the biofilm so as to be able to colonize elsewhere. *Streptococcus mutans* can synthesize an enzyme that can cleave proteins from its own cell surface and thereby detach itself from a mono-species biofilm. Similarly, a protease produced by *Prevotella loescheii* can hydrolyze its own fimbrial-associated adhesin responsible for coaggregation with *S. oralis* as well as binding to fibrin. Bacteria may be able to 'sense' adverse changes in environmental conditions, and these may act as cues to induce the genes involved in active detachment.

SUMMARY

The adhesion of organisms to the 'conditioned' tooth surface is a complex process involving, initially, weak electrostatic attractive forces, followed by a variety of specific molecular interactions between bacterial adhesins and receptors adsorbed to the surface (acquired pellicle). These latter processes together with the synthesis of extracellular polysaccharides (EPS) from, for example, sucrose serve to increase the probability of permanent attachment. EPS also contributes to the plaque matrix. Pioneer species interact directly with the acquired pellicle while subsequent biofilm formation is dependent on intra- and intergeneric coadhesion between bacteria (involving lectin-mediated binding) and the subsequent growth of the attached microorganisms. If conditions become unfavourable, some cells are able to actively detach, providing the opportunity to colonize other sites.

CONSEQUENCES OF BIOFILM FORMATION

Impact on gene expression

Plaque maturation involves the growth of the attached bacteria to produce a structurally- and functionally-organized biofilm. Research on surface-associated growth of microorganisms from a range of habitats has shown that the phenotype of bacteria in a biofilm can differ markedly from that predicted from studies of the same organism in liquid culture. Gene expression may be altered when microorganisms initially make contact with a surface. Genes involved with motility may be repressed while other genes required for attachment or growth on new substrates may be induced or up-regulated (Table 5.1).

Similar surface-associated responses are being identified in plaque bacteria, although the magnitude of the shift in gene expression is often less than that observed for free-living species, perhaps because of the absolute dependence of oral bacteria on a biofilm lifestyle. The exposure of *S. gordonii* to saliva results in the induction of genes (*sspA/B*) that encode for adhesins that can bind to salivary glycoproteins and engage in coaggregation with *Actinomyces* spp. Marked changes in protein profiles following attachment have been identified in *S. mutans* using a whole cell proteomic (protein analysis) approach. During the initial stages of biofilm formation by *S. mutans* (the first two hours following attachment), over 30 proteins were differentially expressed (most were up-regulated but some were down-regulated). There was an increase in the relative synthesis of enzymes involved in carbohydrate catabolism; these might be needed for energy generation, although these molecules are multifunctional and can also act as adhesins when located on the cell surface. In contrast, some glycolytic enzymes involved in acid production were down-regulated in older (3 day) biofilms, while proteins involved in a range of biochemical functions, including protein folding and secretion, amino acid and fatty acid biosynthesis, and cell division, were up-regulated. Of particular significance was the finding of novel proteins of as yet unknown function being expressed by biofilm but not planktonic cells. Genes involved with glucan (*gtfBC*) and fructan (*ftf*) synthesis in *S. mutans* are differentially regulated during biofilm formation. In laboratory models, there was little influence of surface growth on genes involved in exopolymer synthesis during early stages of biofilm formation (<48 hours), but *gtf* expression was markedly up-regulated in older (7 day) biofilms whereas *ftf* activity was repressed. This was interpreted as an indirect effect of biofilm growth on gene expression, probably as a response to changes in local environmental conditions such as sugar concentration or pH as the biofilm matured, rather than due to initial attachment.

Cell–cell signalling

The close proximity of cells with each other in biofilms provides ideal conditions for cell-cell interactions. In addition to more conventional biochemical interactions, there is evidence from microbes in a number of habitats of cell density-dependent growth (quorum sensing), whereby individual cells are able to communicate with, and respond to, neighbouring cells by means of small, diffusible, effector molecules. These include acyl-homoserine lactones produced by Gram negative bacteria and small peptides secreted by Gram positive cells. The peptides are generally detected via two-component signal transduction systems. These cell–cell signalling strategies enable cells to sense and adapt to various environmental stresses, and regulate (and coordinate) the expression of genes that influence the ability of pathogens to cause disease.

The best studied system in oral bacteria is found in *S. mutans*, where quorum sensing is mediated by a competence-stimulating peptide (CSP). This peptide also induces genetic competence in *S. mutans* so that the transformation frequency of biofilm-grown *S. mutans* was 10- to 600-fold greater than for planktonic cells. Lysed cells in biofilms such as plaque could act as donors of DNA, thereby increasing the opportunity for horizontal gene transfer in oral biofilms. CSP is also directly involved in biofilm formation since mutants in some of the genes involved in the CSP signalling system produce defective biofilms. This quorum sensing system also functions to regulate acid tolerance in *S. mutans* in biofilms. When cells are exposed to an acid shock, CSP is released which can initiate a coordinated protective biochemical response by more distant *S. mutans* cells, enabling them to survive a potentially lethal stress.

CSPs are specific for cells of the same species, but other communication systems may function between different genera. Surveys of Gram negative periodontal bacteria suggest that these organisms do not possess the acyl-homoserine lactone signalling molecules detected in environmental bacteria. LuxS genes encode for autoinducer-2 (AI-2), and these have been detected in several genera of oral Gram positive and Gram negative bacteria, implying that AI-2 may be a 'universal language' for interspecies communication in plaque bacteria. Several periodontal bacteria, including *Fusobacterium nucleatum, Prevotella intermedia, Porphyromonas gingivalis* and *Aggregatibacter* (formerly *Actinobacillus*) *actinomycetemcomitans*, secrete a signal related to AI-2. AI-2 is involved in leukotoxin production and iron acquisition in *A. actinomycetemcomitans* and protease (arg-gingipain and lys-gingipain) and haemagglutinin activities in *P. gingivalis*. It has also been shown that *S. gordonii* and *P. gingivalis* can respond to LuxS signals from each other (i.e. they can sense heterologous signals), but the pattern of genes that are regulated by LuxS differs in each species. In LuxS mutants, genes associated with carbohydrate metabolism such as glucosyltransferase and fructanase were down-regulated in the streptococcus while genes relating to haemin acquisition and an arginine-specific protease were up-regulated in *P. gingivalis*.

These findings have led to a quest to understand and identify more of these communication networks. A possible practical outcome from such studies might be the development of analogues of specific signalling molecules that could be used as a novel therapeutic approach to manipulate the properties of oral biofilms. Emerging evidence also suggests that certain members of the resident microflora can also engage in 'cross-talk' with the host, for example, by down-regulating the potential induction of proinflammatory cytokines, thereby actively promoting a harmonious relationship between the normal microflora and the host.

Gene transfer

The close proximity of cell in biofilms provides ideal conditions for horizontal gene transfer. As described above, signalling molecules such as competence-stimulating peptide (CSP) markedly increase the ability of recipient cells to take up DNA. In addition, the transfer of conjugative transposons encoding tetracycline resistance between streptococci has been demonstrated in laboratory biofilm models.

Evidence that horizontal gene transfer can occur in the mouth has come from the discovery that both resident (*S. mitis*, *S. oralis*) and pathogenic (*S. pneumoniae*) bacteria isolated from the naso-pharyngeal area possess genes conferring penicillin resistance that display a common mosaic structure. Similar evidence suggests sharing of genes encoding penicillin-binding proteins among resident oral and pathogenic *Neisseria* spp. These findings suggest that plaque can function as a 'genotypic reservoir' by harbouring transferable mobile elements and genes. Such genetic exchange could have a wide clinical significance given the number of overtly pathogenic bacteria that can appear transiently in the mouth.

Antimicrobial tolerance

Oral bacteria growing as a biofilm such as dental plaque display a markedly reduced sensitivity to antibiotics and antimicrobial agents (Table 5.4), including those used in toothpastes and mouthwashes. For example, the biofilm inhibitory concentration of chlorhexidine and amine fluoride was 300 and 75 times greater, respectively, when *S. sobrinus* was grown as a biofilm compared with the minimum bacteriocidal concentration of planktonic cells. Similarly, antibiotics such as amoxycillin and doxycycline had no effect on the viability of biofilms of *S. sanguinis* when used at MIC levels, and laboratory biofims of *P. gingivalis* displayed increased tolerance to doxycycline and metronidazole. Complete elimination of biofilms sometimes required exposure to 500× MIC for a particular antibiotic, although *S. sanguinis* biofilms were killed following exposure to 10–50× MIC of chlorhexidine.

Table 5.4 Increase in tolerance to antimicrobial agents when oral bacteria are grown as a biofilm.

Bacterium	Antimicrobial agent	Biofilm effect+
Streptococcus sanguinis	chlorhexidine	10 – 50× MIC*
Streptococcus sobrinus	amine fluoride chlorhexidine	75× MBC** 300× MBC
Porphyromonas gingivalis	metronidazole doxycycline amoxycillin	2 – 8× MBC 4 – 64× MBC 2 – 4× MBC

+Biofilm effect = change in sensitivity of cells growing as a biofilm compared to when cells were grown in liquid (planktonic) culture.
*MIC = minimum inhibitory concentration of planktonic cells.
**MBC = minimum bacteriocidal concentration of planktonic cells.

The age of the biofilm can influence the sensitivity of cells to a particular antimicrobial agent. Older biofilms of *S. sanguinis* were less susceptible to chlorhexidine than younger biofilms; the biofilm killing concentration for the former being 200 μg/ml compared with 50 μg/ml for the latter. Similarly, being part of a microbial community can influence the sensitivity of cells to an antibiotic; susceptible organisms can appear resistant if neighbouring cells secrete a neutralizing or drug-degrading enzyme. Bacteria in subgingival plaque can produce sufficient β-lactamase to inactivate penicillin delivered to that site during therapy.

The mechanisms that cause the increased tolerance of biofilm cells to antimicrobial agents are still being investigated, but include (a) limited penetration (diffusion-reaction theory) (Fig. 5.7), (b) inactivation (e.g. by neutralizing enzymes), (c) quenching, (d) unfavourable environmental conditions for activity, (e) slow microbial growth rates, and (d) expression of a novel microbial phenotype (Table 5.1).

STRUCTURE OF MATURE DENTAL PLAQUE

The accumulation of plaque on teeth is the result of the balance between adhesion, growth and removal of microorganisms. The development of plaque in terms of biomass will continue until a critical size is reached. Shear forces will then limit any further

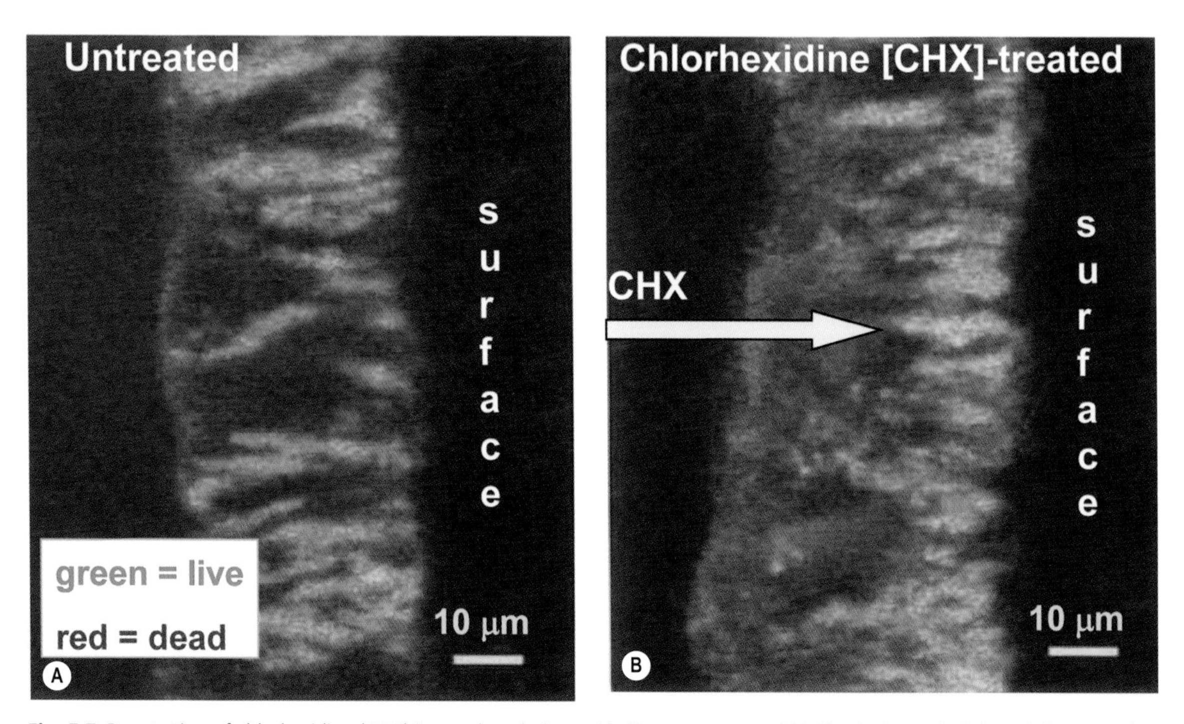

Fig. 5.7 Penetration of chlorhexidine (CHX) into a dental plaque biofilm; an untreated biofilm is shown in (A), and the treated biofilm is shown in (B). The biofilm was visualized with a live/dead stain, in which viable bacteria stain green and dead cells are red. The chlorhexidine has an antimicrobial effect in the outermost layers of dental plaque, but failed to kill cells deeper in the biofilm. Reproduced with permission of Z. Arite.

expansion, but structural development and reorganization may take place continually. Electron microscopy has been used extensively to view dental plaque, the structure of which appeared typically as compressed layers of diverse morphological types of cells that were densely packed together. Pallisaded regions can be seen where filaments and cocci appear to be aligned in parallel at right angles to the enamel surface, while microcolonies, presumably of single cell populations, have also been observed. In addition, horizontal stratification has been described; examples of the ultrastructure of dental plaque are shown in Fig. 5.8.

The early stages of plaque development result in a condensed layer of a limited number of bacterial types. Later, a bulk layer forms which shows less orientation but a higher morphological diversity. This layering has been attributed directly to bacterial succession. In mature plaque, organisms have been seen in direct contact with the enamel due to enzymatic attack on the pellicle. In fissures, impacted food particles can be a common feature of plaque structure. In the gingival crevice, plaque has a thin densely adherent layer on the root surface, with the bulk of the biofilm having a looser structure, especially where it comes into contact with the epithelial lining of the gingival crevice/periodontal pocket. Many bacterial associations have been observed subgingivally in these outer layers, in which cocci are arranged along the length of filamentous organisms, e.g. 'corn-cob', 'test tube brush' or 'rosette' formations (Fig. 5.5, F).

The preparation of material for electron microscopy dehydrates the sample and distorts the natural structure of biofilms. Confocal laser scanning microscopy does not require such sample preparation, and can be used to view specimens in their natural, hydrated state. When dental plaque developed on enamel slices placed in removable devices in the mouth, the architecture of the resultant biofilms had a far more open architecture when viewed by confocal microscopy, with channels or pores penetrating the biofilm. These 'channels' can be filled with extracellular polymers, and this can influence the distribution and movement of molecules in

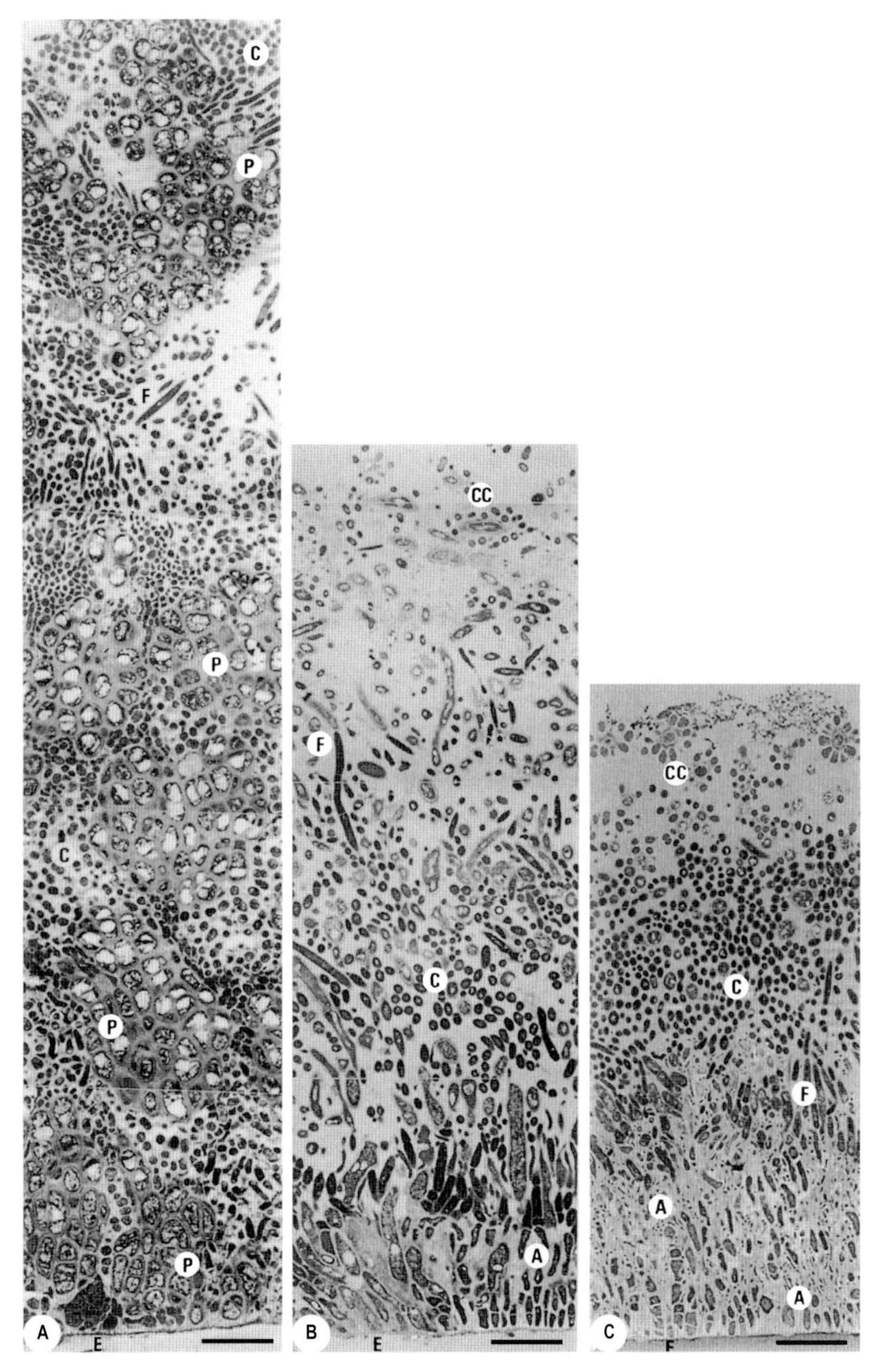

Fig. 5.8 Ultrastructure of 2-week-old dental plaque from three individuals with different patterns of microbial colonization (A–C). C = Gram positive coccal bacteria; F = Gram negative filamentous bacteria; CC = corn-cob formations; P = large, irregular shaped bacteria; E = space remaining after demineralization of enamel. Bar = 5 μm. Published with the permission of Dr B Nyved, Dr O Fejerskov and Munksgaard.

plaque. The use of live/dead stains with confocal microscopy suggests that bacterial vitality may vary throughout plaque, with most viable and active bacteria being present in the central part of the biofilm and lining the channels.

SUMMARY

A biofilm life-style has a direct and indirect impact on gene expression by oral bacteria, with many biofilm-specific genes being expressed. Cells in biofilms also display a decreased sensitivity to antimicrobial agents. Microorganisms in biofilms are in close proximity with one another which facilitates a range of biochemical (antagonistic and synergistic) interactions, as well as opportunities for gene transfer. In addition, attached cells can communicate with one another, and coordinate gene expression, via the production of small diffusible signalling molecules, such as competence-stimulating peptide by *S. mutans*, and autoinducer-2 by a range of oral species. The final outcome is the development of a complex, interactive multi-species, spatially- and functionally-organized biofilm.

BACTERIAL COMPOSITION OF THE CLIMAX COMMUNITY OF DENTAL PLAQUE FROM DIFFERENT SITES

Environmental conditions on a tooth are not uniform. Differences exist in the prevalent nutrients, degree of protection from oral removal forces and in other biological and chemical factors that influence the growth of the resident microflora. These differences will be reflected in the composition of the microbial community, particularly at sites so obviously distinct as the gingival crevice, approximal regions, smooth surfaces, and pits and fissures. The predominant bacterial genera at these sites are shown in Fig. 5.9, while a more detailed description of the microflora at each site is given below.

Fissure plaque

The microbiology of fissure plaque has been determined using either 'artificial fissures' implanted in occlusal surfaces of pre-existing restorations, or by sampling 'natural' fissures. The microflora is mainly Gram positive and is dominated by streptococci, especially extracellular polysaccharide-producing species. In one study, no obligately anaerobic Gram negative rods were found, while others have recovered anaerobes in low numbers such as *Veillonella* and *Propionibacterium* species (Table 5.5). Aerobic and facultatively anaerobic Gram negative species, such as *Neisseria* spp. and *Haemophilus parainfluenzae*, have also been isolated on occasions. A striking feature of the microflora is the wide range of numbers and types of bacteria in the different fissures. In one study, the total anaerobic microflora ranged from 1×10^6 to 33×10^6 colony forming units (CFU) per fissure. Saliva will have a major influence on the biological properties of fissures, and diet may also be a significant factor

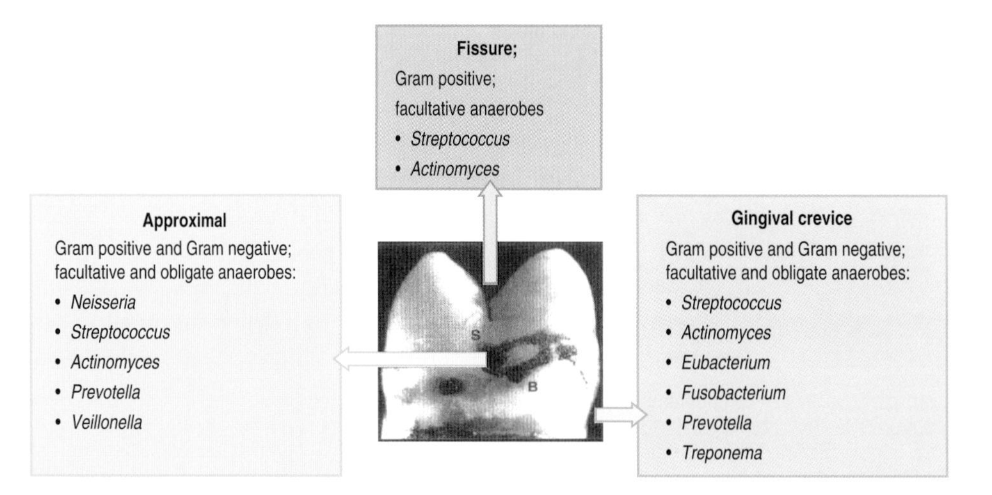

Fig. 5.9 Predominant groups of bacteria found at distinct sites on the tooth surface.

Table 5.5 The predominant cultivable microflora of 10 occlusal fissures in adults.

Bacterium	Median percentage of total cultivable microflora	Range (%)	Percentage isolation frequency
Streptococcus	45	8–86	100
Staphylococcus	9	0–23	80
Actinomyces	18	0–46	80
Propionibacterium	1	0–8	50
Eubacterium	0	0–27	10
Lactobacillus	0	0–29	20
Veillonella	3	0–44	60
Individual species:			
mutans streptococci	25	0–86	70
Streptococcus mitis-group	1	0–15	50
Streptococcus anginosus-group	0	0–3	10
Actinomyces naeslundii	3	0–44	70
Lactobacillus casei	0	0–10	10
Lactobacillus plantarum	0	0–29	10

because impacted food can often be detected. The simpler community found in fissures compared to other enamel surfaces probably reflects a more severe environment. The distribution of bacteria within a fissure has not been studied in detail, although it has been claimed that lactobacilli and mutans streptococci preferentially inhabit the lower depths of a fissure. It is clear from Fig. 5.10 that environmental conditions at the base of the fissure will be very different in terms of nutrient availability, pH, and buffering effects of saliva than areas nearer the plaque surface.

Approximal plaque

The main organisms isolated from a study of approximal plaque are shown in Table 5.6. Although streptococci are present in high numbers, these sites are frequently dominated by Gram positive rods, particularly *Actinomyces* spp. The more reduced nature (low redox potential) of this site compared to that of fissures can be gauged from the higher recovery of obligately anaerobic organisms, although spirochaetes are not usually found. The range and percentage isolation frequency of most bacteria is high, suggesting that each site represents a distinct ecosystem which should be looked at in isolation with regard to the relationship between the resident microflora and the clinical state of the enamel.

The variability of plaque composition was highlighted in a study of several small samples taken from different sites around the contact area of teeth extracted for orthodontic purposes. The recovery and proportions of different groups of bacteria varied according to the location of the sample site around the contact area. The isolation frequency of *S. mutans* and *S. sobrinus* was higher at sub-sites from below the contact area, and this is also the most caries-prone site. Similarly, *A. naeslundii* and *A. odontolyticus* were found more commonly below the contact area, while *Neisseria*, *S. sanguinis* and *S. mitis* biovar 1 were recovered more frequently at sub-sites away from, and to the side of, the contact area. Such variations again emphasize the need for accurate sampling of discrete sites when attempting to correlate the composition of plaque with disease.

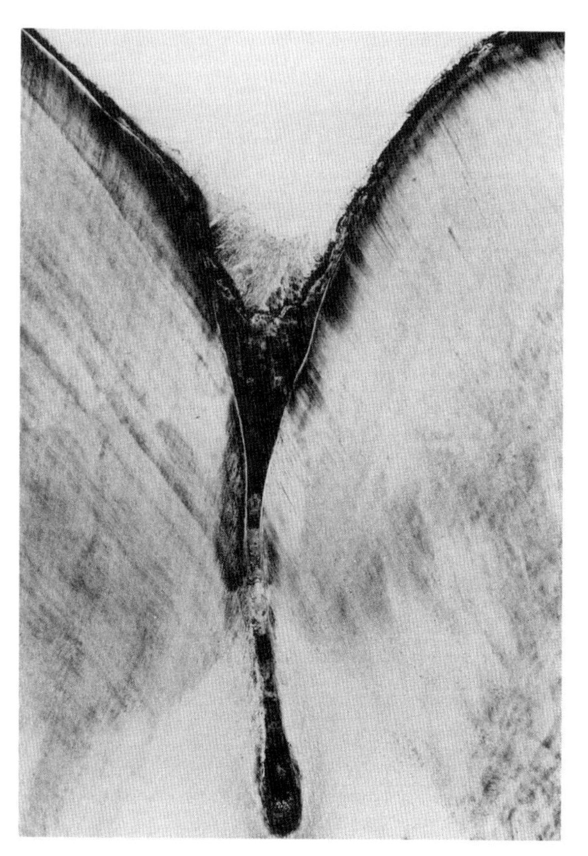

Fig. 5.10 Dental plaque in a fissure on the occlusal surface of a molar. (Magnification approx. × 60.) Published with permission of K. M. Pang.

Gingival crevice plaque

An obviously distinct ecological climate is found in the gingival crevice. This is reflected in the higher species diversity of the bacterial community at this site (Fig. 5.11) although the total numbers of bacteria can be low (10^3–10^6 CFU/crevice). The highest numbers of obligately anaerobic bacteria are cultured from this site, many of which are Gram negative or are *Eubacterium*-like (Table 5.7; Fig. 3.5). Indeed, spirochaetes and anaerobic streptococci are isolated almost exclusively from this site. The ecology of the crevice is influenced by the anatomy of the site and the flow and properties of gingival crevicular fluid (GCF; Ch. 2). Many organisms that are asaccharolytic but proteolytic are found in the gingival crevice; they derive their energy from the hydrolysis of host proteins and peptides, and from the catabolism of amino acids. In disease the gingival crevice enlarges to become a periodontal pocket (Fig. 2.1) and the flow of GCF increases. The diversity of the microflora increases still further in disease and will be described in more detail in Chapter 6.

Among the genera and species associated with the healthy gingival crevice are members of the mitis- and anginosus-groups of streptococci; in addition, Gram positive rods such as *Actinomyces* spp. (*A. odontolyticus, A. naeslundii, A. georgiae*) and *Rothia dentocariosa* can also be found. The most commonly isolated black-pigmented anaerobe in the healthy gingival crevice is *Prevotella melaninogenica* while *P. nigrescens* has also been recovered on occasions. Fusobacteria are among the commonest anaerobes found in the healthy gingival crevice, and capnophilic species such as *Capnocytophaga ochracea* can be isolated.

Molecular studies using culture-independent approaches (e.g. 16S rRNA gene amplification, FISH; Ch. 3) have shown that the subgingival microflora is extremely diverse, even in health. Around 40% of the amplified clones represented novel phylotypes. Human oral TM7 bacteria, of which there are no culturable examples, were detected frequently in samples, and made up around 1% of the total bacteria in healthy subgingival sites (Figs 3.3 and 5.12). A number of spirochaetes were detected, including *Treponema vincentii, T. denticola, T. maltophilum* and *T. lecithinolyticum*, as well as members of the genera *Selenomonas, Prevotella, Capnocytophaga* and *Campylobacter*.

Denture plaque

The microflora of denture plaque from healthy sites (i.e. with no sign of denture stomatitis, Ch. 9) is highly variable as can be deduced from the wide ranges in viable counts obtained for individual bacteria as illustrated in Table 5.8. Differences also occur between the fitting and the exposed surfaces of the denture. In the relatively stagnant area on the denture-fitting surface, plaque tends to be more acidogenic, thereby favouring streptococci (especially mutans streptococci) and sometimes *Candida* spp.. In edentulous subjects, dentures become the primary habitat for mutans streptococci and members of the mitis-group of streptococci. Denture plaque can harbour obligate anaerobes including *A. israelii* and low proportions of Gram negative rods. *Staphylococcus aureus* can be isolated from denture plaque (Table 5.8), and this species is also found commonly in the mucosa of patients with denture stomatitis (Ch. 9).

Table 5.6 The predominant cultivable microflora of approximal plaque.

Bacterium	Mean percentage of total cultivable microflora	Range (%)	Percentage isolation frequency
Streptococcus	23	0.4-70	100
Gram positive rods (predominantly *Actinomyces*)	42	4-81	100
Gram negative rods (predominantly *Prevotella*)	8	0-66	93
Neisseria	2	0-44	76
Veillonella	13	0-59	93
Fusobacterium	0.4	0-5	55
Lactobacillus	0.5	0-2	24
Rothia	0.4	0-6	36
Individual species:			
mutans streptococci	2	0-23	66
Streptococcus sanguinis	6	0-64	86
Streptococcus salivarius	1	0-7	54
Streprococcus anginosus-group	0.5	0-33	45
Actinomyces israelii	17	0-78	72
Actinomyces naeslundii	19	0-74	97

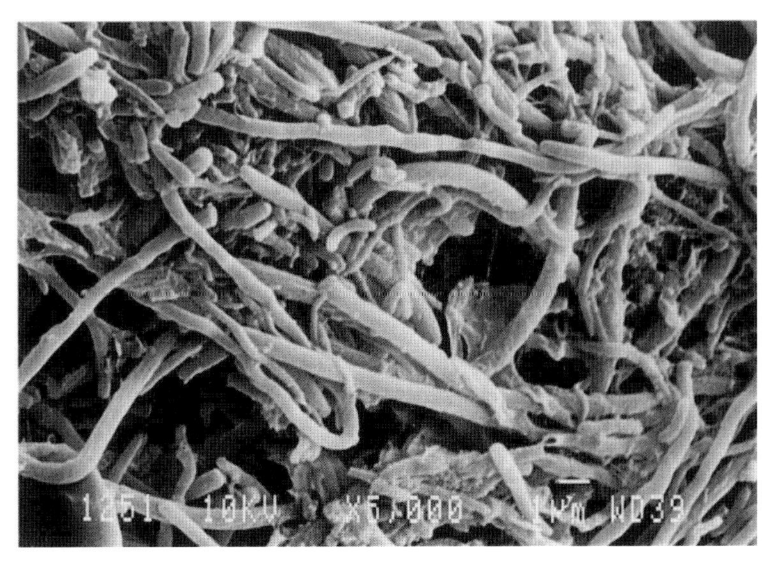

Fig. 5.11 Scanning electron micrograph of subgingival plaque, showing rods, curved rods, filaments and spiral-shaped cells. (Magnification approx. × 5000.) Published with permission of K. M. Pang.

Table 5.7 The predominant cultivable microflora of the healthy gingival crevice.

Bacterium	Mean percentage of total cultivable microflora	Range (%)	Isolation frequency (%)
Gram positive facultatively anaerobic cocci (predominantly *Streptococcus*)	40	2-73	100
Gram positive obligately anaerobic cocci	1	0-6	14
Gram positive facultatively anaerobic rods (predominantly *Actinomyces*)	35	10-63	100
Gram positive obligately anaerobic rods	10	0-37	86
Gram negative facultatively anaerobic cocci (predominantly *Neisseria*)	0.3	0-2	14
Gram negative obligately anaerobic cocci (predominantly *Veillonella*)	2	0-5	57
Gram negative facultatively anaerobic rods	ND*	ND	ND
Gram negative obligately anaerobic rods	13	8-20	100

Samples were taken from the gingival crevice of seven adults humans.
*ND, not detected.

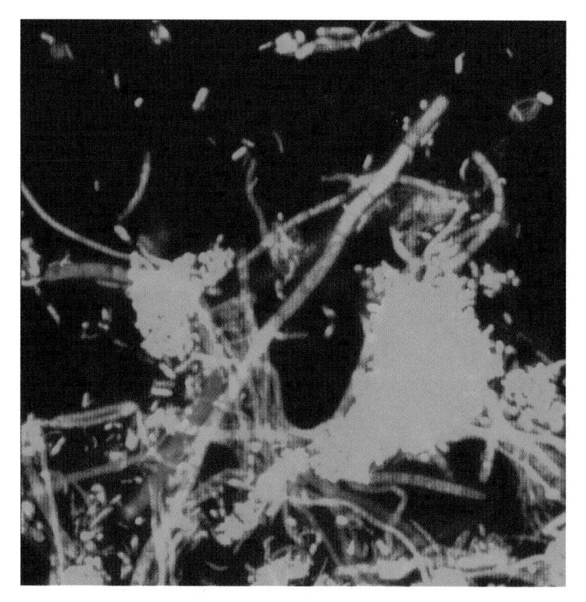

Fig. 5.12 Unculturable bacteria belonging to the TM7 group (blue) in subgingival dental plaque. Reproduced from Ouverney et al, Appl Environ Microbiol 2003 69:6294-6298; with permission from the American Society for Microbiology.

Culture-independent molecular techniques have detected periodontal pathogens such as *Porphyromonas gingivalis, Tannerella forsythia* and *Aggregatibacter actinomycetemcomitans* in the biofilms that develop on the hard palate of dentures in edentulous patients. High numbers of *Actinomyces* spp. and *Capnocytophaga* were also detected.

Dental plaque from animals

There is interest in the microbial composition of dental plaque from animals for two main reasons: (a) to study the influence of widely different diets and lifestyles on the microflora, and (b) to determine the similarity between the microflora of an animal with that of humans to ascertain their relevance as a model of human oral disease. At the genus level, the plaque microflora is similar among animals representing such diverse dietary groups as insectivores, herbivores and carnivores. This emphasizes (a) the significance of endogenous nutrients in maintaining the stability and diversity of the resident microflora, and (b) the specificity of the interaction between this microflora

Table 5.8 The predominant cultivable microflora of denture plaque.

Microorganism	Percentage viable count		Percentage isolation frequency
	Median	Range	
Streptococcus	41	0-81	88
mutans streptococci	<1	0-48	50
S. mitis-group	2	0-30	75
S. anginosus-group	2	0-51	63
S. salivarius-group	0	0-41	38
Staphylococcus	8	1-13	100
S. aureus	6	0-13	88
"S. epidermidis"	0	0-7	13
Gram positive rods	33	1-74	100
Actinomyces	21	0-54	88
A. israelii	3	0-47	63
A. naeslundii	3	0-48	63
A. odontolyticus	1	0-17	63
Lactobacillus	0	0-48	25
Propionibacterium	<1	0-5	50
Veillonella	8	3-20	100
Gram negative rods	0	0-6	38
Yeasts	0.002	0-0.5	63

and the oral ecosystem. Thus, *Actinomyces, Streptococcus, Neisseria, Veillonella,* and *Fusobacterium* are widely distributed in both zoo and non-zoo primates and other animals, and can, therefore, be genuinely considered as autochthonous members of dental plaque (Ch. 4). Following recent taxonomic studies, differences between isolates from man and animals have emerged at the species level. For example, *Streptococcus rattus* and *S. macacae* are isolated exclusively from rodents and primates, respectively, whereas other species of mutans streptococci are found in humans.

PLAQUE FLUID

Plaque fluid is the free aqueous phase of plaque, and can be separated from the microbial components by centrifugation. Analysis of plaque fluid shows it to differ in composition from both saliva and GCF. In particular, the protein content of plaque fluid is higher than that of saliva, as are the concentrations of several important cations including sodium, potassium, and magnesium. Likewise, the levels of albumin, lactoferrin, and lysozyme are greater in plaque fluid than saliva (Table 2.2). A number of enzymes of both bacterial and host (e.g. from polymorphs) origin can be detected in plaque fluid. Specific host defence factors are also found in plaque fluid; sIgA is present at the same concentration as in whole saliva whereas IgG and complement are at higher levels, and are probably derived from GCF. Fluoride binds to plaque components, but is also found free in plaque fluid. Bound fluoride can be released from these components because fluoride concentrations increase in plaque fluid when the pH falls during the bacterial metabolism of fermentable carbohydrates. Acidic products of metabolism are retained in plaque fluid, and a shift in profile from a hetero- to a homofermentative pattern occurs following the intake of dietary sugars.

CALCULUS

Calculus, or tartar, is the term used to describe calcified dental plaque. It consists of intra- and extracellular deposits of mineral, including apatite, brushite, and whitlockite, as well as protein and carbohydrate. Mineral growth can occur around any bacteria; areas of mineral growth can then coalesce to form calculus which may become covered by an unmineralized layer of bacteria. Calculus can occur both supragingivally (especially near the salivary ducts) and subgingivally, where it may act as an additional retentive area for plaque accumulation, thereby increasing the likelihood of gingivitis and other forms of periodontal disease. Calculus can be porous leading to the retention of bacterial antigens and the stimulation of bone resorption by toxins from periodontal pathogens. Over 80% of adults have calculus, and its prevalence increases with age. An elevated calcium ion concentration in saliva may predispose some individuals to be high calculus formers. Once formed, huge removal forces are required to detach calculus; this removal takes up a disproportionate amount of clinical time during routine visits by patients to the dentist. Consequently, a number of dental products are now formulated to restrict calculus formation. These products contain pyrophosphates, zinc salts, or polyphosphonates to inhibit mineralization by slowing crystal growth and reducing coalescence.

MICROBIAL INTERACTIONS IN DENTAL PLAQUE

The close proximity of microorganisms in biofilms facilitates a range of biochemical interactions which can be beneficial to one or more of the interacting populations, while others can be antagonistic (Table 5.9). Examples of synergistic and antagonistic interactions will now be described; other types of interaction, including cell-cell signalling and gene transfer, were described earlier in this Chapter.

Table 5.9 Factors involved in beneficial and antagonistic microbial interactions in dental plaque.

Beneficial (synergistic)	Antagonistic
Enzyme complementation	Bacteriocins
Food chains (food webs)	Hydrogen peroxide
Coadhesion	Organic acids
Cell-cell signalling	Low pH
Gene transfer	Nutrient competition

Synergistic interactions

Although competition for nutrients will be one of the primary ecological determinants in dictating the prevalence of a particular species in dental plaque, bacteria also have to collaborate in order to break down the complex host molecules that act as their primary substrates. Salivary proteins and glycoproteins are the major sources of nitrogen and carbon at healthy sites. Individual species of oral bacteria possess different but overlapping patterns of enzyme activity, so that the concerted action of several species is usually necessary for the complete degradation of host molecules (Figs 5.13 and 5.16). For example, the growth of some organisms will be dependent on others for removing the terminal sugar from

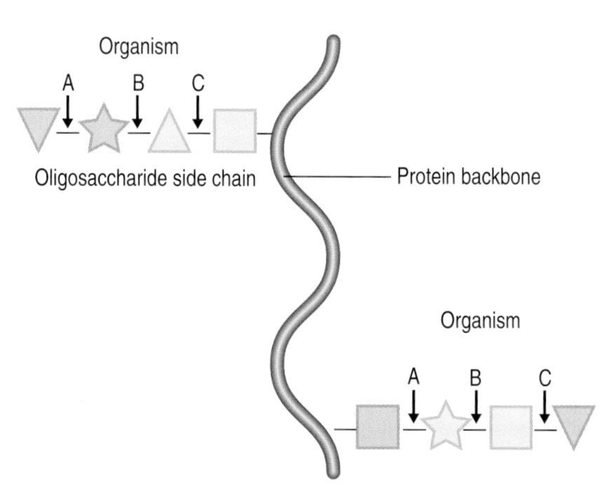

Fig. 5.13 Bacterial cooperation in the degradation of host glycoproteins (enzyme complementation). For example, organism A is able to cleave the terminal sugar of the oligosaccharide side-chain, which enables organism B or D to cleave the penultimate residue, etc.

the oligosaccharide side chain of the glycoprotein to expose a new sugar.

Microbial cooperation in the breakdown of host macromolecules was observed when subgingival bacteria were grown on human serum (used to mimic GCF). Shifts in the microbial composition of the consortia occurred at different stages of glycoprotein breakdown. Initially, carbohydrate side-chains were removed by organisms with complementary glycosidase activities, including *S. oralis*, *E. saburreum* and *Prevotella* spp.. This was followed by the hydrolysis of the protein core by anaerobes such as *P. intermedia*, *P. oralis*, *F. nucleatum*, and to a lesser extent, *Eubacterium* spp.; some amino acid fermentation occurred and the remaining carbohydrate side-chains were metabolized leading to the emergence of *Veillonella* spp.. A final phase was characterized by progressive protein degradation and extensive amino acid fermentation; the predominant species included *Parvimonas micra* (formerly *Peptostreptococcus micros*) and *E. brachy*. Significantly, individual species grew only poorly in pure culture in serum. A consequence of these interactions is that different species avoid direct competition for individual nutrients, and hence are able to co-exist. This type of interaction is an example of protocooperation or mutualism, whereby there is benefit to all participants that are involved in the interaction.

Bacterial polymers are also targets for degradation. EPS synthesized by many plaque bacteria (Table 4.9) can be metabolized by other bacteria in the absence of exogenous (dietary) carbohydrates. The fructan of *S. salivarius* and other streptococci, and the glycogen-like polymer of *Neisseria*, are particularly labile, and only low levels of fructan can be detected in plaque *in vivo*. In addition, mutans streptococci, members of the mitis- or salivarius-groups of streptococci, *A. israelii*, *Capnocytophaga* spp., and *Fusobacterium* spp. possess exo- and/or endo-hydrolytic activity and metabolize streptococcal glucans.

An important nutritional interaction is when the products of metabolism of one organism (primary feeder) become the main source of nutrients for another (secondary feeder). For example, lactate produced from the metabolism of dietary carbohydrates by a range of other species, can be utilised by *Veillonella* spp. and converted to weaker acids. In this way, *Veillonella* spp. can reduce the cariogenic potential of other plaque bacteria; fewer carious lesions were obtained in rats inoculated with either *S. mutans* or *S. sanguinis* and *Veillonella* than in animals mono-infected with either of the streptococci (Fig. 5.14). Strains of *Neisseria*, *Corynebacterium*, and *Eubacterium* are also able to metabolize lactate.

A range of other nutritional interactions between oral bacteria have been described (Fig. 5.15). A mutually beneficial interaction occurs between *S. sanguinis* and *C. rectus*; the anaerobe scavenges inhibitory oxygen, or possibly hydrogen peroxide produced by the streptococcus, while *S. sanguinis* provides *C. rectus* with formate following the fermentation of glucose under carbohydrate-limiting conditions. *Campylobacter rectus* is also able to produce protohaeme for the growth of black-pigmented anaerobes.

Numerous interbacterial nutritional interactions occur in plaque, with the growth of some species being dependent on the metabolism of other organisms. Indeed the diversity of the plaque microflora is due, in part, to:

- the development of such food chains and food webs (Figs 5.14–5.16), and to
- the lack of a single nutrient limiting the growth of all bacterial species.

Bacterial survive by adopting, where possible, alternative metabolic strategies in order to avoid direct competition. Another beneficial interaction among plaque bacteria is coaggregation (coadhesion) which can aid colonization of surfaces and also facilitate metabolic interactions between mutually-dependent strains; this was described earlier in this Chapter.

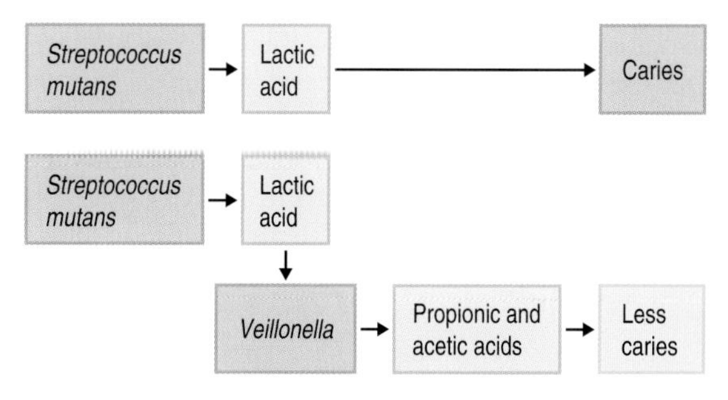

Fig. 5.14 Establishment of a simple food-chain. Bacteria such as *Streptococcus mutans* produce lactate from fermentable sugars that can be metabolized to weaker acids by *Veillonella* spp.; in gnotobiotic animals, this food-chain can reduce the cariogenic potential of these streptococci.

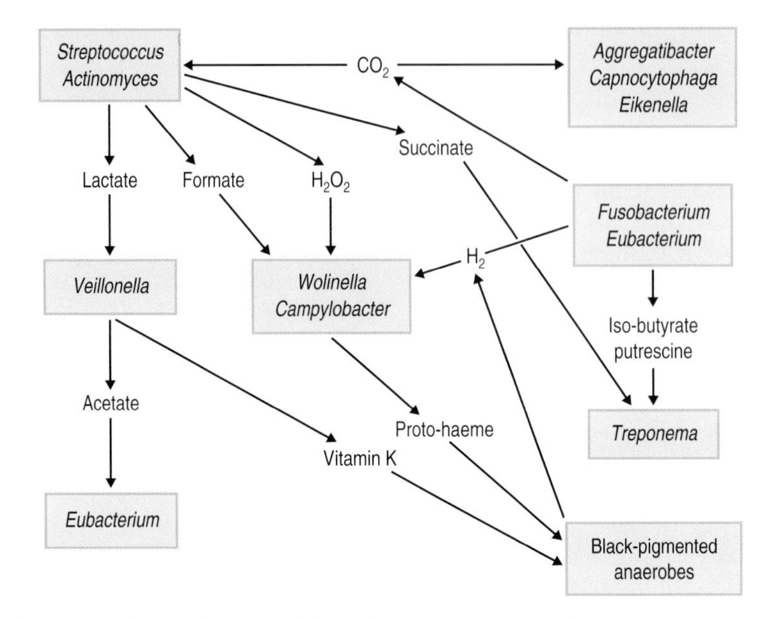

Fig. 5.15 Some potential nutritional interactions (food chains) among plaque bacteria.

Antagonistic interactions

Antagonism is a major contributing factor in determining the composition of microbial ecosystems such as dental plaque (Table 5.9). The production of antagonistic compounds (such as bacteriocins or bacteriocin-like substances, BLIS) can give an organism a competitive advantage when interacting with other microbes. Bacteriocins are relatively high molecular weight proteins that can inhibit the growth of related bacteria while the producer strains are resistant to the action of the bacteriocins they produce. Bacteriocins are produced by most species of oral streptococci (e.g. mutacin by *S. mutans* and sanguicin by *S. sanguinis*), as well as by *C. matruchotii*, black-pigmented anaerobes, and *A. actinomycetemcomitans*; in contrast, *Actinomyces* species are not generally bacteriocinogenic. Although bacteriocins are usually limited in their spectrum of activity, many of the streptococcal bacteriocins are broad spectrum, inhibiting species belonging to Gram positive (including *Actinomyces*) and Gram negative genera. The production of bacteriocins may give strains a competitive advantage during colonization.

Other inhibitory factors produced by plaque bacteria include organic acids, hydrogen peroxide, and enzymes. The production of hydrogen peroxide by members of the mitis-group of streptococci has been proposed as a mechanism whereby the numbers of periodontal pathogens are reduced in plaque to levels at which they are incapable of initiating disease. Some periodontal pathogens (e.g. *A. actinomycetemcomitans*) produce factors inhibitory to oral streptococci, so that certain periodontal diseases (Ch. 6) might result from an ecological imbalance between dynamically-interacting groups of bacteria. The low pH generated from carbohydrate metabolism is also inhibitory to many plaque species, particularly Gram negative organisms and to some streptococci associated with sound enamel. The production of antagonistic factors will not necessarily lead to the complete exclusion of sensitive species. As discussed previously, the presence of distinct microhabitats within a biofilm such as plaque enables bacteria to survive under conditions that would be incompatible to them in a homogeneous environment.

Antagonism will also be a mechanism whereby exogenous (allochthonous) species are prevented from colonizing the oral cavity. For example, some *S. salivarius* strains produce an inhibitor (enocin or salivaricin) active against Lancefield Group A streptococci (*S. pyogenes*). Bacteriocin-producing strains may prevent colonization of the mouth by this pathogen in a manner similar to that proposed for streptococci in the pharynx. It has been claimed that *S. salivarius* is more frequently isolated from the throats of children who do not become colonized following exposure to Group A streptococci than from those who do become infected. In New Zealand, children can be deliberately implanted with bacteriocin-producing strains of *S. salivarius* to reduce infections by Group A streptococci; this process is termed '**replacement therapy**'. These, and other inhibitory bacteria, are being considered for future use as oral **probiotics**. Thus, microbial interactions will play a major role in determining both the final composition and the pattern of development of the plaque microflora.

DENTAL PLAQUE AS A MICROBIAL COMMUNITY

Numerous studies have shown that oral bacteria do not behave randomly during the formation of dental plaque. Plaque forms in an organized manner via physicochemical and specific intermolecular, adhesin-receptor interactions, followed later by interbacterial coadhesion, metabolic interactions and cell–cell communication. These interactions produce a spectrum of ecological niches (metabolic functions; Ch. 1), and produce a number of distinct benefits for the component microorganisms enabling the survival and growth of fastidious species by:

- the synergistic catabolism of complex host macromolecules so that substrates can be utilized that would be recalcitrant to degradation by individual species,
- modulation of local environmental conditions (pH, oxygen tension, redox potential), thereby enabling the growth of obligate anaerobes in an overtly aerobic habitat, and of pH-sensitive bacteria during periods of low pH, and
- efficient nutrient and energy cycling via cross-feeding and food webs.

Great metabolic diversity exists within the plaque microflora, ranging from organisms that can catalyze the initial splitting of complex host polymers into smaller units, to those such as sulphate-reducing bacteria and methanogens that gain energy from the utilization of simple end products of metabolism (Fig. 5.16). The recent detection of these latter groups of organism in plaque confirmed that this biofilm acts as a true microbial community, since it is capable of fully exploiting the total energetic

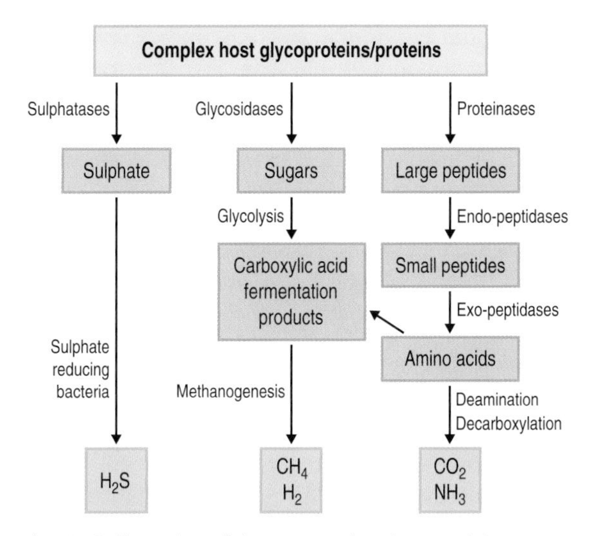

Fig. 5.16 Illustration of the concerted and sequential breakdown of complex host substrates by communities of oral bacteria with complementary enzyme activities.

potential of the available nutrients. In such a microbial community, the metabolic efficiency of the whole is greater than that of the sum of the individual species since substrate utilization involves both the concerted and sequential catabolism of these complex molecules. Growth of such a community as a biofilm confers additional benefits since cells are protected from the host defences, antimicrobial agents and from other hostile factors; for example, a sensitive organism can be rendered 'resistant' by neighbouring cells expressing inactivating or neutralizing enzymes such as β-lactamase, IgA-protease or catalase. In addition, the closely coupled physical and metabolic interactions leave few niches unfilled thereby reducing the likelihood of colonization by exogenous microbes, and contributing to the natural microbial stability of the microflora of plaque (microbial homeostasis; see next section).

SUMMARY

The overall benefits of a microbial community lifestyle to the component species are:

- an extended habitat range,
- increased substrate diversity and metabolic efficiency, and
- increased protection from host defences and environmental stresses.

For some groups of interacting consortia of organisms, the community life-style also increases their pathogenic potential (**pathogenic synergism**). Groups of organisms are able to cause disease that would be unable to do so in pure culture; examples include most periodontal diseases (Ch. 6) as well as abscesses (Ch. 7). In these polymicrobial infections, organisms that are not involved directly in tissue destruction can play vital roles in the disease process. Some organisms can support those with a more obvious pathogenic role by, for example, providing protection from host defences (e.g. by the production of IgA proteases), modifying the local environment (e.g. consuming oxygen and lowering the redox potential), providing key nutrients (e.g. via food chains or by contributing to the catabolism of complex host molecules), and by inactivating inhibitors (e.g. β-lactamase production to neutralize penicillins).

An overview of some of potential interactions in a microbial community such as dental plaque is shown in Fig. 5.17.

MICROBIAL HOMEOSTASIS IN DENTAL PLAQUE

Despite its microbial diversity, the composition of dental plaque at any site is characterized by a remarkable degree of stability or balance among the component species. This stability is maintained in spite of the host defences, and despite the regular exposure of the plaque community to a variety of modest environmental stresses. These stresses include diet, the regular challenge by exogenous species, the use of dentifrices and mouthwashes containing antimicrobial agents (Ch. 6), and changes in saliva flow and hormone levels (Fig. 5.18). The ability to maintain community stability in a variable environment has been termed **microbial homeostasis.** This stability stems not from any metabolic indifference among the components of the microflora but results rather from a balance of dynamic microbial interactions, including both synergism and antagonism. When the environment is perturbed, self-regulatory mechanisms (homeostatic reactions) come into force to restore the original balance. An essential component of such mechanisms is negative feedback, whereby a change in one or more organisms results in a response by others to oppose or neutralize such a change. There is a tendency for homeostasis to be greater in microbial communities with a higher species diversity.

Despite the microbial diversity of dental plaque, homeostasis does breakdown on occasions. The main causes for this are listed in Table 5.10, and can be divided into either:

- deficiencies in the immune response, or
- other (non-immune) factors.

The host defences, together with the resident microflora, serve to maintain microbial homeostasis

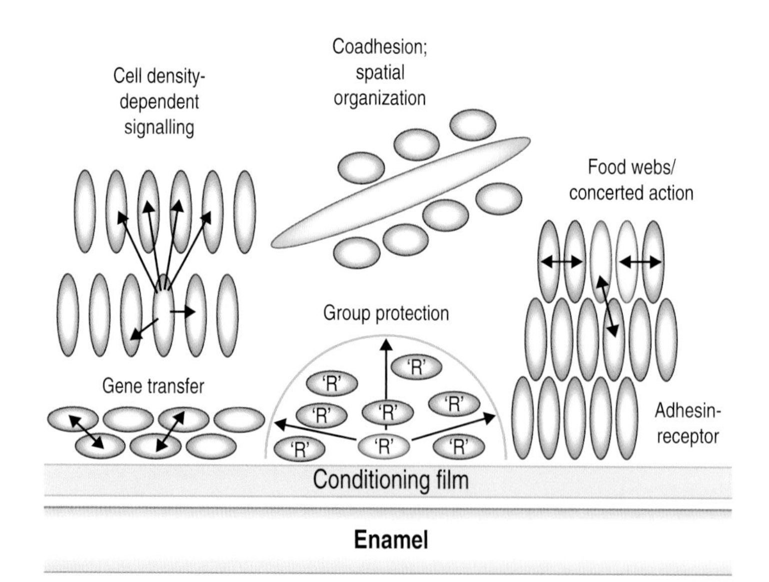

Fig. 5.17 Schematic representation of the types of interaction that occur in a microbial community, such as dental plaque, growing as a biofilm.

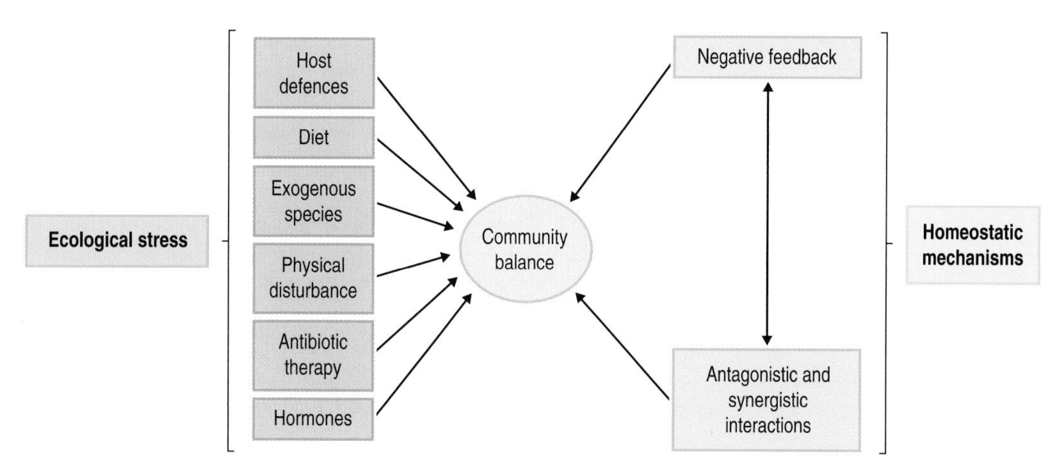

Fig. 5.18 Factors involved in the maintenance of microbial homeostasis in the mouth.

Table 5.10 Factors responsible for the breakdown of microbial homeostasis in dental plaque.

Immunological factors	Non-immunological factors
sIgA-deficiency	Xerostomia
Neutrophil dysfunction	Antibiotics
Chemotherapy-induced myelosuppression	Dietary carbohydrates/low pH
Infection-induced myelosuppression (e.g. AIDS)	Increased GCF flow Oral contraceptives

in plaque (and on other oral surfaces), and together they act synergistically to prevent colonization by exogenous species and the invasion of host tissues by opportunistic pathogens. Therefore, treatment strategies, including the use of antibiotics, should avoid irreversible damage to the resident oral microflora so as to retain the beneficial properties of dental plaque and the microflora of other oral sites.

The remainder of this book will be devoted to describing the consequences of the breakdown of microbial homeostasis in the mouth, and describe the aetiology of the major oral diseases.

CHAPTER SUMMARY

Dental plaque is a microbial biofilm with a high species diversity found on the tooth surface, embedded in polymers of salivary and bacterial origin. The development of dental plaque is an example of autogenic succession whereby microbial factors influence the pattern of the development of the microflora. The formation of dental plaque can be divided arbitrarily into a number of distinct stages. These include the adsorption of host and bacterial molecules to form the acquired pellicle, passive transport of bacteria to the pellicle-coated tooth surface, a reversible phase involving van der Waals attractive forces and electrostatic repulsion, an irreversible phase involving specific intermolecular interactions between bacterial adhesins and host receptors, coadhesion of bacteria to already attached organisms, matrix synthesis, and cell division leading to confluent growth and biofilm formation. Some organisms in plaque produce signalling molecules enabling cells to communicate with one another and coordinate their activity. The properties of bacteria in a biofilm are different to those of planktonically-grown cells. Gene expression can be altered on a surface, while cells in biofilms are more tolerant of antimicrobial agents.

The pioneer species that form the plaque biofilm include members of the mitis-group of streptococci, haemophili, and *Neisseria* species; many of the streptococci produce an IgA protease. The composition of the climax community of plaque shows variations at different sites on the tooth surface due to differences in their biological properties. The microbial community of fissures is less diverse than that of approximal sites and the gingival crevice. Obligate anaerobic bacteria form a significant part of the microflora from these latter two sites, so special precautions are necessary when sampling and processing plaque from these areas in order to maintain the viability of the resident microorganisms.

The balance of the microflora at a site remains reasonably stable unless severely perturbed by an environmental stress. Such a stable microflora is also able to prevent exogenous species from colonizing. This stability (termed microbial homeostasis) is due, in part, to a dynamic balance of microbial interactions, including synergism and antagonism. Synergistic interactions include coadhesion, the development of food-chains, and metabolic cooperation when degrading complex host and bacterial polymers. Antagonism can be due to the production of bacteriocins, hydrogen peroxide, organic acids and a low pH. The spatial heterogeneity of a biofilm such as plaque can lead to the coexistence of species that would be incompatible with one another in a homogeneous environment. Dental plaque functions as a true microbial community; the interactions of the component species results in a metabolic efficiency and diversity that is greater than the sum of its constituent species. Dental plaque must never be regarded as a constant, static ecosystem: a consideration of the points raised throughout this chapter serve to emphasize its dynamic nature.

FURTHER READING

Allison DG, Gilbert P, Lappin-Scott HM, Wilson M (eds) 2000 Community structure and co-operation in biofilms. Society for General Microbiology Symposium 59. Cambridge University Press, Cambridge.

Carlsson J 2000. Growth and nutrition as ecological factors. In: Kuramitsu HK, Ellen RP (eds) Oral bacterial ecology. The molecular basis. Horizon Scientific Press, Wymondham, p 67-130.

Gilbert P, Maira-Litran T, McBain AJ, Rickard AH, Whyte FW 2002 The physiology and collective recalcitrance of microbial biofilm communities. Adv Microb Physiol 46:203-255.

Hall-Stoodley L, Costerton JW, Stoodley P 2004 Bacterial biofilms: from the natural environment to infectious diseases. Nat Rev Microbiol 2:95-108.

Hannig M 2002 The protective nature of the salivary pellicle. Int Dent J 52: 417-423.

Jenkinson HF, Lamont RJ 2005 Oral microbial communities in sickness and in health. Trends Microbiol 13:589-595.

Kolenbrander PE, Andersen RN, Blehert DS et al 2002 Communication among human oral bacteria. Microbiol Molec Biol Revs 66: 486-505.

Kolenbrander PE, Palmer RJ, Rickard AH et al 2006 Bacterial interactions and successions during plaque development. Periodontology 2000 42:47-79.

Kroes I, Lepp PW, Relman DA 1999 Bacterial diversity within the human subgingival crevice. Proc Nat Acad Sci USA 96:14547-14552.

Larsen T 2002 Susceptibility of *Porphyromonas gingivalis* in biofilms to amoxicillin, doxycycline and metronidazole. Oral Microbiol Immunol 17:267-271.

Marsh PD, Nyvad B 2008 The oral microflora and biofilms on teeth. In: Fejerskov O, Kidd EAM (eds) Dental caries. The disease and its clinical management, 2nd Edition Blackwell Munksgaard, Oxford, p 163-187.

Newman HN, Wilson M (eds) 1999 Dental plaque revisited. Oral biofilms in health and disease. BioLine, Cardiff.

Paster BJ, Bosches SK, Galvin JL et al 2001 Bacterial diversity in human subgingival plaque. J Bacteriol 183:3770-3783.

Socransky SS, Haffajee AD 2002 Dental biofilms: difficult therapeutic targets. Periodontol 2000 28:12-55.

Suntharalingam P, Cvitkovitch DG 2005 Quorum sensing in streptococcal biofilm formation. Trends Microbiol 13:3-6.

Verran J 2005 Malodour in denture wearers: an ill-defined problem. Oral Dis 11 Suppl 1:24-28.

Wilson M, Devine D (eds) 2003 Medical implications of biofilms. Cambridge University Press, Cambridge.

Wood SR, Kirkham J, Marsh PD et al 2000 Architecture of intact natural human plaque biofilms studied by confocal laser scanning microscopy. J Dent Res 80:1436-1440.

Chapter | 6 |

Plaque-mediated diseases – dental caries and periodontal diseases

RELATIONSHIP OF PLAQUE BACTERIA TO DISEASE: GENERAL PRINCIPLES

Preventative and curative regimens for caries and periodontal diseases would be more precise if the particular microorganism(s) causing the disease could be identified. Historically, for any microbe to be considered responsible for a given condition, Koch's postulates were applied:

1. The microbe should be found in all cases of the disease with a distribution corresponding to the observed lesions.
2. The microbe should be grown on laboratory media for several subcultures.
3. A pure subculture should produce the disease in a susceptible animal.

An additional postulate has since been added:

4. A high antibody titre to the microbe should be detected during infection; this may provide protection on subsequent reinfection.

Despite extensive sampling of plaque in health and disease, together with data from infection studies using germ-free animals, no single microbe has been found which completely satisfies Koch's postulates for plaque-mediated diseases. The groups of organisms associated with caries and periodontal diseases will be described in later sections; however, these 'pathogens' can often be detected at healthy sites, albeit in lower numbers. Thus, alternative versions of Koch's postulates have been devised to explain the role of individual bacteria from plaque in caries or periodontal diseases:

1. A microbe should be present in sufficient numbers to initiate disease.
2. The microbe should generate high levels of specific antibodies.
3. The microbe should produce relevant virulence factors.
4. The microbe should cause disease in an appropriate animal model.
5. Elimination of the microbe should result in clinical improvement.

RELATIONSHIP OF PLAQUE BACTERIA TO DISEASE: CONTEMPORARY PERSPECTIVES

There have been two main schools of thought on the role of plaque bacteria in the aetiology of caries and periodontal diseases. The **'Specific Plaque Hypothesis'** proposed that only a few species out of the diverse collection of organisms comprising the resident plaque microflora, are actively involved in disease. This proposal has been valuable because it focussed efforts on controlling disease by targeting preventative measures and treatment against a limited number of organisms. On occasions, however, disease occurs in the apparent absence of these putative pathogens, while these organisms may be recovered from healthy sites. This led to the **'Non-Specific Plaque Hypothesis'** being proposed, in which disease is considered to be the outcome of the overall activity of the total plaque microflora. In this way, a heterogeneous mixture of microorganisms could play a role in disease. In some respects, the arguments about the relative merits of these hypotheses may be about semantics, since plaque-mediated diseases are essentially mixed culture (**polymicrobial**) infections, but in which only certain (perhaps specific!) species are able to predominate. The arguments then centre around the definitions of the terms specific and non-specific. If not actually specific, then the diseases certainly show evidence of specificity.

Recently, an alternative hypothesis has been proposed (the **'Ecological Plaque Hypothesis'**) that reconciles the key elements of the earlier two hypotheses. In brief, the ecological plaque hypothesis proposed that the organisms associated with disease may also be present at sound sites, but at levels too low to be clinically relevant. Disease is a result of a shift in the balance of the resident microflora due to a response to a change in local environmental conditions (Fig. 6.1). For example, repeated conditions of low pH in plaque following frequent sugar intake favours the growth of acid-producing and acid-tolerating species that cause caries, while the inflammatory response to dental plaque accumulation around the gums results in an increased flow in gingival crevicular fluid that can provide a source of different nutrients that favours the growth of the proteolytic and obligately anaerobic bacteria that predominate in periodontal disease. Importantly, therefore, prevention can be achieved not only by the direct inhibition of the causative bacteria but also by the 'removal' or 'neutralization' of the forces that drive the selection of these organisms. These theories will be discussed later in more detail.

RELATIONSHIP OF PLAQUE BACTERIA TO DISEASE: IMPLICATIONS FOR STUDY DESIGN

Two types of epidemiological survey have been designed to determine the role of plaque bacteria in

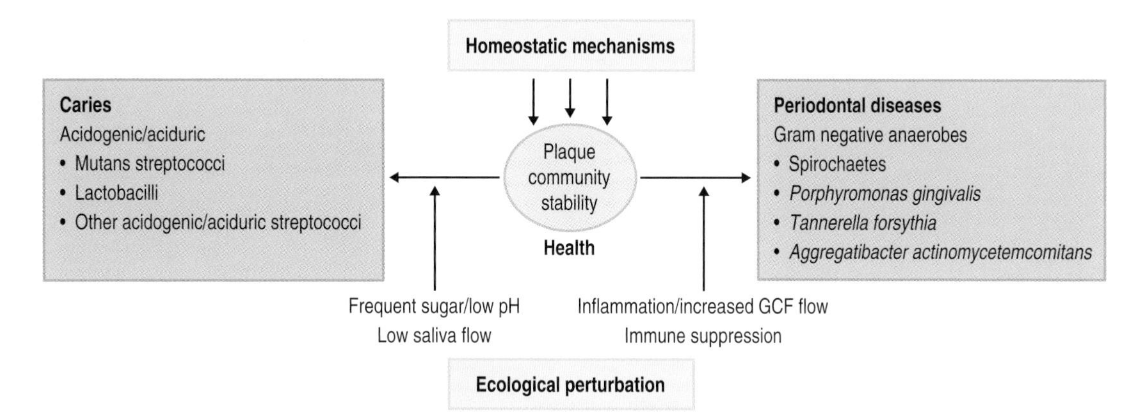

Fig. 6.1 Ecological shifts in the dental plaque microflora in health and disease.

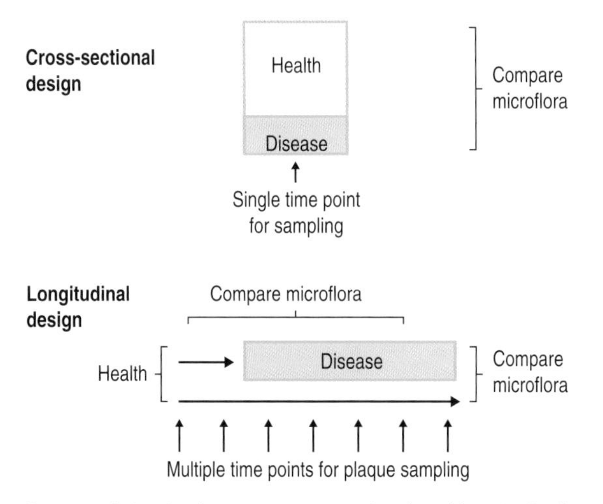

Fig. 6.2 Distinction between cross-sectional and longitudinal study designs to investigate the role of dental plaque bacteria in caries or periodontal diseases.

human disease (Fig. 6.2). In **cross-sectional surveys**, predetermined surfaces in a population are sampled at a single time point, and the plaque microflora is related to the caries or periodontal status of the site at that time. However, with this type of study, it cannot be determined for certain whether the species that are isolated at the time when disease is diagnosed caused the decay or inflammation, or arose because of it. Only 'associations' can be derived from this study design, but they have the advantage that large numbers of sites/people can be analysed, and different patient groups, age groups, tooth surfaces, diets, intervention strategies, etc. can be compared. Likewise, it cannot be determined whether the site, at the time of sampling, was progressing, arrested, or healing, and each phase may have a different microflora. In order to overcome these difficulties, **longitudinal studies** have been designed in which initially clinically healthy sites are sampled at regular intervals over a set time period (Fig. 6.2). Sites are selected on the basis of previous epidemiological surveys from which it can be predicted that a statistically relevant number of sites should suffer disease within the time span of the study. The microflora can then be compared: (a) before and after the diagnosis of disease, and (b) between those sites that became diseased and those that remained healthy throughout the study, so that true **cause-and-effect** relationships can be established. A consequence of this approach is that, for practical reasons, resources permit that only a limited number of individuals can be followed for prolonged periods.

Superimposed on the challenges of study design outlined above are those associated with the sampling and microbiological analysis of plaque (Ch. 4). The plaque microflora is diverse, and disease is not due to colonization by exogenous (non-oral) species (such events might be more easy to recognise), but to changes in the relative proportions of members of the resident microflora. Traditional culture techniques can recover, at present, only about 50% of the microflora (Ch. 3), and so the role of potentially significant organisms could be under-estimated or missed using these approaches. Furthermore, irrespective of the methods used, there are wide inter-subject variations in the composition of the plaque microflora (Ch. 5), so that when data are averaged from numerous individuals, clear associations between bacteria and disease can be obscured. Similarly, the composition of dental plaque can vary over relatively small distances. This can pose difficulties during longitudinal studies since, ideally, the same location should be resampled on each occasion. In addition, there is the possibility that regular sampling could distort the subsequent re-establishment of plaque. Despite these problems of study design and methodology, much progress has been made, and the major findings will now be discussed in the following sections.

Dental caries

In industrialized societies, caries affects the vast majority of individuals. Caries of enamel surfaces is particularly common up to the age of 20 years, whereas, in later life, root-surface caries is an increasing problem due to gingival recession exposing the vulnerable cementum to microbial colonization. Dental caries can be defined as the localized destruction of the tissues of the tooth by bacterial fermentation of dietary carbohydrates. Cavities begin as small demineralized areas below the surface of the enamel (Fig. 6.3); once enamel has been affected, caries can progress through the dentine and into the pulp (Fig. 6.4). Demineralization of the enamel is caused by acids, particularly lactic acid, produced from the microbial fermentation of dietary carbohydrates. Lesion formation involves dissolution of the enamel and the transport of the calcium and phosphate ions away into the surrounding environment. The initial stages of caries are reversible and remineralization can occur, particularly in the presence of fluoride.

EVIDENCE FOR CARIES AS AN INFECTIOUS DISEASE

In his famous Chemico-Parasitic Theory, Miller (1890) suggested that oral bacteria converted dietary carbohydrates into acid which solubilized the calcium phosphate of the enamel to produce a caries lesion. Although Clarke isolated an organism (which he called *Streptococcus mutans*) from a human caries lesion in 1924, definitive proof for the causative role of bacteria came only in the 1950s and 1960s following experiments with germ-free animals. Pioneering experiments showed that germ-free rats developed caries when infected with bacteria described then as enterococci. Evidence for the transmissibility of caries came from studies on hamsters. Caries-inactive animals had no caries even when fed a highly cariogenic (i.e. sucrose-rich) diet. Caries only developed in these animals when they were caged with or ate the faecal pellets of a group of caries-active hamsters. Further proof came when streptococci, isolated from caries

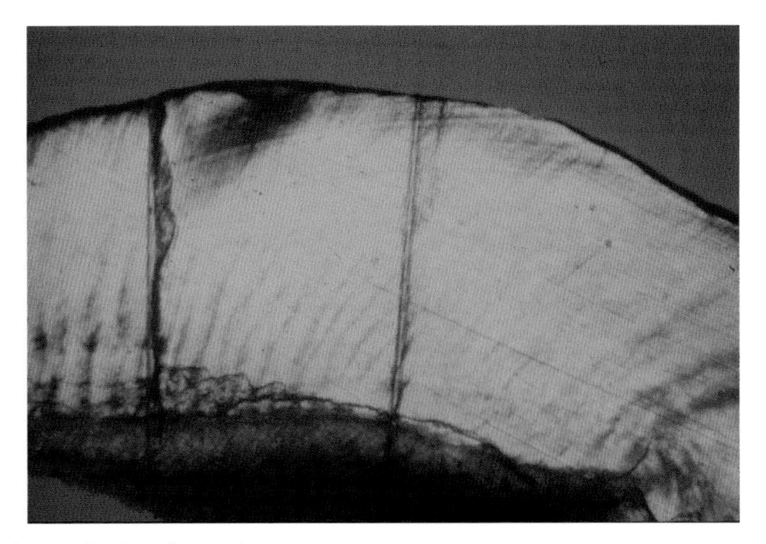

Fig. 6.3 Sub-surface demineralization of enamel.

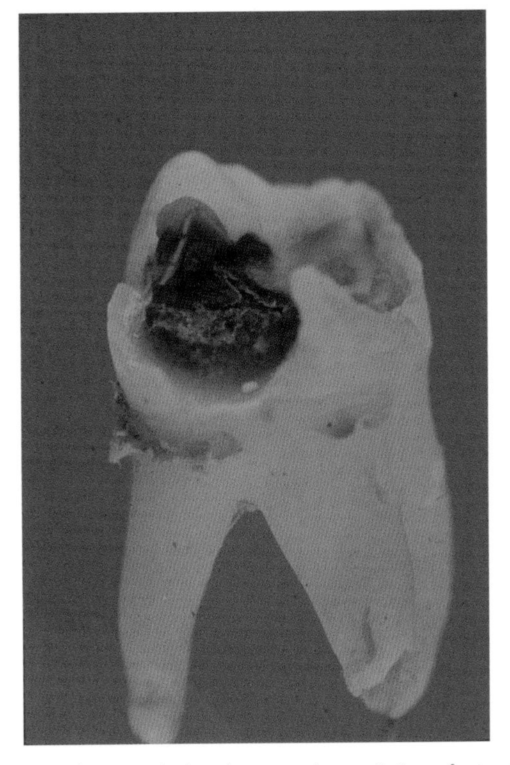

Fig. 6.4 Photograph showing extensive cavitation of a tooth.

lesions in rodents, caused rampant decay when inoculated into the oral cavity of previously caries-inactive hamsters, while animals treated with appropriate antibiotics did not develop caries. The importance of diet became apparent when the colonization and production of caries by most streptococcal populations occurred only in the presence of sucrose.

Mutans streptococci can cause caries of smooth surfaces, as well as in pits and fissures, in hamsters, gerbils, rats and monkeys fed on cariogenic diets, and these are the most cariogenic group of bacteria found. Other bacteria, including members of the mitis-, anginosus-, and salivarius groups of streptococci, *Enterococcus faecalis, Actinomyces naeslundii, A. viscosus* and lactobacilli, can also produce caries under conducive conditions in some animals, although the lesions are usually restricted to fissures. The ability of mutans streptococci to cause dental caries has also been confirmed during vaccination studies. Immunization of rodents or primates fed a cariogenic (high sugar) diet with whole cells or specific antigens of *S. mutans* and *S. sobrinus* led to a reduction in the number of these organisms in plaque and a decrease in the number of caries lesions when compared with control animals. Subsequent experiments using defined mutants helped to confirm the importance of traits such as the production of intracellular and extracellular polysaccharides from sucrose to the cariogenic potential of mutans streptococci (see later; Table 6.5).

AETIOLOGY OF HUMAN ENAMEL CARIES

Unlike the studies of animals, any relationship between particular oral bacteria and caries in humans must be derived by indirect means in epidemiological surveys (see above). Patients on long-term, broad-spectrum antibiotic therapy frequently exhibit a reduced caries experience, while epidemiological surveys of different human populations have found a strong (but not exclusive) association between mutans streptococci and caries.

Natural history of dental caries

Cavitation is the final stage of enamel caries (Fig. 6.4); it is preceded by a clinically-detectable small lesion, known as a 'white spot', and before that by subsurface demineralization, which can only be detected by histological techniques (Fig. 6.3). Not all white-spot lesions progress to cavitation; in some studies only about half of these early lesions penetrated the dentine after 3-4 years. White spot lesions do not just arrest, but can even remineralize, a process that is enhanced by fluoride. Enamel caries often occurs in teeth shortly after eruption (hence, its historical association with young people), and some teeth and surfaces are more vulnerable than others. The prevalence of caries is highest on the occlusal surfaces of first and second molars, and lowest on the lingual surfaces of mandibular teeth. The risk to approximal surfaces is intermediate to those described above. With the reduction in the incidence of dental caries in the young, it is predicted that caries risk for some surfaces will now extend over the life-time of an individual. If confirmed, this trend would have important implications for caries prevention strategies. Some individuals are more caries prone than others, and this may be related to their diet (e.g. frequency of sugar intake), lack of optimum saliva flow (e.g. flow is severely reduced in xerostomia patients), and low exposure to fluoride.

Microbiology of enamel caries

Buccal and lingual **smooth surfaces** are easy to clean and generally suffer from decay only rarely.

However, they are easy to study for experimental purposes, both in terms of clinical diagnosis and in plaque sampling. Higher proportions (10–100 fold) of mutans streptococci have been found on white-spot lesions on smooth surfaces compared with adjacent sound enamel. As stated earlier, such an association does not prove a causal relationship and the actual proportions of mutans streptococci are often low. Suspensions of plaque from white-spot lesions produce a lower pH minimum and a faster rate of pH-fall than plaque from sound enamel.

Fissures on occlusal surfaces (Figs 2.2 and 5.10) are the most caries-prone sites. Caries can develop rapidly on these surfaces, and it is at these sites that the strongest association between mutans streptococci and dental decay has been found. In one cross-sectional study, 71% of carious fissures had viable counts of mutans streptococci that were >10% of the total cultivable plaque microflora, whereas 70% of the fissures that were caries free at the time of sampling had no detectable mutans streptococci. An inverse relationship between mutans streptococci and *S. sanguinis* is frequently observed. In a longitudinal study of North American children, the proportions of mutans streptococci, *S. sanguinis* and lactobacilli were monitored before and at the time of caries development in occlusal fissures. The subjects were divided into several groups according to their previous caries experience and to their caries activity during the study. The proportions of mutans streptococci increased significantly at the time of diagnosis of most lesions. However, mutans streptococci were only a minor component of the plaque from five fissures which became carious. Counts of lactobacilli were significantly higher at these sites and, it was concluded, that these were probably responsible for lesion formation. A subsequent longitudinal study confirmed these findings, and demonstrated an even stronger relationship between mutans streptococci and caries initiation (Table 6.1), whereas lactobacilli, when present, were strongly associated with sites requiring restoration. Thus, there was a strong correlation between mutans streptococci and fissure decay, although lesions could also develop at some sites in the apparent absence of this group of bacteria. There were also surfaces where mutans streptococci appeared to persist in moderately high numbers without any evidence of detectable caries.

A major prospective study of young Swiss children (7–8 years) specifically examined the question as to whether colonization by mutans streptococci was a risk factor for caries in fissures (and on smooth surfaces). Both fissures and smooth surfaces of first permanent premolars that suffered demineralization without cavitation were heavily colonized with mutans streptococci (10^4-10^5 colony forming units [CFU]/ml of sample) around 12–18 months prior to the clinical diagnosis of the lesion. The proportions of mutans streptococci appeared to increase markedly 6-9 months prior to lesion detection to reach 11–18% and 10–12% of the total streptococcal microflora of fissures and smooth surfaces, respectively. This study demonstrated that colonization and an increase in proportions of mutans streptococci preceded lesion formation by about six months. As with other studies of caries, however, several sites had high counts of mutans streptococci (>20% of the total streptococcal count) but no

Table 6.1 Mean proportions of mutans streptococci (MS) and lactobacilli (L) on teeth in schoolchildren (7–8 years old) who remained caries free or who developed a caries lesion during a longitudinal study

Time (months) before caries diagnosis	Mean bacterial proportions in fissure plaque					
	Caries sites		Filled sites		Caries free sites	
	MS	L	MS	L	MS	L
0	29	8	–	–	9	2
6	25	8	15	3	17	1
12	16	1	20	2	9	3
18	9	<1	16	1	11	1

Data taken from: Loesche WJ et al, Infect Immun 1984 46: 765-772.

evidence of caries. Larger lesions (with cavitation) were found only at a relatively few sites. In five out of six carious fissures, the median count of mutans streptococci rose from 10^2 to $>10^4$ CFU/ml sample around 12 months prior to lesion detection; this represented a final mean proportion of 18% of the total streptococcal count. The remaining carious fissure had no detectable mutans streptococci at any time during the study, again illustrating that species other than mutans streptococci can play a role in lesion formation on occasions. An additional feature of the design of this study was that some sites were diagnosed with a lesion which subsequently remineralized. Some of these sites had levels of mutans streptococci greater than 20% of the streptococcal microflora, and yet the lesion remineralized within 12 months. During this period, the levels of mutans streptococci fell markedly between 6 and 9 months prior to the diagnosis of the reversal. Overall, however, this study provided convincing data on the important role of mutans streptococci in the initiation of dental caries.

A challenge for studies of **approximal** surfaces lies with the difficulty in accurately diagnosing early lesions, and with the fact that plaque samples are inevitably removed from the whole interproximal area, including that overlying sound enamel as well as carious enamel. The microflora can vary markedly at different sites around the contact area between teeth, irrespective of whether a lesion is developing, so that specific associations can sometimes be obscured. Early cross-sectional studies found a positive correlation between elevated levels of mutans streptococci and lesion development. Many of these studies, however, were limited in scope, and only monitored a few types of microorganism, and sometimes only mutans streptococci. In order to combat this, a limited number of longitudinal studies have been performed. A less clear cut association was found in a survey of English schoolchildren, aged 11–15 years. Mutans streptococci could be found in high numbers prior to demineralization at a number of sites, but lesions also appeared to develop on occasions in the apparent absence of this group of bacteria. Mutans streptococci were also present at other sites in equally high numbers for the duration of the study without any diagnosis of caries. There was evidence that the isolation frequency and proportions of mutans streptococci increased after, rather than before, the first radiographic detection of some lesions, especially in those that progressed deeper into the enamel, suggesting that the composition of the microflora might shift as the lesion progresses through the tooth (microbial succession; Ch. 4).

Similar findings were found in a study of Dutch army recruits, aged 18–20 years. Mutans streptococci were isolated from 40% and 86% of sites from caries-free and caries-active recruits, respectively. Marked differences in the distribution of individual species were found; *S. mutans* (serotype *c*) strains were isolated from both groups whereas *S. sobrinus* (serotype *d*) was recovered almost exclusively from caries-active recruits (Table 6.2). The prevalence of the combined species of mutans streptococci also showed a direct but not unique correlation with the progression of a lesion into the dentine. Again, relatively high proportions of mutans streptococci persisted at some tooth surfaces without caries progression while on occasions caries could develop in their apparent absence.

A major limitation of traditional culture approaches is that around 50% of the oral microflora cannot as yet be grown in the laboratory, and so molecular methods have been developed to characterize the complex communities in the mouth (Chs 3 and 4). A more diverse microflora

Table 6.2 Prevalence of mutans streptococci at approximal tooth surfaces with and without caries progression

	Total number of tooth surfaces	The number of sites with mutans streptococci at proportions of*:		
		0%	0–5%	>5%
Caries progression	14	1†	3	10
No caries progression	41	21	17	3

*The number of sites in which mutans streptococci were detected at a particular percentage of the total cultivable microflora.
†Number of tooth surfaces.

has been reported when these methods have been applied to sites with caries, and novel taxa have been described. One study confirmed the relationship of *S. sanguinis* with sound enamel and *S. mutans* and lactobacilli with caries lesions, but additionally found *Actinomyces gerencseriae* and other *Actinomyces* spp. to be implicated in caries initiation and *Bifidobacterium* spp. with advanced lesions. Another study used molecular approaches to investigate the microbial diversity of plaque from teeth with lesions at different stages of disease. They found 10% of subjects with rampant caries in the secondary dentition did not have detectable levels of *S. mutans*. In lesions where mutans streptococci could not be detected, there were high levels of lactobacilli, low pH tolerating non-mutans streptococci and *Bifidobacterium* spp.. High levels of *Actinomyces* species and non-mutans streptococci were found in early (white spot) lesions, while mutans streptococci and lactobacilli, together with *Propionibacterium* and *Bifidobacterium* spp. dominated advanced (deep dentine) lesions. The data supported the ecological plaque hypothesis in that shifts in the bacterial composition of plaque were seen between healthy sites and those with lesions of increasing severity, and the organisms associated with caries were all acid producing species.

Rampant caries can occur in particular subgroups of people who are especially prone to decay, such as xerostomic patients (who have a markedly reduced salivary flow rate due to radiation treatment for head and neck cancer), those with Sjögren's syndrome, or as a side-effect of medication. These patients also generally consume soft diets, with a high sucrose content, and may often suck 'candies' to relieve their symptoms. Longitudinal studies of patients undergoing radiation treatment showed large increases in the numbers and proportions of mutans streptococci and lactobacilli in plaque and saliva. Other species associated with sound enamel, such as *S. sanguinis*, *Neisseria* spp. and Gram negative anaerobes, decreased during this period.

'Nursing-bottle' caries is the extensive and rapid decay of the maxillary anterior teeth associated with the prolonged and frequent feeding of young infants with bottles or pacifiers containing formulas with a high concentration of fermentable carbohydrate. Plaque bacteria receive an almost continuous provision of substrates from which they can make acid. Such prolonged conditions of low pH are conducive, and indeed selective, for mutans streptococci and lactobacilli, and proportions of mutans streptococci in plaque can reach >50% of the microflora. Other studies have reported elevated levels of *S. mutans*, *Actinomyces israelii*, lactobacilli, *Veillonella* spp. (presumably reflecting high concentrations of lactate; see Ch. 5), and *C. albicans* (which also tolerates acidic conditions) in nursing caries lesions.

Caries can re-occur beneath and around previous restorations (**recurrent or secondary caries**), and treatment of this accounts for a large proportion of the restorative needs of the adult population. Secondary dentinal involvement is of particular concern because it can be difficult to diagnose non-invasively, and it poses the threat of pulpal inflammation and infection (see later). Mutans streptococci and lactobacilli have been isolated in high numbers from recurrent caries while a more diverse microflora has been isolated when dentine is affected (see later).

Numerous studies have shown mutans streptococci to be important cariogenic bacteria; they generally appear in the mouth once teeth have erupted, although mutans streptococci have been detected in pre-dentate infants. The mother is the main source of these bacteria; additional factors that correlate with *S. mutans* colonization are sweetened drinks taken by infants to bed, frequent exposure to sugar, snacking, and sharing of foods with adults, whereas non-colonization is associated with toothbrushing and multiple courses of antibiotics. This information can play an important part in developing appropriate caries control strategies.

SUMMARY

Enamel caries is associated with a shift in the balance of the microflora of dental plaque. The isolation frequency and proportions of acid-producing and acid-tolerating species, especially mutans streptococci and lactobacilli, are higher at sites with caries. No single species is uniquely associated with dental caries, so that caries can occur on occasions in the apparent absence of mutans streptococci, while these organisms can sometimes persist at sites without evidence of demineralization.

Microbiology of root surface caries

The reduction in enamel caries in industrialized societies has resulted in large proportions of the public retaining their teeth into later life. Gingival recession occurs in old age exposing the susceptible cementum surface of the root to microbial colonization; root surfaces can also become exposed due to mechanical injury or to periodontal surgery (e.g. following scaling and root planing). These cementum surfaces are even more vulnerable than enamel to demineralization by plaque acids. The prevalence of root surface caries increases with age; approximately 60% of individuals aged 60 years or older now have root caries or fillings.

Experimental animal studies

Direct evidence for the role of oral microorganisms in root-surface caries came from early studies with animals in which filamentous bacteria were observed invading the root surfaces of hamsters and causing caries. Human isolates of *Actinomyces naeslundii* were then shown to cause root surface caries in germ-free rats and hamsters, as were pure cultures of mutans streptococci and strains belonging to the mitis- and anginosus-groups of streptococci.

Human studies

Early studies were designed around the findings from the first animal experiments, and focused on the role of Gram positive filamentous bacteria, especially *Actinomyces* spp., in root surface caries. Among the organisms isolated from lesions were *Rothia dentocariosa, Actinomyces naeslundii* and *A. odontolyticus*; in some studies, mutans streptococci were also associated with root surface caries.

Subsequent studies have tended to confirm a stronger association between mutans streptococci and lactobacilli with root surface caries. In a major longitudinal survey in Canada, although no direct correlation between specific bacteria and root caries was found, the presence of mutans streptococci and lactobacilli on root surfaces was predictive for the subsequent development of a lesion. Other studies have attempted to subdivide the lesions into initial (or 'soft') and advanced (or 'hard'). Several groups reported higher proportions (often around 30% of the total cultivable microflora) of mutans streptococci at the initial lesion (Table 6.3), sometimes in association with lactobacilli. Lactobacilli have occasionally been found at arrested (hard, black-coloured) lesions. Following improvements to the classification of *Actinomyces* spp., the predominant species isolated from infected dentine of active root caries lesions are *A. israelii* > *A. gerencseriae* > *A. naeslundii* > *A. odontolyticus* > *A. georgiae*.

In situ devices have been worn by volunteers to study the microflora of actively-progressing root surface caries lesions. In one study, elderly subjects (mean age: 70 years) carried root surface specimens from human molars on their partial dentures for 3 months. After this period, the predominant plaque microflora was determined and the integrity of the experimental root surface was measured by highly sensitive techniques (quantitative microradiography). Although the composition of the microflora showed distinct individual differences, plaque samples from surfaces showing the highest loss of mineral were dominated either by (a) *A. naeslundii*, or (b) a combination of mutans streptococci and lactobacilli. Plaque from root surfaces with less pronounced mineral loss harboured a more complex microflora including *Actinomyces* spp., mutans streptococci, *S. mitis* biovar 1, *Veillonella* spp., Gram negative rods, and low numbers of lactobacilli.

Table 6.3 Mean percentage viable counts (and percentage isolation frequencies in parentheses) of some plaque bacteria from root surfaces, with and without caries

Bacterium	**Sound root surface**	**Root surface caries**	
		Initial (soft)	**Advanced (hard)**
Mutans streptococci	2 (84)	29 (92)	8 (92)
Streptococcus sanguinis	19 (96)	11 (97)	22 (85)
Actinomyces naeslundii	12 (90)	11 (85)	13 (96)

The recent application of more sophisticated approaches to sampling plaque has given new insights into the relationship between the composition of the microflora and lesion development. One study used a specially designed device to lift plaque from discrete areas directly into reduced transport fluid to preserve the viability of obligately anaerobic bacteria. The caries status of these precise sampling sites was then assessed by a variety of sensitive techniques including contact microradiography, and light and electron microscopy. In this way, the surface directly beneath the plaque that had been sampled could be reliably classified as being a sound, active or arrested carious root lesions. Regardless of the degree of mineralization, the microflora from these root surfaces was more diverse than had previously been reported, and resembled that associated with gingivitis (see later). On all surfaces, *Actinomyces* were the predominant group of bacteria, especially *A. naeslundii, A. odontolyticus* and *A. gerencseriae*. Arrested lesions had significantly lower numbers of bacteria than either sound surfaces or active lesions. Gram negative species formed around 50% of the microflora on sound and active carious surfaces, with *Prevotella* spp. (particularly *P. nigrescens*) being highly prevalent. Other Gram negative bacteria, including *Capnocytophaga* spp., *Campylobacter* spp. and *Leptotrichia buccalis*, were preferentially isolated from plaque overlying active lesions. This may be because a number of these species are sufficiently saccharolytic to demineralize cementum and dentine, while others are proteolytic, and could hydrolyze the dentine collagen matrix. These data suggest that (a) caries initiation on root surfaces can have a polymicrobial aetiology, and (b) bacterial succession occurs during the development of root surface lesions.

Molecular and culture approaches have been used to characterize the microbial community of carious dentine. The predominant bacteria recovered by anaerobic cultivation included a novel *Propionibacterium* spp., *Olsenella profusa* and *Lactobacillus rhamnosus*. Even more novel taxa were detected when DNA was extracted directly from the lesions, amplified by PCR, and bacterial identification was based on 16S rRNA gene sequence analysis (Chs 3 and 4). Forty four taxa were detected by the molecular approach alone, of which 31 had never been described previously (although they were generally close relatives of cultivable species). The predominant taxa identified by the molecular methods included *S. mutans*, lactobacilli and *Rothia dentocariosa*.

SUMMARY

Root surface caries is common in older age groups when the cementum becomes exposed and susceptible to microbial colonization. While mutans streptococci and lactobacilli are common at sites with root surface caries, the microflora can be complex from deeper lesions. Infected dentine has high proportions of *Actinomyces* spp., as well as a diverse range of proteolytic and obligately anaerobic species that may be involved in the degradation of dentine.

Bacterial invasion of dentine and root canals

Dentine can be invaded:

(a) by direct progression of an enamel caries lesion;

(b) from caries of the root surface (see above);

(c) from a periodontal pocket via lateral or accessory canals (Fig. 6.5),

(d) as a result of fracture or trauma during operative procedures, or

(e) as a result of secondary or recurrent caries (see above).

Scaling and root planing can predispose some root surfaces to bacterial invasion by exposing dentine tubules; in addition, bacteria may lodge in injured pulp following a transient bacteraemia (anachoresis) (Fig. 6.5).

The microbial community from the advancing front of a dentinal lesion is diverse and contains many facultatively- and obligately-anaerobic Gram positive bacteria belonging to the genera *Actinomyces, Bifidobacterium, Eubacterium, Lactobacillus, Parvimonas* (formerly *Peptostreptococcus*), *Propionibacterium* and *Rothia*. Streptococci are recovered less frequently, but when mutans streptococci have been isolated they can be one of the predominant members of the community. Gram negative bacteria such as *Prevotella, Porphyromonas*, and *Fusobacterium* spp. can also be isolated but they are generally present only in low numbers.

The microflora found in the dentine and pulp of periodontally-diseased human teeth is also diverse and may be derived predominantly from the subgingival area. Numerous Gram positive and Gram negative species have been identified; some are more prevalent in the dentine (e.g. *A. odontolyticus, Bifidobacterium* spp.), some predominate in the pulp (e.g. black-pigmented anaerobes),

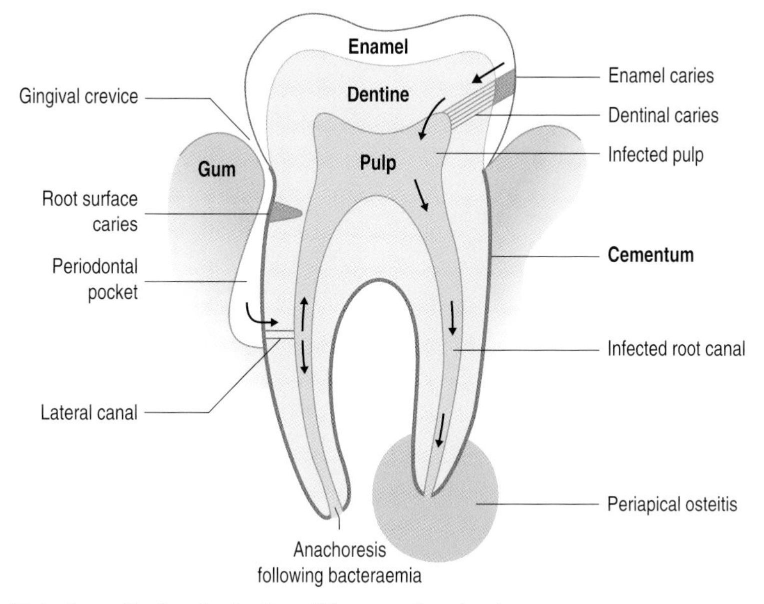

Fig. 6.5 Progression of infections affecting the tooth and its supporting structures.

while others are found equally at both sites (e.g. *A. naeslundii, Veillonella* spp., *F. nucleatum*). Dentine collagen is denatured and modified during the caries process, and becomes more susceptible to breakdown by non-specific proteases, and this explains the presence of both acidogenic and proteolytic bacteria.

Bacteria in the dentine tubules obtain their nutrients from dentinal fluid, which contains glycoproteins such as IgG, albumin and fibrinogen. When streptococci come into contact with exposed type I collagen there is up-regulation of specific genes that enhances cell adhesion and growth. For example, *S. gordonii* increases expression of the adhesin, antigen I/II, and long chains of streptococci develop along collagen fibrils.

Once bacteria are in the pulp, inflammation can occur which may result eventually in necrosis of the root canal. A further consequence is that microorganisms can invade and destroy tissue surrounding the apex of the root, producing a spreading or localized infection (Fig. 6.5). Diverse mixed culture of bacteria are cultured, including black-pigmented anaerobes (*Prevotella intermedia, Prevotella melaninogenica, Porphyromonas endodontalis, P. gingivalis*), and *Prevotella dentalis, Campylobacter sputorum, Eubacterium* spp. and *Parvimonas* (formerly *Peptostreptococcus*) spp.. Some of these species (*P. endodontalis, P. dentalis*) are found almost exclusively in infected root canals and abscesses of endodontal origin. Another study of necrotic pulps found *Propionibacterium, Eubacterium* and *Fusobacterium* spp. to be the predominant bacteria, with *Bifidobacterium, Lactobacillus, Actinomyces* and *Veillonella* spp. as minor components. Certain bacterial combinations are associated with endodontic clinical symptoms, e.g. *Parvimonas micra* (formerly *Peptostreptococcus micros*), *Porphyromonas* and *Fusobacterium* are linked with pain.

The treatment of infections of the root canal (endodontics; Ch. 7) involves the removal of infected and dead tissue both mechanically and by irrigation, sometimes accompanied by treatment with antimicrobial agents to reduce the microbial community to a level where the cavity can be restored effectively.

MICROBIOLOGICAL TESTS TO PREDICT CARIES ACTIVITY

Microbiological tests have been used in an attempt to predict sites or individuals at risk of caries. These usually involve the estimation of the numbers of mutans streptococci in either plaque or saliva samples by plate counts in the laboratory, or by semi-quantitative, commercially-available, chair-side tests. There is now the promise of rapid molecular methods to detect cariogenic bacteria. Although a strong positive correlation has been found between levels of mutans streptococci and caries experience on a group or population level, the association is less clear cut for individuals. This is not surprising given that caries is a multi-factorial disease (Fig. 1.1), and clinical studies indicate that the relationship between mutans streptococci and caries is not absolute.

The best predictor of future caries is the current caries status of the individual. In such cases, patients with a high incidence of caries can be assumed to have not only the relevant microflora but also the appropriate risk factors (cariogenic diet, impaired saliva flow, etc.) conducive to lesion formation. In such patients, microbiological tests based on counts of mutans streptococci can give a high positive predictive value, while in other subjects the positive prediction is only around 40–50%. Generally, the absence of mutans streptococci is a stronger indicator of low caries risk than is the presence of these bacteria for high risk.

The most valuable use of salivary microbiological tests can be in young children (e.g. under the age of four years), because this could identify infants at risk of subsequent disease. Such tests can also be useful in monitoring high-risk patients, such as those wearing orthodontic bands, and also xerostomic patients. The tests can also be used in a secondary role to monitor patient compliance in terms of dietary control, or in motivating patients by giving them tangible evidence of events in their own mouth.

PATHOGENIC DETERMINANTS OF CARIOGENIC BACTERIA

Determinants of cariogenicity are often linked to sugar metabolism (Table 6.4). Mutants defective in various aspects of sucrose metabolism have been compared in terms of their relative cariogenicity in animal models (Table 6.5). Strains of *S. mutans* defective in insoluble glucan synthesis were unable to colonize teeth as effectively as the parent strains, and caused fewer smooth surface caries lesions in an animal (rat) model. The synthesis of intracellular storage compounds enables *S. mutans* to continue making acid even in the absence of dietary carbohydrates. Mutants defective in intracellular polysaccharide (IPS) synthesis produced fewer caries lesions than parent strains when inoculated in pure cultures in gnotobiotic rodents. Mutants of *S. mutans* defective in either lactic dehydrogenase or fructosyltransferase (Ch. 4) activity are also markedly less cariogenic in rat caries models while, in contrast, fructanase was shown not to be essential for virulence.

Distinctive characteristics of cariogenic bacteria are:

- the ability to rapidly transport sugars when in competition with other plaque bacteria,
- the rapid conversion of such sugars to acid, and
- the ability to maintain these activities and grow even under extreme environmental conditions, such as at a low pH.

Few oral bacteria are able to tolerate acidic conditions for prolonged periods, but most strains of mutans streptococci and lactobacilli are not only able to remain

Table 6.4 Characteristics of mutans streptococci that contribute to their cariogenicity

Property	Comment
Sugar transport	High and low affinity transport systems operating over a wide range of conditions to ensure substrate uptake, even under extreme environments, e.g. low pH.
Acid production	An efficient glycolytic pathway rapidly producing low terminal pH values in plaque.
Aciduricity	Cells have specific biochemical attributes enabling them to survive, metabolize and grow at low pH values.
Extracellular polysaccharide (EPS) production	EPS contributes to the plaque matrix, consolidates attachment of cells, and may localize acidic fermentation products.
Intracellular polysaccharide (IPS) production	IPS utilization allows acid production to continue in the absence of dietary sugars.

Table 6.5 The use of mutants of mutans streptococci to determine traits linked to cariogenicity

Trait	Property of mutant	Effect on cariogenicity*
glucosyltransferase**	decreased colonization and plaque formation	reduced
fructosyltransferase	loss of extracellular fructan	none
fructanase	no breakdown of extracellular fructans	none
IPS production	no intracellular glycogen	reduced
antigen 1/11	decreased ability to adhere	none
enzyme II (PTS)	decreased sucrose transport	none
lactic dehydrogenase	no lactic acid production	reduced
"aciduricity"***	reduced tolerance of low pH	reduced

*If a mutation did not lead to a reduction in caries, it does not necessarily mean that the trait is not important in cariogenicity. It may reflect the fact that the particular trait is not essential for caries in an animal model; also, mutans streptococci often have more than one mechanism for a particular function, e.g. adherence.
**mutations in *gtfB* and *gtfC*, , but not in *gtfD*, led to a reduction in cariogenicity.
***this mutant was not fully characterized.

viable (survive) at a low pH, but are able to continue to metabolize and multiply, i.e. they are **acidogenic** (strongly acid producing) and **aciduric** (acid-loving). Microbial survival in acidic environments depends on the cell maintaining a favourable intracellular pH despite sharp fluctuations in external pH (Ch. 4), and *S. mutans* achieves this by a number of specific mechanisms (Table 4.8). Some strains of other species also display an acid tolerant phenotype, including members of the anginosus-, mitis- and salivarius-groups of streptococci, while there can be variation in acid tolerance even among strains of *S. mutans*.

The importance that the combination of acidogenicity and acidurity confers on potentially cariogenic bacteria was shown in the laboratory using mixed culture competition studies. At a constant pH 7, *S. mutans* and *L. casei* were non-competitive and were only minor components (<1%) of a microbial community, even when exposed to daily pulses of fermentable sugar (glucose). When the pH was allowed to fall after a glucose pulse, *S. mutans* and *L. casei* gradually increased in proportions until they eventually dominated (>50%) the mixed culture at the expense of acid sensitive species associated with enamel health (e.g. *S. gordonii, N. subflava*). As the proportions of the acidogenic/aciduric populations rose, so the rate and extent of the pH-fall increased. The final numbers of *S. mutans* and *L. casei* was shown to be inversely proportional to the environmental pH – i.e. their counts became higher as the culture pH became lower.

RE-EVALUATION OF THE MICROBIAL AETIOLOGY OF DENTAL CARIES

A consistent feature of most of the clinical studies already described has been the occasional but consistent finding of carious sites from which no mutans streptococci can be isolated. This suggests that bacteria other than mutans streptococci can make a contribution to demineralization. Bacteria isolated from such plaque samples have been compared in their ability to lower the pH of laboratory media. While strains of *S. mutans* produced a final pH in the region of 3.95–4.10, a range of other streptococci achieved terminal values of pH 4.05–4.50. These strains are often numerically dominant, and belong to the mitis-group (especially *S. mitis, S. oralis* and *S. gordonii*), salivarius-group and anginosus-group of streptococci. Similarly, when the rates of acid production were compared, mutans streptococci were generally faster at low environmental pH values, but other streptococci had greater rates at pH 7.0 and pH 6.0. Such findings reinforce the view that although mutans streptococci are clearly key causative organisms in enamel caries, other bacteria can contribute to, and modulate, the strength of the cariogenic challenge at a site. The converse situation is also not uncommon, where mutans streptococci are found in high numbers but in the apparent absence of any demineralization of the underlying enamel. This may be due to the presence of lactate-consuming species (e.g. *Veillonella*), or to the production of alkali at low pH (e.g. ammonia production by urease or arginine deiminase activities of bacteria such as *S. salivarius* and *S. sanguinis*, respectively).

These findings allow a model to be constructed to explain the changes in the ecology of dental plaque that lead to the development of a caries lesion. Cariogenic bacteria may be found naturally in dental plaque, but at neutral pH, these organisms are weakly competitive and are present only as a small proportion of the total plaque community. In this situation, with a conventional diet, the levels of such potentially cariogenic bacteria are clinically insignificant, and the processes of de- and remineralization are in equilibrium. If the frequency of fermentable carbohydrate intake increases, then plaque spends more time below the critical pH for enamel demineralization (approximately pH 5.5; Fig. 2.3). The effect of this on the microbial ecology of plaque is two-fold. Conditions of low pH favour the proliferation of mutans streptococci and lactobacilli, and tip the balance towards demineralization. Greater numbers of mutans streptococci and lactobacilli in plaque result in more acid being produced at even faster rates, thereby enhancing demineralization still further. Other bacteria could also make acid under similar conditions, albeit at a slower rate, but would contribute to the initial stages of demineralization, or could cause lesions in the absence of other (more overt) cariogenic species in a susceptible host. If aciduric species were not present initially, then the repeated conditions of low pH coupled with the inhibition of competing organisms might increase the likelihood of colonization by mutans streptococci or lactobacilli. This sequence of events would account for the lack of total specificity in the microbial aetiology of caries and explain the pattern of bacterial succession observed in many clinical studies. This model forms the basis of the **'ecological plaque hypothesis'** (Fig. 6.6). In this hypothesis, caries is a consequence of changes in the natural balance of the resident plaque microflora brought about by an alteration in local environmental conditions (e.g. repeated conditions of high sugar and low plaque pH). The hypothesis also acknowledges the dynamic relationship that exists between the microflora and the host, so that the impact of alterations in key host factors (such as saliva flow) on plaque composition is taken into account. This is of great significance for caries prevention since implicit in the hypothesis is the concept that disease can be controlled not only by targeting directly the putative pathogens (e.g. by inhibition of mutans streptococci by antimicrobial agents) but also by interfering with the factors that are driving the deleterious shifts in the balance of the microflora (e.g. lowering the acid challenge by reducing the frequency of sugar intake, or by promoting the use of snacks containing sugar substitutes). These, and other caries preventive strategies, will be discussed in a later section.

The ecological plaque hypothesis also defines aetiological agents in a different way. Rather than just focussing on the role of particular named

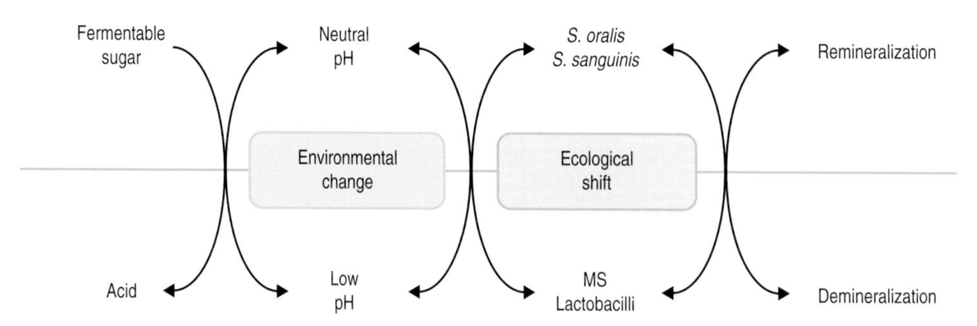

Fig. 6.6 A schematic representation of the ecological plaque hypothesis in relation to the aetiology of dental caries. Frequent metabolism of fermentable sugars in dental plaque produces regular and prolonged conditions of low pH; this environmental change in plaque favours the growth of acid-tolerating bacteria (such as mutans streptococci, MS, and lactobacilli) at the expense of species associated with sound enamel. Such a change in the microflora predisposes a surface to demineralization. Disease could be prevented by not only targeting the putative pathogens, but also by interfering with the factors driving their selection.

organisms in disease, the ecological plaque hypothesis attempts to **define the involvement of microbes on the basis of their properties or functions**. Thus, cariogenic bacteria are acidogenic and aciduric; such properties will not be unique to a single species in the same way that toxin production can be specific to a medical pathogen such as *Clostridium tetani* (the aetiological agent of tetanus), and could vary among strains of a particular species. Indeed, there will be a spectrum of pathogenic potential among many species of plaque bacteria and even among strains within a species. In general, however, the organisms that are optimally equipped biochemically to be acidogenic and aciduric belong to the mutans streptococci (these strains also produce glucans that contribute to the plaque matrix, and they store fermentable intracellular polysaccharides (IPS) produced from sucrose) and lactobacilli, and these organisms are consistently isolated in elevated numbers from caries lesions, but other strains of bacteria will contribute to a degree that is proportional to their acidogenic/aciduric phenotype.

FURTHER READING – DENTAL CARIES

Aas JA, Griffen AL, Dardis SR et al 2008 Bacteria of dental caries in primary and permanent teeth in children and young adults. J Clin Microbiol 46:1407-1417.

Becker MR, Paster BJ, Leys EJ et al 2002 Molecular analysis of bacterial species associated with childhood caries. J Clin Microbiol 40:1001-1009.

Bowden GHW 2000 The microbial ecology of dental caries. Microb Ecol Health & Dis 12:138-148.

Brailsford SR, Shah B, Simons D et al 2001 The predominant aciduric microflora of root-caries lesions. J Dent Res 80:1828-1833.

Burne RA 1998 Oral streptococci....products of their environment. J Dent Res 77:445-452.

Gomes BP, Pinheiro ET, Gade-Neto CR et al 2004 Microbiological examination of infected dental root canals. Oral Microbiol Immunol 19:71-76.

Fejerskov O, Kidd EAM (eds) 2008 Dental caries. The disease and its management, 2nd edn. Blackwell, Oxford.

Lang NP, Hotz PR, Gusberti FA, Joss A 1987 Longitudinal clinical and microbiological study on the relationship between infection with *Streptococcus mutans* and the development of caries in humans. Oral Microbiol Immunol 2:39-47.

Loesche WJ, Eklund S, Earnest R, Burt B 1984 Longitudinal investigation of bacteriology of human fissure decay: epidemiological studies in molars shortly after eruption. Infect Immun 46:765-772.

Love RM, Jenkinson HF 2002 Invasion of dentinal tubules by oral bacteria. Crit Rev Oral Biol Med 3:171-183.

Marchant S, Brailsford SR, Twomey AC et al 2001 The predominant microflora of nursing caries lesions. Caries Res 35:397-406.

Munson MA, Banerjee A, Watson TF, Wade WG 2004 Molecular analysis of the microflora associated with dental caries. J Clin Microbiol 42:3023-3029.

Nyvad B, ten Cate JM, Robinson C (eds) 2004 Cariology in the 21st century. State of the art and future perspectives. Caries Res 38:168-329.

Schüpbach P, Osterwalder V, Guggenheim B 1995 Human root caries: microbiota in plaque covering sound, carious and arrested carious root surfaces. Caries Res 29:382-395.

Periodontal diseases

The term 'periodontal diseases' embraces a number of conditions in which the supporting tissues of the teeth are attacked. Periodontal diseases are common in developed countries, and are a leading cause of tooth loss (Ch. 1). In periodontal diseases, the junctional epithelium at the base of the gingival crevice migrates down the root of the tooth to form a periodontal pocket (Fig. 6.5). This is partly as a result of direct action by the microorganisms themselves, but mainly as a result of the indirect, but potentially damaging, side-effects of a de-regulated inflammatory response mounted by the host in response to plaque accumulation.

ECOLOGY OF THE PERIODONTAL POCKET: IMPLICATIONS FOR PLAQUE SAMPLING

As discussed in Chapters 2, 4 and 5, the ecology of the gingival crevice is different to that of other sites in the mouth; it is more anaerobic and the site is bathed in gingival crevicular fluid (GCF). In disease, the crevice becomes a pocket, and the Eh (oxidation-reduction potential; Ch. 2) falls to low levels (i.e. it is highly anaerobic), while the flow of GCF is increased by 147% in gingivitis and by up to 30 fold in periodontitis. While GCF delivers humoral and cellular defence factors to combat the microbial insult, it also provides a number of proteins and glycoproteins that serve as novel substrates for bacterial metabolism, e.g. iron and haeme-containing molecules such as transferrin and haemoglobin. Unlike dental caries, many of the bacteria associated with periodontal diseases are asaccharolytic (i.e. cannot metabolize carbohydrates for energy) but are proteolytic. A consequence of proteolysis is that the pH in the pocket during disease becomes slightly alkaline (pH 7.4–7.8) compared to near neutral values in health (ca. pH 6.9). The growth and enzyme activity of periodontal pathogens such as *Porphyromonas gingivalis* is enhanced by alkaline growth conditions. Likewise, the temperature of the periodontal pocket can increase slightly during inflammation. These changes in environment affect gene expression and alter the competitiveness of periodontal pathogens such as *P. gingivalis*, thereby changing the natural balance (homeostasis) of the subgingival microflora to favour the growth of proteolytic, and often Gram negative, anaerobes (Fig. 6.1).

The flow of GCF can remove microorganisms not attached firmly to a surface. The cementum surface of the tooth is colonized by Gram positive bacteria belonging to the genera *Streptococcus* and *Actinomyces*. Many putative periodontal pathogens (*Prevotella*, *Porphyromonas*, *Fusobacterium* spp.) can attach to this layer of cells by coaggregation/coadhesion (Ch. 5). Likewise, black-pigmented anaerobes and *Parvimonas micra* (formerly *Peptostreptococcus micros*) may persist in the pocket due to their ability to adhere to crevicular epithelial cells. Indeed, their attachment to these cells is markedly enhanced when the epithelium has been treated with proteases of bacterial or host origin.

When attempting to determine the microflora of a periodontal pocket, care has to be taken to preserve the viability of the obligately anaerobic species during the sample taking, dispersing, diluting and cultivation of the sample (Ch. 4). Ideally, the sample should be taken from the base of the pocket, near the advancing front of the lesion in order to avoid removing organisms that are not associated with tissue destruction, and which might obscure any association between specific bacteria and disease activity. Also, it is often difficult to diagnose periodontal diseases accurately, so not all studies are comparing identical pathological conditions. Furthermore, it is not clear whether chronic periodontitis progresses at (a) a continuous slow rate, or (b) by distinct periods of disease activity over relatively short periods of time, followed by phases of quiescence or even repair. This would have implications for sampling strategies, since it would be necessary to remove plaque only during periods of disease activity. The use of rigorous plaque recovery approaches, together with the application of molecular techniques has led to the discovery of organisms never before described.

EVIDENCE FOR MICROBIAL INVOLVEMENT IN PERIODONTAL DISEASES

Germ-free animal studies

Germ-free animals rarely suffer from periodontal disease, although, on occasions, food can be impacted in the gingival crevice producing inflammation. Inflammation is much more common and severe when specific bacteria, particularly some of those isolated from human periodontal pockets, are used in pure culture to infect these animals. These bacteria include streptococci and *Actinomyces* spp. but are more commonly Gram negative, for example, *Aggregatibacter* (formerly *Actinobacillus*), *Prevotella*, *Porphyromonas*, *Capnocytophaga*, *Eikenella*, *Fusobacterium* and *Selenomonas* spp.. Furthermore, periodontal diseases are arrested when an antibiotic active against the particular microbe is administered to the infected animal.

Human studies

Classical experiments have demonstrated that the accumulation of plaque around the gingival margin reproducibly induces an inflammatory response in the tissues in 10–20 days. Removal of plaque results in resolution of the inflammatory response. Similarly, plaque control and antibiotic treatment studies have confirmed the role of microorganisms in human disease. These latter types of studies, however, can give no information as to whether disease results from the activity of (a) a single, or only a limited number of species (the '**specific plaque hypothesis**'); or (b) any combination of a wider range of plaque bacteria (the '**non-specific plaque hypothesis**') (see earlier).

In order to test these hypotheses, a large number of cross-sectional epidemiological studies have been performed on patients with particular forms of periodontal disease (Fig. 6.2). As with dental caries, a disadvantage of this type of study is that true 'cause-and-effect' relationships can never be determined. Microorganisms that appear to predominate at diseased sites might be present as a result of the disease, rather than having actually initiated it. With the exception of gingivitis, longitudinal studies (which do not suffer from this drawback) are not usually possible because of the lengthy natural history of most forms of periodontal disease and the difficulties in predicting subjects and sites likely to be affected. Recently, as with dental caries, the '**ecological plaque hypothesis**' has been applied to explain the aetiology of periodontal disease. This hypothesis proposes that changes in local environmental conditions in the subgingival region (e.g. the increased flow of GCF that occurs during inflammation, and the resultant increases in pH and temperature) favour the growth of the proteolytic and obligately anaerobic species (many of which are Gram negative) at the expense of those bacteria seen in health. This results in a shift in the overall balance of the subgingival microflora, thereby predisposing a site to disease; this hypothesis will be described in relation to periodontal diseases in more detail later in this Chapter.

MICROBIOLOGY OF PERIODONTAL DISEASES

The classification of periodontal diseases has changed to reflect increased knowledge of the natural history of these diseases; in the new classification scheme, there is less emphasis on the rate of disease progression or on the age of the patient. The main types of periodontal disease are: (a) gingival diseases, (b) chronic periodontitis, (c) necrotizing forms of periodontal diseases, and (d) aggressive periodontitis. Chronic and aggressive periodontitis can be localized or generalized, and there can be modifiers of chronic periodontitis such as diabetes, smoking, certain medications and HIV infection. Periodontitis can also occur as a manifestation of systemic diseases, for example, as a result of haematological disorders (e.g. neutropaenia and leukaemia) or genetic disorders, many of which affect neutrophil function (e.g. Papillon–Lefèvre syndrome, Chediak–Higashi syndrome). There are other rare forms of periodontal diseases that will not be covered in this Chapter that are due to developmental and acquired deformities and conditions, or to endodontic lesions.

In periodontal diseases, there is a shift in the balance of the normal subgingival microflora (Fig. 6.1). The healthy gingival crevice has substantial proportions of Gram positive, facultatively anaerobic bacteria such as *Streptococcus* and *Actinomyces* species together with some obligately anaerobic bacteria (Table 5.7). The most commonly isolated black-pigmented anaerobe in the healthy gingival crevice is *Prevotella melaninogenica* although *P. nigrescens* has also been recovered on occasions; *Porphyromonas gingivalis* is rarely isolated from healthy sites. Molecular studies using culture-independent approaches (e.g. 16S rRNA amplification; FISH) have shown that the subgingival microflora is extremely diverse, even in health. A number of spirochaetes can be detected, including *Treponema vincentii*, *T. denticola*, *T. maltophilum* and *T. lecithinolyticum*, as well as

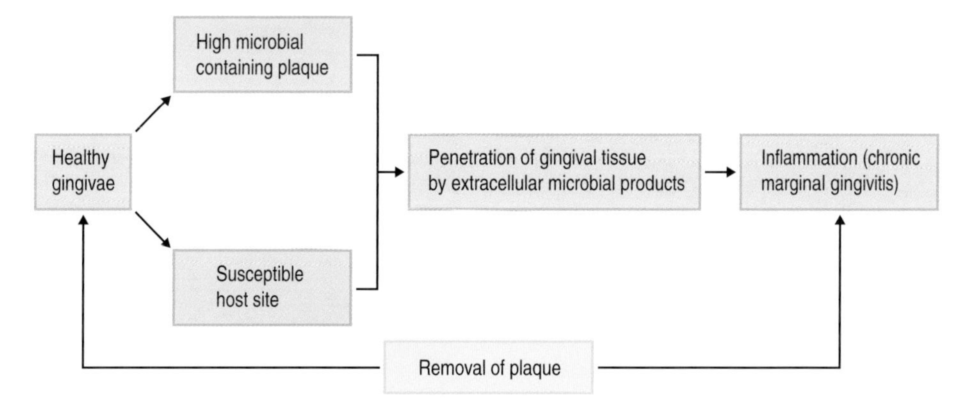

Fig. 6.7 Schematic diagram of the aetiology of chronic gingivitis.

members of the *Selenomonas, Prevotella, Capnocytophaga* and *Campylobacter* genera. Around 40% of amplified clones represented novel phylotypes. Human oral TM7 bacteria, of which there are no culturable examples, were detected frequently in samples, and made up around 1% of the total bacteria in healthy subgingival sites (Figs 3.3 and 5.12).

Gingivitis

Chronic marginal gingivitis is a non-specific, reversible inflammatory response to dental plaque involving the gingival margins. If good oral hygiene is restored, gingivitis is usually eradicated and the tissues becomes clinically normal again (Fig. 6.7). Estimates of the incidence of gingivitis are difficult to determine but probably the whole dentate population is affected by this condition at some stage. Generally, gingivitis is regarded as resulting from a non-specific proliferation of the normal gingival crevice microflora due to poor oral hygiene. Gingival diseases can also be modified by systemic factors. The clinical signs are exaggerated and the gingivae are more oedematous and inflamed in individuals undergoing hormonal disturbances (e.g. during puberty or pregnancy). Certain drug therapies (e.g. immunosuppressive drugs) can also result in gingivitis.

The observation in the 1960s that gingivitis develops in a predictable and reproducible manner in volunteers who refrain from oral hygiene permitted the design of longitudinal studies (Fig. 6.2) to determine the bacteriological events that lead to disease. The microflora associated with gingivitis is more diverse and differs in overall composition from that found in health. There is an increase (10–20 fold) in plaque mass, and there is a shift from the streptococci-dominated plaque of gingival health (Ch. 5) to one in which *Actinomyces* spp., capnophilic (especially *Capnocytophaga* spp.) and obligately anaerobic Gram negative bacteria predominate.

The potential diversity of the subgingival microflora, and the difficulties associated with data analysis, can be gauged from the results of two comprehensive microbiological culture studies. Around 160 different bacterial groups (taxa) were cultivated from four young adults participating in an experimental gingivitis study, while more than 100 non-spirochaetal taxa were isolated from 21 children and adults with naturally-occurring gingivitis. In the former study, of the 166 taxa isolated, 73 showed a positive correlation with gingivitis, 29 were negatively correlated while the remainder either showed no correlation or were regarded as being present as a result of gingivitis. This last conclusion emphasizes the value of longitudinal studies. Despite the variability in the composition of the microflora between subjects, certain trends emerged from these studies. The microflora became more diverse with time as gingivitis developed although none of the taxa from either study were uniquely associated with gingivitis. However, some organisms that were found only rarely in health were found more commonly in gingivitis.

Not all sites with gingivitis progress to more serious forms of periodontal disease, but it is accepted that gingivitis must precede periodontitis. Certainly, some species that predominate in periodontitis, but which are not detectable in the healthy gingiva, have been found as a small percentage of the microflora in gingivitis. This suggests that environmental conditions which develop during gingivitis (e.g. bleeding, increased flow of GCF) may favour the growth of species implicated in periodontitis.

Chronic periodontitis

This is the most common form of advanced periodontal disease affecting the general population, and is a major cause of tooth loss after the age of 25 years. In the USA, about one third of adults suffer from the disease at some time during their life. It differs from chronic gingivitis in that in addition to the gingivae being involved, there is loss of attachment between the root surface, the gingivae and the alveolar bone, and bone loss itself may occur (Fig. 6.8), giving an increased depth on probing (Fig. 6.9), and

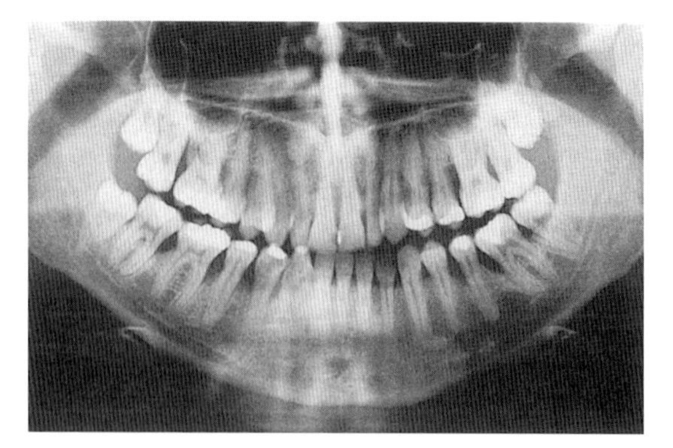

Fig. 6.8 Radiograph of chronic periodontitis showing extensive bone loss.

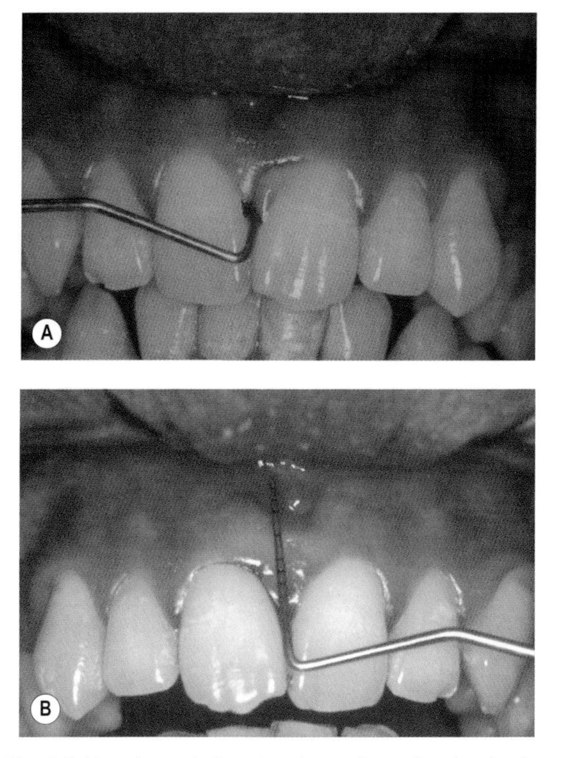

Fig. 6.9 Use of a periodontal probe to determine the depth of a pocket: (A) the probe *in situ*; (B) the probe removed and overlain on the tissues to show the extent of the loss of attachment.

bleeding. In contrast to gingivitis, these pathological changes are irreversible. Under the current classification scheme, periodontitis can be either **localized** (i.e. only certain sites are affected), or **generalized**. Factors that enhance plaque retention or impede plaque removal, such as subgingival calculus, overhanging restorations or crowded teeth, can predispose towards chronic periodontitis.

Early studies of plaque associated with chronic periodontitis relied on microscopically-observed, qualitative morphological descriptions of the microorganisms present. Dark-field microscopy showed that many of the bacteria in plaque from patients with deep pockets were motile (probably *Campylobacter rectus* and *Selenomonas sputigena*) and spiral-shaped (e.g. *Treponema* spp.). Attempts have been made to use the presence of these morphotypes as the basis of a cheap and rapid test for use in the clinic to monitor the status of a pocket or effectiveness of treatment. Difficulties have arisen because many putative pathogens cannot be recognised on the basis of their cell morphology alone. Immunological and oligonucleotide probes specific for targeted pathogens can now be used to detect selected bacteria directly in plaque samples without the need for lengthy cultural procedures; other molecular approaches have been used to detect currently 'unculturable' taxa (Chs 3 and 4).

Table 6.6 Some of the predominant bacteria that have been commonly cultured from sites with chronic periodontitis in adults

Gram positive	Gram negative
Eubacterium brachy	*Tannerella forsythia*
Eubacterium nodatum	*Fusobacterium nucleatum*
Mogibacterium timidium	*Porphyromonas gingivalis*
Parvimonas micra	*Prevotella intermedia*
Peptostreptococcus stomatis	*Prevotella loescheii*
Parvimonas micra	*Dialister pneumosintes*
	Campylobacter rectus
	Treponema spp.

Numerous cross-sectional microbiological culture studies have been performed on different patient groups with pockets of varying depths from numerous geographical regions. All studies agree that the cultivable microflora is diverse and is composed of large numbers of obligately anaerobic Gram negative rod and filament-shaped bacteria, many of which are asaccharolytic (unable to gain energy from the catabolism of carbohydrates) but proteolytic. These bacteria are often difficult to recover and identify in the laboratory and there is often conflicting evidence as to which organisms are the primary pathogens. Some of the bacteria that have been implicated from cultural studies are listed in Table 6.6.

Studies have implicated certain clusters or complexes of bacteria with disease. In a series of studies, over 13 000 subgingival plaque samples from nearly 200 subjects were screened for the presence of 40 preselected target bacterial species using a molecular approach (a DNA–DNA checkerboard hybridization technique). Five clusters were identified (Fig. 6.10); the 'red complex' was found most frequently in deeper periodontal pockets, and consisted of *Tannerella forsythia*, *Porphyromonas gingivalis*

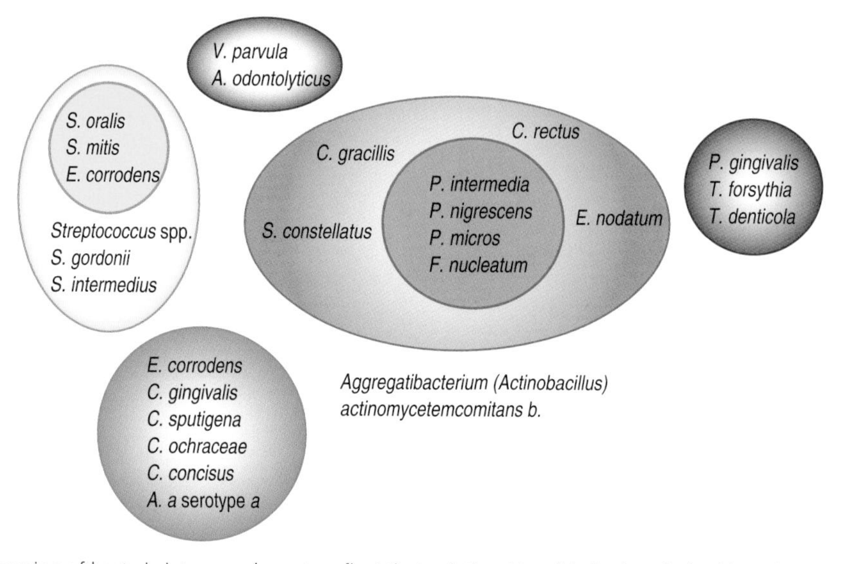

Fig. 6.10 The grouping of bacteria into complexes to reflect their relationship with the host in health and periodontal disease. The 'red complex' is found most frequently in deep periodontal pockets, and their presence was usually preceded by members of the 'orange complex'. Members of the 'yellow', 'green' and 'purple' complexes were generally associated with healthy sites.

and *Treponema denticola*, and their presence was often preceded by members of the orange complex, which was also often found in deeper pockets, but was more diverse in membership. In contrast, species of the yellow, green and purple complexes, together with *A. naeslundii*, were considered to be 'host compatible', and were generally associated with healthy sites. *Aggregatibacter* (formerly *Actinobacillus*) *actinomycetemcomitans* serotype *b* did not fall within a complex, and is associated more with aggressive periodontitis (see later). Thus, chronic periodontitis appears to result from the activity of mixtures of interacting bacteria, and therefore has a polymicrobial aetiology. There is a progressive change in the composition of the microflora from health and gingivitis to periodontitis. This change involves not only the emergence of apparently previously undetected species, but also modifications to the numbers, or proportions, of a variety of species already present.

Two theories have been proposed to explain the emergence of previously undetected species. It may be due to the selective growth (enrichment) of a microorganism that is present in health in only very low numbers, due to a change in the environment during disease. Alternatively, it might be due to the exogenous acquisition of periodontal pathogens from other diseased sites or subjects. The recent application of sensitive molecular approaches has identified low levels of many of the putative pathogens at healthy sites, while evidence of transmission of organisms such as *P. gingivalis* and *A. actinomycetemcomitans* between spouses has been obtained. However, in either situation, a major change to the ecology of the habitat has to occur in order to enable low levels of an organism to outcompete the existing members of the resident microflora and reach clinically significant proportions within the subgingival biofilm. The most likely environmental changes capable of causing such a shift in the microflora are associated with the host inflammatory response (Fig. 6.11). The increased flow of gingival crevicular fluid (GCF) not only introduces components of the host defences but also a range of novel nutrients that selects for the growth of asaccharolytic, anaerobic bacteria. This proteolytic metabolism leads to a rise in local pH, which also favours the growth of many of the bacteria that predominate in periodontitis (Fig. 2.4).

The application of molecular methods to characterize the subgingival microflora of sites with chronic periodontitis has further emphasized the diversity of bacteria found in these sites (Table 6.7). A large proportion of clones identified by 16S rRNA gene sequencing belong to novel phylotypes, some of which have no cultivable representatives. Some studies have detected unculturable

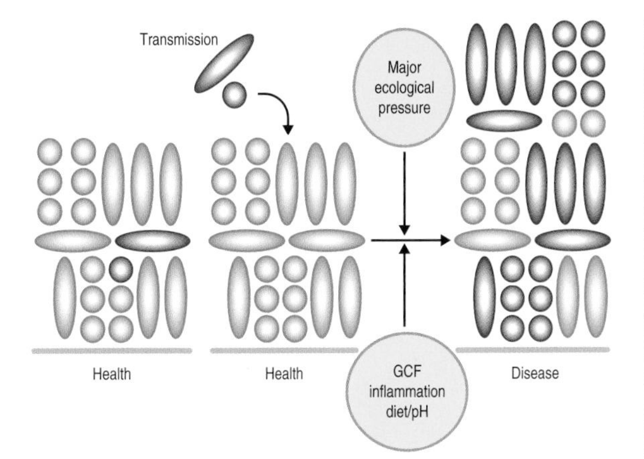

Fig. 6.11 Schematic representation of factors driving shifts in the balance of the microflora in health and periodontal diseases. The microflora of dental plaque is distinct in health and disease. Potential pathogens (shown in red) may be present in low numbers in plaque at healthy sites or transmitted in low numbers from other sites. A major ecological pressure is necessary for such pathogens to outcomplete other members of the resident microflora (green) and achieve the numerical dominance needed for disease to occur.

examples of *Treponema* spp. (Fig. 6.12) or members of the Obsidian Pool, OB11, and TM7 phylotypes (Fig. 3.3). Within the TM7 group, the oral clone I025 was detected in only 1/18 samples from healthy sites but was found in 38/58 samples from periodontally-diseased sites. Other strains that have been recovered almost exclusively from diseased sites include *Treponema socranskii, Filifactor alocis, Dialister pneumosintes, Porphyromonas gingivalis* and *Porphyromonas endodontalis* (Table 6.7). These types of culture-independent studies are changing our views on the role of bacteria in disease. Such studies have confirmed that complex consortia can be isolated from sites with advanced disease, and that poorly classified organisms that are currently difficult or impossible to grow in the laboratory can predominate in deep pockets. It has yet to be determined whether these organisms are playing an active role in disease or are there as a consequence of tissue destruction. In the future it may be possible to screen for the presence of these disease-associated complexes using probes in DNA microarray or DNA–DNA checkerboard hybridization formats. Such studies may enable a clearer association of certain consortia with disease to be discerned, and facilitate improved diagnosis and treatment monitoring.

SUMMARY

Gingivitis is a reversible condition associated with an increase in plaque mass. There is little evidence to implicate specific bacteria with the onset of inflammation, although the complexity of the microflora increases, and there is a shift away from a Gram positive-dominated community to one with larger numbers of Gram negative obligate anaerobes. Some sites progress to chronic periodontitis in which the gingival crevice deepens to become a periodontal pocket, and there is loss of attachment and bone loss; tissue destruction is irreversible. The microflora becomes even more diverse; culture-based studies have confirmed the shift to a Gram negative, obligately anaerobic microflora, with complexes containing mixtures of species such *as Porphyromonas gingivalis, Tannerella forsythia* and a range of spirochaetes being commonly isolated from deep pockets. Culture-independent approaches have detected a large number of novel phylotypes, including taxa that cannot yet be cultivated ('unculturables').

Necrotizing periodontal diseases

Both necrotizing ulcerative gingivitis and necrotizing ulcerative periodontitis are included in this category. It is not clear whether these are separate diseases or are part of a single disease process. Both conditions can be manifestations of underlying systemic problems such as HIV infection, and they can be linked to emotional stress and tobacco smoking.

Necrotizing ulcerative gingivitis (NUG), also described as Vincent's disease, trench mouth, or acute necrotizing gingivitis, is a severe form of necrotizing inflammation of the interdental papillae, accompanied by spontaneous gingival bleeding and intense pain. It is characterized clinically by the formation of a grey pseudomembrane on the gingivae which easily sloughs off revealing a bleeding area beneath it. NUG can often be diagnosed by the characteristic halitosis (bad breath) it produces. NUG is a true infection and, unlike chronic gingivitis, microorganisms can be seen invading the host gingival tissues. In smears of the affected tissues the invading microbes resemble spirochaetes and fusiform bacteria (fuso-spirochaetal complex; Fig. 6.13). Early electron microscopic investigations showed that the invading microorganisms consisted primarily of large and intermediate-sized spirochaetes which were present in the lesions in high numbers and in advance of other microorganisms.

Table 6.7 Bacteria detected directly in subgingival plaque by 16S rRNA sequencing, and implicated in chronic and necrotizing periodontal diseases

Named species	Novel phylotype
Fusobacterium animalis	TM7 (clone I025)
Atopobium parvulum	*Deferribacteres* clones
Atopobium rimae	*Selenomonas* clone
Cantonella morbi	*Desulfobulbus* clone
Dialister pneumosintes	*Megasphaera* clone
Treponema socranskii	*Treponema* clones
Eubacterium saphenum	*Eubacterium* clone
Eubacterium nodatum	
Slackia exigua	
Abiotrophia adiacens	
Filifactor alocis	
Gemella haemolysans	
Streptococcus constellatus	
Campylobacter gracilis	
Campylobacter rectus	
Haemophilus parainfluenzae	
Tannerella forsythia	
Porphyromonas gingivalis	
Porphyromonas endodontalis	

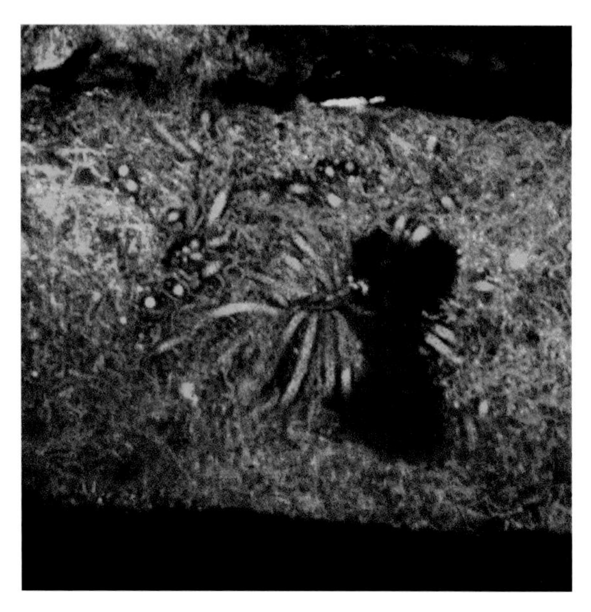

Fig. 6.12 Unculturable *Treponema* species detected in subgingival plaque by fluorescent in situ hybridization (FISH). Red: *Treponema* spp; green: other bacteria. Courtesy of Dr Annette Moter and produced with permission. (see text on Fig 3.3A).

A heterogeneous collection of microorganisms has been isolated from ulcerated sites. Various spirochaetes (*Treponema* spp.) were found in high numbers (approximately 40% of the total cell count), but in view of the fuso-spirochaetal pattern characteristically observed by microscopy, the most unusual finding was the relatively low numbers of *Fusobacterium* spp. and the high proportions of *Prevotella intermedia*, which averaged 3 and 24% of the total cultivable microflora, respectively. More recent studies have used culture independent approaches (16S rRNA gene sequencing; FISH), and these have confirmed the predominance of a diverse range of *Treponema* species in lesions, many of which cannot be cultivated, but showed that the 'fusiform' bacteria could belong to a broader range of genera including *Leptotrichia*, *Capnocytophaga* and *Tannerella* in addition to *Fusobacterium* spp.. Clones from other non-culturable phylotypes were also detected, e.g. *Deferribacteres*. One study also detected increased levels of *Porphyromonas gingivalis*, *Selenomonas sputigena* and *Actinomyces gerencseriae* in NUG. Metronidazole is effective in eliminating the fuso-spirochaetal complex from infected sites and this is associated with rapid clinical improvement.

Necrotizing ulcerative periodontitis is a painful condition that affects a small proportion of HIV-positive subjects. Molecular (culture-independent) approaches detected a wide range of bacteria including *Bulleida extructa*, *Dialister*, *Fusobacterium*, *Selenomonas*, *Veillonella*, members of the TM7 phylum, and anaerobic streptococci, while surprisingly some of the more common organisms isolated from periodontal diseases in HIV-negative patients (e.g. *P. gingivalis*) were not recovered.

Aggressive periodontitis

Previously, patients that were diagnosed as having 'Localized Juvenile Periodontitis' (LJP), 'Generalized Juvenile Periodontitis' or 'Early Onset Periodontitis' are now described as suffering from

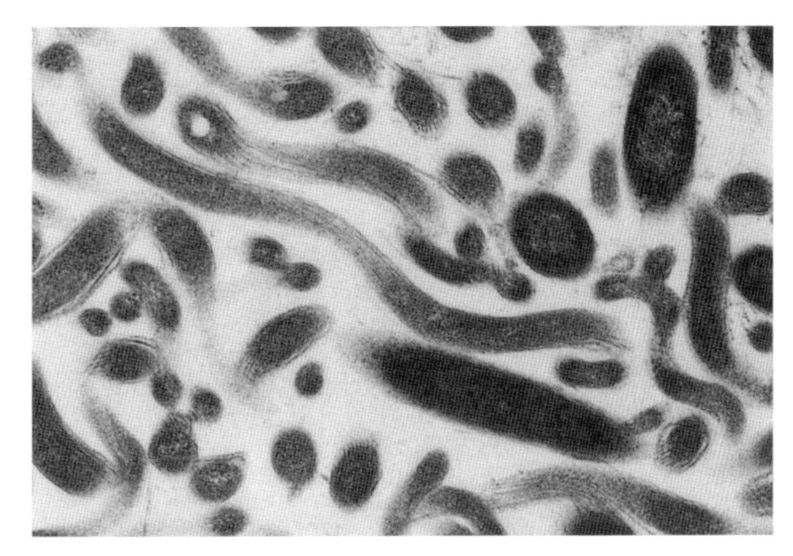

Fig. 6.13 Electron micrograph of a sample from necrotizing ulcerative gingivitis (NUG) showing spirochaetes.

aggressive periodontitis (the age-related terminologies have been discarded) which can either be localized or generalized.

Aggressive periodontitis is a rare condition (affecting only around 0.1% of the susceptible age group) which usually occurs in adolescents. The disease appears to start around puberty, is more common in girls, cases often cluster in families, and loss of attachment is rapid. Aggressive periodontitis also shows some racial predispositions, being slightly more common in people of West African and Asian origin. Two forms of the disease have been described. In localized aggressive periodontitis there is a distinct pattern of alveolar bone loss that is characteristically localized, for as yet unknown reasons, to the first permanent molars and the incisor teeth (Fig. 6.14). In contrast, a generalized form has been described in which many teeth are affected. The majority of patients with aggressive periodontitis have a variety of functional abnormalities of neutrophils. These abnormalities have been associated with signal transduction pathways, and there is reduced chemotaxis and phagocytosis, but increased superoxide radical production. This deficiency is coupled with, or is a direct cause of, the presence of relatively high numbers of *Aggregatibacter* (formerly *Actinobacillus*) *actinomycetemcomitans*. The microflora of plaque from patients with aggressive periodontitis is relatively sparse, considering the severity and rapidity of the tissue destruction and bone loss. There are relatively few microorganisms present (approximately 10^6 CFU/pocket) belonging to only a limited number of species, and the majority of these are capnophilic (CO_2-loving) Gram negative rods. In some culture studies, *A. actinomycetemcomitans* could be recovered from 97% of affected sites and comprise up to 70% of the cultivable microflora. However, *A. actinomycetemcomitans* can be detected using molecular techniques in low numbers quite commonly at healthy sites in some communities. For example, its prevalence was 13% in Finland and 20–25% in urban USA, perhaps again emphasizing the key role of the need for a susceptible host; furthermore *A. actinomycetemcomitans* could not be recovered from some sites with the disease. Nevertheless, affected individuals tend to have elevated serum antibody titres to this microorganism, while its reduction or elimination results in a resolution of disease activity; recurrence of the disease is usually related to the reappearance of *A. actinomycetemcomitans*. These findings have important implications in treatment design because tetracycline is effective in eliminating *A. actinomycetemcomitans* from infected pockets, and resolving the clinical condition. This is in contrast to other forms of chronic inflammatory periodontal disease when metronidazole might be chosen because of its specific action against obligately anaerobic bacteria. Tetracycline does not always lead to complete elimination of *A. actinomycetemcomitans* from the pocket, and the combination of metronidazole and amoxycillin has been found to be particularly effective in these

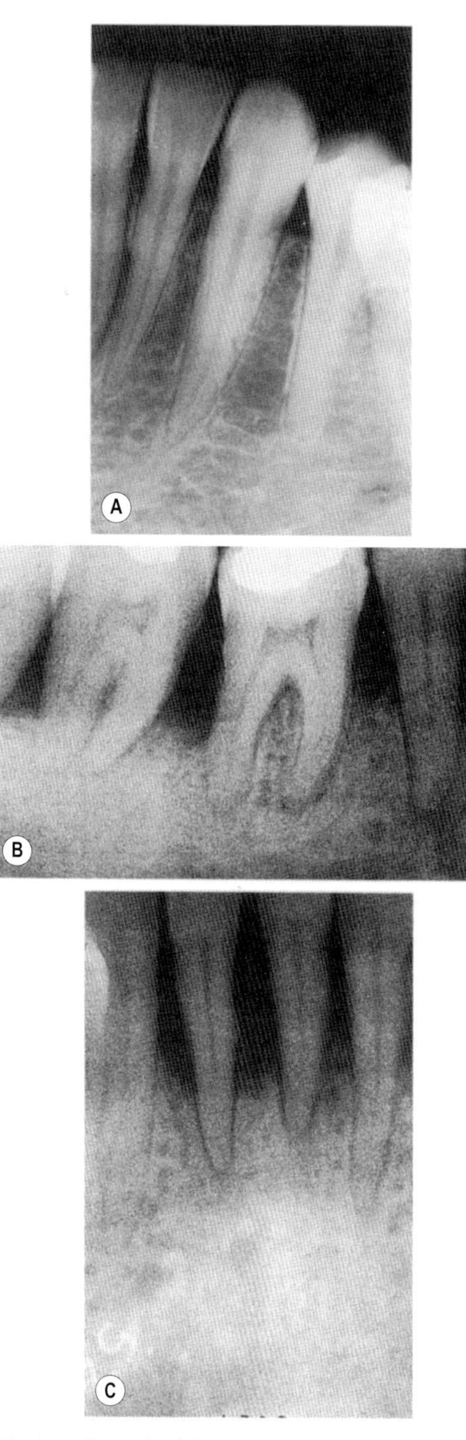

Fig. 6.14 Radiograph of (A) normal periodontium, and (B) and (C) localized aggressive periodontitis, showing bone loss.

situations, particularly when combined with scaling and root planing.

Five serotypes (*a–e*) of *A. actinomycetemcomitans* have been described, and more than one serotype can be found in the mouth of an individual. Strains of *A. actinomycetemcomitans* produce a range of virulence factors, including a powerful leukotoxin (i.e. a protein toxic for polymorphs), LPS (endotoxin, which can stimulate bone resorption), and cell surface associated material, which also induces resorption of bone. In addition, *A. actinomycetemcomitans* produces enzymes with the ability to degrade collagen, as well as other, less well-defined factors, that modulate the activity of the host defences. *A. actinomycetemcomitans* can also invade gingival connective tissues. Generally, serotype *b* strains are more common in aggressive periodontitis. Intra-family transmission of strains may occur, and molecular studies have provided evidence for the existence of virulent clones. The JP2 clone overproduces the leukotoxin and is found endemically in people from Morocco and other parts of North West Africa. The presence of this JP2 clone in plaque significantly raises the risk of adolescents suffering from aggressive periodontitis (the risk increases 18-fold compared to subjects without *A. actinomycetemcomitans*, although this risk is reduced if sites harbour both JP2 and non-JP2 clones).

In contrast to most other forms of periodontal disease, therefore, localized aggressive periodontitis appears to result from the activity of a relatively specific microflora dominated by a single species. As stated above, sites have been found in which *A. actinomycetemcomitans* is not necessarily the predominant microorganism, which is analogous to the situation described earlier with respect to dental caries and the presence of mutans streptococci. In these pockets, small spirochaetes, *Eikenella corrodens*, *Wolinella* sp. and *Fusobacterium nucleatum* are often numerous.

In a study of generalized aggressive periodontitis, *Treponema* species were closely associated with disease (including morphotypes that could not be cultured but which could be distinguished by microscopy), as were *F. nucleatum*, lactobacilli, several species of *Eubacterium*, *Parvimonas* spp., *Prevotella intermedia* and *Selenomonas* spp.. The role, and therefore the significance, of most of these bacteria in disease has yet to be determined.

SUMMARY

Necrotizing ulcerative periodontitis is a painful, condition which has a fuso-spirochaetal aetiology. Culture and molecular studies have detected a range of *Treponema* spp. and fusiform bacteria invading gingival tissues. Aggressive periodontitis is rare and is associated with functional abnormalities of neutrophils. Plaque from affected sites is sparse but, in the localized form of the disease, often contains *Aggregatibacter actinomycetemcomitans*, strains of which produce a powerful leukotoxin. The presence of the JP2 clone is a major risk factor for subsequent disease, and is found in adolescents originating from North West Africa.

Other periodontal diseases

Acute, or exaggerated, forms of gingivitis can arise due to a variety of predisposing factors or circumstances including HIV infection, diabetes, pregnancy, puberty, menstruation, stress, or the use of oral contraceptives.

Pregnancy gingivitis

The exaggerated gingivitis seen in pregnancy is linked to an increase in the proportions of the black-pigmented anaerobe, *P. intermedia*, during the second trimester, possibly due to the increased levels of steroid hormones in GCF.

Acute streptococcal gingivitis

This condition affects the gingivae which can result in severe illness. The gingivae become red, swollen and full of fluid (oedematous), the temperature is raised and the regional lymph nodes are also enlarged. Lancefield Group A streptococci (*S. pyogenes*) can be isolated from the affected gingivae. This disease is usually preceded by a sore throat and hence it is possible that there is a direct spread of *S. pyogenes* from throat to gingivae.

Acute herpetic gingivitis

The majority of infectious cases of gingivitis are bacterial in origin but occasionally viral gingivitis is seen, predominantly in young people. The commonest form is acute herpetic gingivitis, the causative agent of which is Herpes simplex type 1 (HSV-1). Acute herpetic gingivitis is seen usually in children and appears as ulcerated swellings of the gingivae which are acutely painful. The symptoms may persist for 7 to 21 days and herpetic lesions may concomitantly be present on lips or any area of the oral mucosa. The diagnosis is usually made on clinical criteria although cytological smears and cytopathic effects following culture have been used for confirmation; direct immunofluorescence is also used for diagnosis. Antiviral agents (e.g. acyclovir and penciclovir) can be effective treatments.

Diabetes mellitus-associated gingivitis

The relationship between diabetes and periodontal disease may be bi-directional. Both conditions stimulate the release of pro-inflammatory cytokines that have a direct effect on the periodontal tissues. In general, patients with diabetes have more severe episodes of gingivitis compared with healthy controls, especially in younger subjects whose condition is poorly controlled. Many of the host response traits that confer susceptibility in periodontal disease in otherwise healthy individuals are exaggerated in diabetics. Susceptibility traits include neutrophil dysfunction, altered cross-linking and glycosylation of collagen, defective secretion of growth factors and subsequent impaired healing. Diseased sites have higher proportions of *Capnocytophaga*, and other periodontal pathogens including *P. gingivalis* and spirochaetes. Sometimes, non-oral bacteria (e.g. staphylococci) have been isolated. These changes in microflora may reflect a compromised host defence. Periodontal disease may increase insulin resistance in diabetic patients. Periodontal pathogens may raise pro-inflammatory mediators that result in insulin resistance and an increase in blood glucose, thereby predisposing individuals to develop type 2 diabetes. Mechanical treatment of periodontitis, when combined with antimicrobial agents, can improve glycaemic control.

HIV-associated periodontal disease

The impaired immune response in HIV patients can result in colonization of subgingival sites by opportunistic oral pathogens, such as *Gemella*, *Dialister*, *Streptococcus* and *Candida* spp.. Classical periodontal pathogens, such as *P. gingivalis*, *T. forsythia* and spirochaetes are not necessarily prevalent.

Noma (cancrum oris)

Noma is a severe gangrenous disease that causes a rapid necrotizing destruction of soft and hard tissue of the face, including bone. Noma was often fatal before the use of antibiotics such as metronidazole. The classic form of the disease affects young children, although immunocompromized adults can also be affected; the disease is characterized by a strong putrid odour. Noma is most common in Africa, but is also reported in parts of Latin America and Asia. The WHO estimated that about 200 000 children under 6 years of age contract noma each year; consequently, noma has been declared a priority by WHO. Risk factors include malnutrition, poor oral hygiene and a compromized immune system due to, for example, infection with measles, malaria or HIV. The disease process may involve three stages: (a) a staging period, where infection, e.g. measles, results in a lowered host resistance, and the appearance of oral lesions; (b) an infection period, where some trigger activates a polymicrobial infection, and (c) a tissue invasion and destruction phase, during which an acute ulcerative condition progresses to oro-facial gangrene, which is life-threatening. *Fusobacterium necrophorum*, which can be acquired from domesticated livestock, has been isolated from some advanced noma lesions, and has been proposed as the trigger organism for the development of Cancrum oris; infected children are often in regular close contact with animals. Evidence of oral Herpes virus, especially cytomegalovirus, has been found in noma patients, and it has been suggested that such an infection could lower local immunity leading to overgrowth by bacterial pathogens. Culture-based studies have recovered *P. intermedia*, streptococci and *Actinomyces* spp, as well as opportunistic pathogens such as staphylococci and pseudomonads, from lesions. A culture-independent study detected a diverse range of bacteria including 25 phylotypes that had never previously been grown in the laboratory. Bacteria that were unique to noma lesions included members of the genera *Eubacterium*, *Porphyromonas* and *Treponema*; species more commonly isolated from soil were also detected, and this might reflect the fact that advanced noma lesions are open to the environment. Treatment focuses on improving overall health (e.g. nutritional rehabilitation), administration of broad spectrum antibiotics and, when possible, introduction of oral hygiene; reconstructive surgery is often necessary once healing is complete.

PATHOGENIC MECHANISMS IN PERIODONTAL DISEASE

Periodontal diseases are characterized by the progressive destruction of the supporting tissues of teeth in the apparent absence (at least in the early stages) of significant tissue invasion. Tissue damage, therefore, must also be mediated by surface components and extracellular products of bacteria (Table 6.8). These bacterial products can cause destruction of gingival tissue by two mechanisms. In one, damage results from the *direct* action of bacterial enzymes and cytotoxic products of bacterial metabolism. In the other, bacterial components are only *indirectly* responsible, and tissue destruction is the inevitable side effect of a subverted and exaggerated host inflammatory response to plaque antigens; this has been termed 'bystander damage' (Fig. 6.15).

There is also an hypothesis proposing a role for herpes viruses in destructive periodontal diseases. Herpes simplex virus, human cytomegalovirus and Epstein–Barr virus type 1 nucleic acids have been detected in lesions from aggressive types of periodontitis. These viruses can infect various host cells, including polymorphonuclear leukocytes, macrophages and lymphocytes, and they induce the expression of potentially tissue-damaging cytokines and chemokines. In this way, it is proposed that these viruses could reduce the effectiveness of the local host defences, thereby giving certain subgingival bacteria the opportunity to escape from homeostasis and reach clinically-significant levels. The tissue tropism of herpes virus infections may explain the localized pattern of tissue destruction seen in some forms of periodontitis, while the reactivation of these viruses may explain the episodic nature of tissue destruction.

Indirect pathogenicity

Any subgingival plaque bacterium could be considered to be playing a role in tissue destruction via the indirect pathogenicity route if they contribute to an inflammatory host response. Bacterial antigens can penetrate the crevicular epithelium and stimulate either humoral or cell mediated immunity. Humoral immunity results in the synthesis of immunoglobulins, which activate the complement cascade that leads to inflammation and the generation of prostaglandins. Prostaglandins are inflammatory

Table 6.8 Bacterial factors implicated in the aetiology of periodontal diseases

Stage of disease		Bacterial factor
Attachment to host tissues		Surface components, e.g. 'adhesins' Surface structures, e.g. fimbriae
Multiplication at a susceptible site		Protease production to obtain nutrients Development of food chains Inhibitor production, e.g. bacteriocins
Evasion of host defences		Capsules and slimes PMN-receptor blockers Leukotoxin Immunoglobin-specific proteases Complement-degrading proteases Suppresser T cell induction
Tissue damage	(a) direct	**Enzymes** 'Arginine-specific' proteases (gingipain) Collagenase Hyaluronidase Chondroitin sulphatase **Bone resorbing factors** Lipoteichoic acid Lipopolysaccharide (LPS) Capsule Surface-associated material. **Cytotoxins** Butyric and propionic acids Indole Amines Ammonia Volatile sulphur compounds
	(b) indirect	Inflammatory response to plaque antigens (see text).

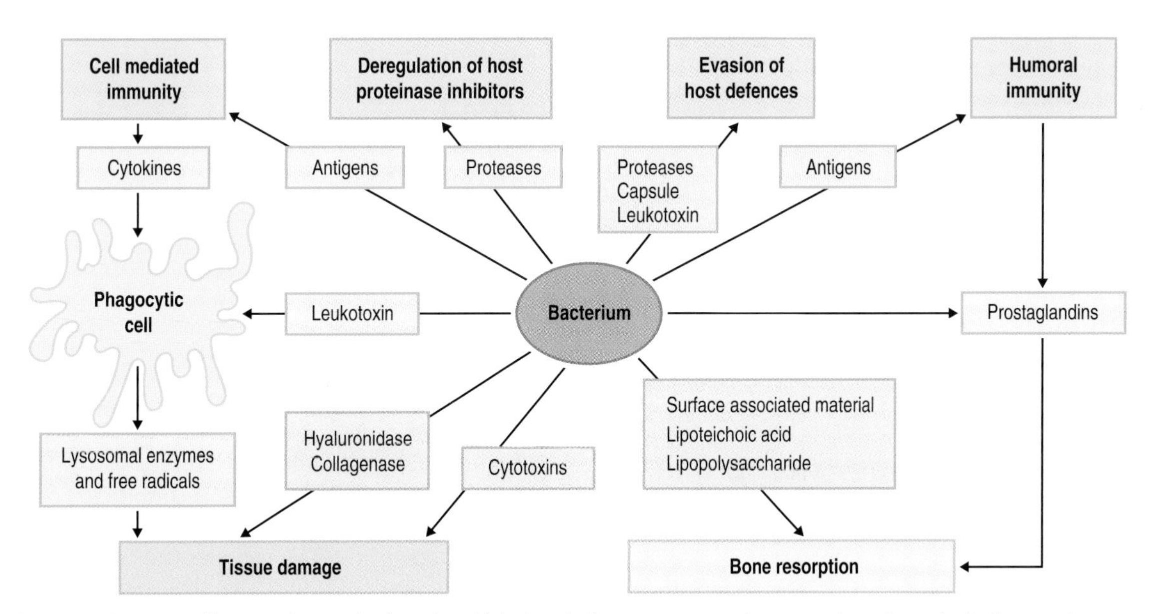

Fig. 6.15 Diagram to illustrate the mechanisms by which dental plaque can cause damage to host tissues by indirect and indirect routes of pathogenicity.

mediators, and can stimulate bone resorption. Levels of prostaglandins in GCF correlate with periodontal status, and can act as molecular predictors of attachment loss. In contrast, cellular immunity leads to the release of cytokines from activated T-lymphocytes, and these modulate macrophage activity. Activated macrophages release cytokines such as tumour necrosis factor-alpha (TNF-α), interferon gamma (IFN-γ), and interleukin-1 (IL-1). Both IL-1 and TNF-α can induce collagenase release from a variety of connective tissue cells, including fibroblasts, and cause bone resorption and tissue damage.

Important host tissue cells in the gingival crevice include the pocket epithelium and the periodontal ligament. These cells are made up of collagen and glycosaminoglycan (GAG) molecules linked to a protein core. The main proteoglycans of the gingivae and periodontal ligament are hyaluronic acid, heparin sulphate, dermatan sulphate and chondroitin sulphate 4. These proteoglycans can be degraded by elastase and cathepsin B; both enzymes are present in the inflamed gingival crevice, and are probably derived from polymorphs, macrophages and fibroblasts. Mast cells can be found migrating through the junctional epithelium and into the pocket, and can release histamine and other vaso-active molecules, as well as a range of proteases.

Many host cells in the gingival crevice also contain proteinase inhibitors such as α-1-proteinase inhibitor and α-2-macroglobulin, which are responsible for inactivating proteases in host tissues, thereby enabling the host to control the potentially destructive forces of the inflammatory response. As will be discussed in the next section, bacterial proteases can degrade these important control molecules, leading to further 'bystander damage' to tissues. Tissue damage in active periodontal disease is due in part, therefore, to a deregulated and subverted immune response.

Direct pathogenicity

The putative pathogens produce a range of potential virulence factors that enable them to:

(a) colonize and multiply at subgingival sites,

(b) evade or inactivate the host defences,

(c) induce tissue damage and, on occasions,

(d) invade host tissues.

These virulence factors will be described in the following sections.

Colonization and multiplication

Periodontal pathogens are able to attach to and colonize the subgingival surfaces via bacterial adhesins that interact with specific receptors (Chs 4 and 5). These receptors may be located either on the root surface or on gingival epithelial cells, or the pathogens may coadhere to already attached Gram positive bacteria such as streptococci and *Actinomyces* spp.. Some of these putative pathogens produce a range of proteases (e.g. *Porphyromonas gingivalis* produces gingipains with a specificity for either arginine or lysine residues: arg- and lys-gingipains, respectively) and glycosidases in order to obtain nutrients from the catabolism of host molecules; often several species with complementary enzyme profiles combine to break down these complex molecules (Ch. 4). Bacteria such as *P. gingivalis* also possess haemagglutination and haemolytic activities, which may be a means of targeting appropriate substrates for the release of essential cofactors for growth, such as haemin, from host molecules. The arg-gingipains of *P. gingivalis* (see later) cleave proteins to leave exposed arginine residues, which in turn can act as receptors for its own fimbriae, thereby facilitating colonization by the exposure of 'cryptitopes' (Ch. 4). The gingipains of *P. gingivalis* can also contribute to nutrition by generating the vascular permeability enhancement factor, bradykinin, either through a direct action on kininogen or via activation of pre-kallikrein, resulting in the entry of elevated levels of plasma proteins (which can act as nutrients) into the pocket. The lys-gingipain also plays an essential role in nutrition by obtaining haemin from haemoglobin. The concerted action of arg- and lys-gingipains is necessary for the production of the black pigment layer on the surface of *P. gingivalis* (micro-oxo bishaem layer), that protects cells against oxidative damage.

Evasion and/or inactivation of the host defences

Phagocytic cells form the main defence strategy by the host against periodontal pathogens. Many strains of *A. actinomycetemcomitans* produce a powerful leukotoxin able to lyse human neutrophils, monocytes and a sub-population of lymphocytes, whilst other cell types (e.g. epithelial and endothelial cells, fibroblasts, erythrocytes) are resistant. The leukotoxin belongs to the RTX (repeats-in-toxin) family of bacterial pore-forming cytolysins; *Campylobacter rectus* also produces a leukotoxin. The JP2 clone of

A. actinomycetemcomitans serotype *b* overproduces the leukotoxin by up to 20 times that seen in other strains, and its presence is a significant risk factor for localized aggressive periodontitis. The same clone has not been isolated from Caucasians or from healthy individuals, giving rise to the speculation that this might represent a specific, and highly infectious, clone of a periodontal pathogen.

Periodontal pathogens can produce a range of molecules that cause tissue damage by inducing host cells to produce pro-inflammatory cytokines. These molecules, termed 'modulins', include lipopolysaccharides and other less well defined cell wall components. Other bacterial components can inhibit the chemotaxis of polymorphonuclear leukocytes (PMNs), and interfere with their ability to kill bacteria or phagocytose cells. Bacteria, including *A. actinomycetemcomitans*, also exert an immunosuppressive effect, perhaps mediated by cell surface proteins, while *P. gingivalis*, possesses a capsule, which protects cells against phagocytosis. *Aggregatibacter actinomycetemcomitans*, *T. forsythia*, *P. gingivalis*, and other pathogens may also evade the host defences by invading epithelial cells (Ch. 4; Fig. 4.6).

The proteases of *P. gingivalis* play a critical role in deregulating the host control of the inflammatory response, and in evading the action of other components of the immune system. Arg-gingipain can inactivate both complement (e.g. by degrading C3 and C5) and antimicrobial peptides (Ch. 2); a range of proteases can also degrade immunoglobulins (IgA, IgG and IgM) and interfere with the respiratory burst of neutrophils, reducing the likelihood of opsonization. The maintenance of tissue homeostasis, and the coordination of the innate and adaptive immune response, is dependent on a complex intercellular signalling network mediated by cytokines. Components of *P. gingivalis* can stimulate the production of pro-inflammatory cytokines such as TNF-α and IL-1, but arg-and lys-gingipain can subvert this host response by degrading these key molecules and enzymically modifying others. Arg-gingipain can also inactivate the two major plasma protease inhibitors, α_1-antitrypsin and α_2-macroglobulin, thereby reducing the ability of the host to regulate the scale and ferocity of the inflammatory response. Expression and activity of these enzymes is up-regulated by environmental changes (e.g. by increases in local pH and haemin concentration) that occur during the transition from a normal gingival crevice to a periodontal pocket. Other periodontal pathogens, including *Tannerella forsythia* and *Treponema denticola*, also produce proteases with arginine-x specificity. Thus, some periodontal pathogens can subvert and deregulate the host's attempt to control subgingival plaque so that 'by-stander' tissue damage occurs, while the influx of potential nutrients is increased so that their growth is selectively enhanced.

Tissue-damaging enzymes and metabolites

Members of the subgingival microflora produce enzymes that may play a direct role in the damage of host tissues in the periodontal pocket. For example, *P. gingivalis* has been shown to produce collagenases that can degrade collagen, although the majority of collagenase activity in GCF is host-derived. Once denatured, collagen may be broken down by bacterial proteases with a broader specificity. Other enzymes produced by subgingival bacteria that may damage tissue matrix molecules directly include hyaluronidase, chondroitin sulphatase, and glycylprolyl peptidase. These enzymes can also be detected on outer membrane vesicles of Gram negative bacteria such as *P. gingivalis*; these vesicles can be shed from the bacterial cell surface during growth, enhancing the likelihood of tissue penetration by these enzymes. Once the integrity of the epithelium is impaired, the increased penetration of cytotoxic bacterial metabolites such as indole, amines, ammonia, volatile sulphur compounds (e.g. methyl mercaptan, H_2S), and butyric and propionic acids can induce further damage. *Fusobacterium nucleatum* is the most commonly isolated species in periodontal pockets, and it produces large concentrations of butyrate and volatile sulphur compounds. Bone loss is a feature of advanced forms of periodontal disease (Fig. 6.8); bone resorption can be induced by molecules from periodontal pathogens (e.g. LPS, lipoteichoic acid and surface-associated proteins).

Invasion

Microbial invasion of host tissues occurs in necrotizing ulcerative gingivitis (NUG), where there is superficial invasion of the gingival connective tissues by spirochaetes. Invasion also occurs in other forms of periodontal disease, e.g. localized aggressive periodontitis, advanced chronic periodontitis, and in HIV-associated periodontal disease. The persistence of putative pathogens such as *P. gingivalis* in health may be linked to their ability to invade host cells and survive in this privileged site, out of the reach of the host defences.

The invasion of gingival tissue by *A. actinomycetemcomitans* shows some similarities to other intracellular pathogens, such as *Shigella flexneri* and *Listeria monocytogenes*, but there are also unique features, especially with respect to cell-to-cell spread. Contact between *A. actinomycetemcomitans* and a host cell triggers effacement of the microvilli, formation of 'craters' on the host cell surface, and rearrangement of host cell actin at the site of entry. Bacteria appear to enter the host cell through ruffled apertures on the cell surface, and entry occurs in a host-derived, membrane-bound vacuole. The host-derived vacuolar membrane that initially surrounds the internalized bacterial cells soon disappears and cells of *A. actinomycetemcomitans* grow rapidly intracellularly, and spread to neighbouring cells by using host cell microtubules. These protrusions contain cells of *A. actinomycetemcomitans*, and interconnect with other host cells, enabling cell-to-cell spread of the bacteria to occur.

SUMMARY

The interaction between the developing subgingival microflora and the host's immune and inflammatory response is a critical determinant in the balance between health/tissue homeostasis and destructive periodontal disease. Bacterial enzymes, including lys-gingipain, are essential to sustain microbial growth by acquiring essential nutrients from host molecules such as haemoglobin. Tissue damage can arise via direct (e.g. the action of bacterial enzymes such as collagenase and hyaluronidase, and cytotoxic metabolites such as butyrate and ammonia) and indirect (by-stander damage due to a de-regulated host response) routes. Bacterial proteases play a critical role in the subversion of the host response. These proteases can degrade components of the host defences (immunoglobulins, complement, regulatory proteins), as well as inhibitors produced by the host to regulate host proteases involved in inflammation. Similarly, by destroying regulatory proteins, bacterial proteases can activate the kallikrein–kinin pathway that increases vascular permeability, ensuring an increased supply of nutrients into the gingival crevice. Some periodontal pathogens also evade the host defences by capsule production, or by invading epithelial cells. In this way, the balance can shift in favour of accelerated microbial growth, thereby invoking a further frustrated response by the host when trying to control the microbial assault on the subgingival tissues.

PATHOGENIC SYNERGISM AND PERIODONTAL DISEASE

One of the most consistent features of the microbiology of periodontal diseases is the isolation of complex consortia (complexes) of bacteria from diseased sites (Fig. 6.10). In particular, in chronic periodontitis, the composition of these mixtures can differ considerably both between and within studies of patients presenting with apparently similar clinical features.

For the establishment of disease, organisms must gain access to and adhere at a susceptible site, multiply, overcome or evade the host defences, and then produce or induce tissue damage (see previous section). A large number of virulence traits are needed for each stage in the disease process (Table 6.8), and it is unlikely that any single microorganism will produce all of these factors optimally or in every situation. Thus, tissue destruction is probably a result of consortia of interacting bacteria. In this way, periodontal diseases are a particularly striking example of a **polymicrobial infection,** whereby microorganisms that are individually unable to satisfy all of the requirements necessary to cause disease, combine forces to do so (**pathogenic synergism**). Thus, although only a few species (e.g. *Porphyromonas gingivalis, Treponema* spp.) produce enzymes that cause tissue damage directly, the persistence of these 'primary pathogens' in the pocket may be dependent on other organisms to provide means of attachment (e.g. receptors for coaggregation on *Streptococcus* and *Actinomyces* spp.), or essential nutrients for growth (e.g. vitamin K, protohaeme, succinate) via food webs and food chains (Ch. 5). Similarly, the bacteria that support the growth of the 'primary pathogens' may also require other organisms to suppress or inactivate the host defences, or to inhibit competing organisms (e.g. by bacteriocin production) to ensure their survival. Bacteria could also have more than one function in the aetiology of periodontal disease and a schematic diagram illustrating this pathogenic synergism is shown in Fig. 6.16. Our ability to interpret results from future microbiological studies of periodontal disease would be greatly enhanced if we knew more about the role (or niche; Ch. 1) of particular species in the disease process. In a polymicrobial infection such as periodontal disease, a microorganism could still be highly significant without necessarily having the potential to cause tissue

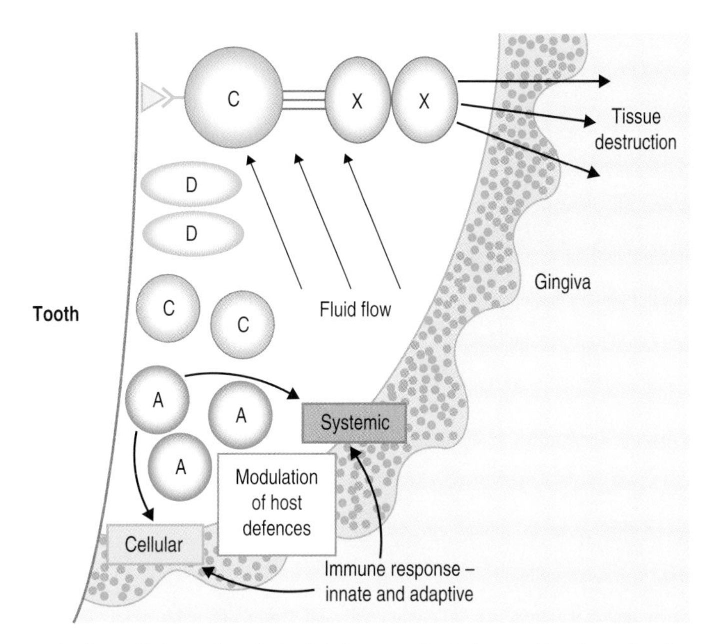

Fig. 6.16 Pathogenic synergy in the aetiology of periodontal diseases. Bacteria capable of causing tissue damage directly (e.g. species X) may be dependent on the presence of other cells (e.g. organisms C and D) for essential nutrients or attachment sites so that they can grow and resist the removal forces provided by the increased flow of GCF. Similarly, both of these groups of bacteria may be reliant for their survival on other organisms (e.g. A and C) to modulate the host defences. Individual bacteria may have more than one role (e.g. organism C) in the aetiology of disease.

destruction directly (and satisfy Koch's postulates), while in other pockets, different bacteria could fill identical roles.

AETIOLOGY OF PERIODONTAL DISEASE – CONTEMPORARY PERSPECTIVE

The predominant bacteria found in the various types of periodontal disease are different to those that are prevalent in the healthy gingival crevice. One of the most intriguing questions in periodontology, therefore, concerns the reservoir and source of these potential periodontal pathogens. Some periodontopathic bacteria can attach to mucosal surfaces, and a range of putative periodontal pathogens (including black-pigmented anaerobes, *Capnocytophaga* spp., spirochaetes and *Fusobacterium* spp., etc) can be isolated from the dorsum of the tongue and from tonsils. Recently, *P. gingivalis*, *T. forsythia* and *A. actinomycetemcomitans* were detected in 23%, 11% and 30%, respectively, of tongue samples from young children. Most species were detected more frequently from tongue rather than plaque samples, confirming that the tongue may act as a reservoir for these periodontal pathogens. Some pathogens may also persist by invading buccal epithelial cells (Fig. 4.6).

In general, the putative periodontal pathogens are non-competitive with other members of the resident subgingival microflora at healthy sites, and remain at low levels; such levels would not be clinically significant. If plaque is allowed to accumulate beyond levels that are compatible with health, then the host mounts an inflammatory response. The flow of GCF is increased, and this introduces into the crevice not only components of the host defences but also complex host molecules (e.g. transferrin, haemoglobin, etc.) that can be catabolized and used as a nutrient source by the proteolytic Gram negative anaerobes that predominate in advanced periodontal lesions. This metabolism leads to an increase in local pH and a fall in the redox potential (i.e. the pocket becomes slightly alkaline and more anaerobic). These changes in the local environment will up-regulate some of the virulence factors associated with these putative pathogens (e.g. protease activity by *P. gingivalis*), and favour their growth at the expense of the species associated with gingival health (i.e. increase the competitiveness of the potential pathogens). This can lead to a shift in the proportions of the resident subgingival microflora (Fig. 6.1). This is analogous to the increases in mutans streptococci and *Lactobacillus* spp. seen prior to caries development following the repeated ingestion of dietary carbohydrates.

Evidence for these bacterial population shifts has come from laboratory studies. The growth of subgingival plaque on human serum (used to mimic GCF) led to the selection of species associated with periodontal destruction, such as black-pigmented anaerobes, anaerobic streptococci, *Fusobacterium* spp. and spirochaetes; most of these species could not be detected in the original samples. Likewise, in the laboratory, a rise in pH from 7.0 to 7.5 (as can occur during inflammation) allowed the proportions of *P. gingivalis* to rise from <1% to >99% of a microbial community of black-pigmented anaerobes. If similar events occur in a pocket, then periodontal diseases can be regarded as endogenous infections, caused by an imbalance in the composition of the resident microflora at a site, due to an alteration in the ecology of the local habitat. This view is formulated in the '**ecological plaque hypothesis**', which describes the dynamic relationship between the resident microflora and the host in health and disease in ecological terms (Fig. 6.17). A consequence of this hypothesis is that disease can be prevented not only by targeting the putative pathogens, but also by interfering with the environmental factors that drive the changes in the balance in the microflora, e.g. such as by reducing the severity of the inflammatory response, or by altering the redox potential of the pocket to prevent the growth of the obligate anaerobes. Other relevant changes in the local environment that could perturb the host-microbe balance could come from trauma, an alteration in the immune status of the host (e.g. during systemic disease or after drug therapy), or from tobacco smoking.

Transmission of *P. gingivalis* and *A. actinomycetemcomitans* can occur among family members, with parents and children sharing identical strains. Likewise, some married couples have the same clonal types of *P. gingivalis* and *A. actinomycetemcomitans* indicating that these species can be transmitted between spouses (Ch. 4). Therefore, treatment might also require elimination or suppression of putative periodontal pathogens from their primary oral reservoirs. However, even if a pathogen is acquired from another individual, it will be present initially at only low cell levels. As described earlier, a major ecological disturbance will have to occur at a site if these putative pathogens are going to be able to out-compete the other members of the plaque microflora, and achieve numerical dominance and clinical significance (Fig. 6.11).

Destructive disease is the outcome of a complex interplay of interactions between the host and the altered microbial challenge (Fig. 6.18). This interplay can be considered to occur between several discrete, interactive compartments: (a) the microbial challenge, (b) the immune and inflammatory response of the host, and (c) connective tissue and bone metabolism. These interactions are influenced by disease modifiers, which may be genetic (e.g. neutrophil defects) or environmental (e.g. tobacco smoking) factors. The clinical signs reflect the sum of these interactions, and the severity of the disease can feed back to influence the microbial challenge,

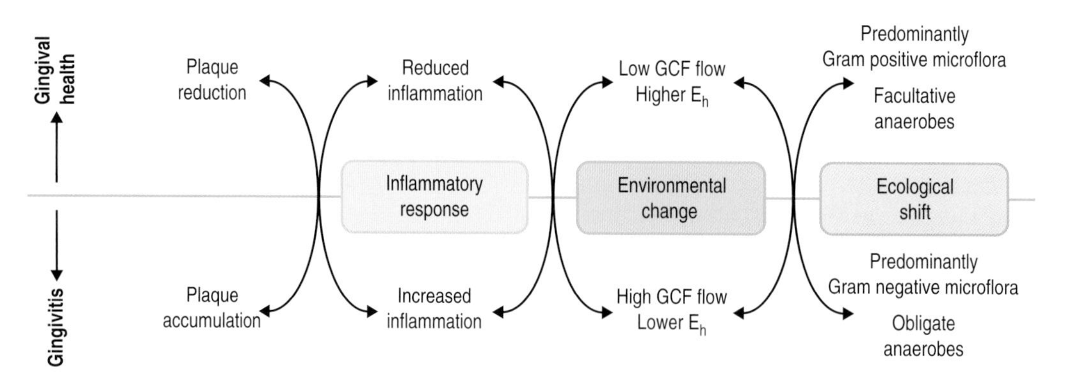

Fig. 6.17 A schematic representation of the 'ecological plaque hypothesis' in relation to periodontal disease. Plaque accumulation produces an inflammatory host response; this causes changes in the local environmental conditions which favour the growth of proteolytic and anaerobic Gram negative bacteria. Disease could be prevented by not only targeting the putative pathogens, but also by interfering with the factors driving their selection.

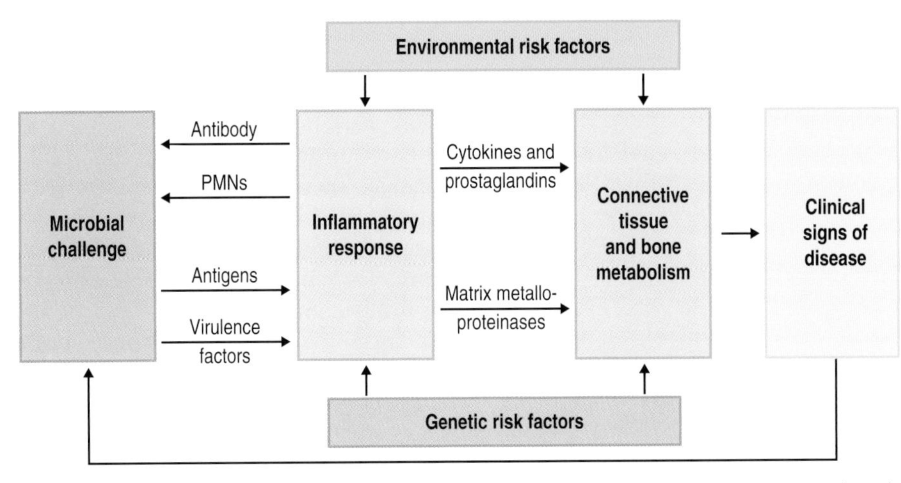

Fig. 6.18 A schematic representation of the interrelationships between the host and dental plaque in periodontal disease.

as described above in the 'ecological plaque hypothesis' (altered pH, increased supply of nutrients). The bacteria most adapted to the changing environmental conditions will be selected and, as described in an earlier section, this can lead to the up-regulation of virulence factor production (e.g. arg-gingipains). In this way, there is **a continual spiralling escalation of the inflammatory challenge followed by an increasingly more destructive host response**.

At the boundary of the microbe and host response compartments, the microbial challenge is countered by the innate and adaptive immune response. The outcome of this confrontation is the critical determinant in determining whether the microbial challenge will be contained, or whether destructive disease will ensue. An effective host response can control plaque, although this might manifest itself as mild inflammation to the gingivae, but there is no permanent soft or hard tissue destruction. In contrast, a subverted or de-regulated response will influence the signalling pathways between the immune and inflammatory compartment and that of the connective tissue and bone metabolism compartment (Fig. 6.18). Increases in locally acting inflammatory mediators may activate host cells (stromal cells), which in turn stimulate the production of host matrix metalloproteinases and other components of the tissue remodelling machinery. Ultimately, this can lead to the development of a deep periodontal pocket, destruction of the supporting connective tissue, and, eventually, to loss of bone.

SUMMARY

Periodontal diseases are the result of the complex interplay between the host and the subgingival microflora. If plaque mass increases beyond levels compatible with health, the host mounts an inflammatory response. If this response is insufficient to control plaque, then previously minor components of the subgingival microbial community can be enriched due to the resultant changes in the pocket environment (e.g. increased supply of proteinaceous nutrients in GCF; rise in pH; fall in redox potential). The emerging proteolytic microflora can deregulate the inflammatory response, resulting in re-modelling of the subgingival tissues, which can eventually lead to pocket formation and bone loss. Treatment focuses on plaque removal, or on altering the pocket environment to suppress pathogen growth.

PREDICTORS OF DISEASE ACTIVITY

The increased understanding of the complex interactions that exist between host cells and the subgingival microflora has raised the possibility that markers or predictors of disease activity might exist that are more sensitive than existing crude indices, such as changes in probing depth. Some of these have been discussed in various sections throughout this Chapter, and include:

(a) sensitive and rapid tests for detecting putative pathogens (e.g. using immunological or oligonucleotide probes in a variety of formats). Given the polymicrobial nature of the microbial challenge, it is likely that 'complexes' of implicated bacteria may need to be measured to indicate the risk of a site to suffer from destructive disease. In the future, DNA microarrays that are capable of rapidly detecting the full complement of the oral microflora in health and disease (i.e. >700 taxa) may be used to determine the profile of culturable and non-culturable microorganisms at any site. The probes used in these microarrays can be spotted on to microscope slides, and read by automated scanners.

(b) detection of selected enzymes in subgingival plaque or in GCF. Synthetic substrates can be degraded to a coloured product by 'diagnostic' enzymes of microbial or host origin. For example, benzoyl arginine naphthylamine (BANA) is hydrolyzed by the arginine-specific proteases produced by *P. gingivalis*, *T. forsythia* and *T. denticola*, and has been incorporated into a rapid diagnostic kit. This test has been shown to be highly sensitive and specific at detecting enzyme activity, and in clinical studies, the test was capable of predicting sites at risk of attachment loss.

(c) detection of inflammatory mediators or tissue breakdown products in GCF. Paper strips can collect GCF from control and inflamed sites, and host enzymes can be measured (e.g. metallo-proteinases such as collagenase; cysteine proteinases such as cathepsin; serine proteinases including elastase); for example, levels of aspartate aminotransferase have correlated with gingival inflammation. Commercial chair-side tests are being developed to measure some of these enzymes. Tissue degradation products, including glycosaminoglycans, as well as prostaglandins and cytokines, could also be measured in GCF.

Such tests could help with the diagnosis of a site, the monitoring of treatment, or possibly predict those sites at risk of future breakdown. The use of these tests will require an understanding of the biological basis of the test, and the data obtained will be complex and need careful interpretation.

PERIODONTAL HEALTH AND GENERAL HEALTH

Evidence suggests that an association exists between periodontal disease and the general health of an individual, particularly with respect to cardiovascular and respiratory diseases, diabetes mellitus and a risk of pre-term labour and low birth weight infants. The hypothesis to explain this association is as follows. Periodontal diseases represent an inflammatory response by the host to the build up of dental plaque; these subgingival biofilms contain large numbers of Gram negative species which (a) possess LPS and other potentially inflammatory cell surface components, and (b) shed toxic metabolites and other molecules, which induce prostaglandins and pro-inflammatory cytokines. The periodontium has a large surface area for contact between the host and the subgingival microflora, and, because it is so vascular, this site can act as a potential systemic source of inflammatory mediators which could affect distant sites in the body.

Oral microorganisms, including periodontal pathogens, can enter the blood stream during transient bacteraemias, where they may play a role in systemic disease. The link between oral bacteria (especially streptococci) and infective endocarditis (Ch. 8) is irrefutable, but research has also suggested that periodontal bacteria may be an added risk factor for cardiovascular disease. Several microorganisms, including *Chlamydia pneumoniae* and cytomegalovirus, have been implicated in the infectious aetiology of atherosclerosis. Molecular techniques have also detected DNA from oral Gram negative bacteria in nearly half of the atheromatous plaques that have been sampled in some studies. The bacteria detected included *T. forsythia*, *P. gingivalis*, *P. intermedia* and *A. actinomycetemcomitans* but further research is needed in this area. Similarly, microorganisms associated with periodontal diseases may give rise to aspiration pneumonia in susceptible patients since anaerobic bacteria found in periodontal pockets have been isolated from infected lungs.

Some recent human epidemiological studies and animal experiments have demonstrated that periodontal diseases could represent a previously unrecognised and clinically significant risk factor for pre-term labour or low birth weight babies. This could be either as a direct consequence of pre-term labour or due to premature rupture of membranes, although this has not been confirmed in all population groups. In some studies that did find an association, elevated levels of *T. forsythia* were reported in the plaque of women with pre-term, low birth weight babies compared with women with normal births. Elevated levels of prostaglandins have also been found in the GCF of mothers with pre-term, low birth weight babies.

In this important clinical area, there is a need for further large, well-controlled investigations in diverse but homogeneous population groups, in which the statistical analyses are adequately adjusted for other life-style confounding risk factors (smoking, alcohol consumption, maternal education, etc). Longitudinal, prospective studies are also needed to determine whether the observed periodontal disease is causal for these medical sequelae. The outcome of intervention studies, in which the impact of periodontal treatment on the subsequent development of systemic disease is monitored, will be crucial in confirming the impact of oral disease on general health.

FURTHER READING – PERIODONTAL DISEASE

Aas JA, Barbuto SM, Alpagot T et al 2007 Subgingival plaque microbiota in HIV positive patients. J Clin Periodontol 34:189-195.

Booth V, Downes J, van den Berg J, Wade WG 2004 Gram-positive anaerobic bacilli in human periodontal disease. J Periodont Res 39:213-220.

Curtis MA, Slaney JM, Aduse-Opoku J 2005 Critical pathways in microbial virulence. J Clin Periodontol 32 (Suppl 6) 28-38.

Demmer RT, Desvarieux M 2006 Periodontal infections and cardiovascular disease: the heart of the matter. J Am Dent Assoc 137(suppl)14S-20S.

Eley BM, Manson JD 2004 Periodontics, 5th edn. Wright, Oxford.

Haubek D, Ennibi O-K, Poulsen K, Vaeth M, Poulsen S, Kilian M 2008 Risk of aggressive periodontitis in adolescent carriers of the JP2 clone of *Aggregatibacter (Actinobacillus) actinomycetemcomitans* in Morocco: a prospective longitudinal cohort study. Lancet 371(9608):237-242.

Kilian M, Frandsen EVG, Haubek D, Poulsen K 2006 The etiology of periodontal disease revisited by population genetic analysis. Periodontol 2000 42:158-179.

Lamster IB, Ahlo JK 2007 Analysis of gingival crevicular fluid as applied to the diagnosis of oral and systemic diseases. Ann N Y Acad Sci 1098:216-229.

Nishihara T, Koseki T 2004 Microbial etiology of periodontitis. Periodontology 2000 36:14-26.

Paster BJ, Bosches SK, Galvin JL et al 2001 Bacterial diversity in human subgingival plaque. J Bact 183:3770-3783.

Paster BJ, Falkler WA Jr, Enwonwu CO 2002 Prevalent bacterial species and novel phylotypes in advanced noma lesions. J Clin Microbiol 40:2187-2191.

Paquette DW, Brodala N, Nichols TC 2007 Cardiovascular disease, inflammation, and periodontal infection. Periodontol 2000 44:113-126.

Raghavendran K, Mylotte JM, Scannapieco FA 2007 Nursing home-associated pneumonia, hospital acquired pneumonia and ventilator-associated pneumonia: the contribution of dental biofilms and periodontal inflammation. Periodontol 2000 44:164-177.

Slots J 2007 Herpes viral-bacterial synergy in the pathogenesis of human periodontitis. Curr Opin Infect Dis 20:278-283.

Socransky SS, Haffajee AD 2005 Periodontal microbial ecology. Periodontology 2000 38:135-187.

Tanner ACR, Izard J 2006 *Tannerella forsythia*, a periodontal pathogen entering the genomic era. Periodontology 2000 42:88-113.

Vergnes JN, Sixou M 2007 Preterm low birth weight and maternal periodontal status: a meta analysis. Am J Obstet Gynecol 196:135.e1-7.

Approaches for controlling plaque-mediated diseases

Mechanical removal of plaque by efficient oral hygiene procedures can almost completely prevent plaque-mediated diseases. Plaque control can be achieved by conventional oral hygiene measures such as toothbrushing and flossing, which can be augmented by professional prophylaxis during routine visits to the dentist. Plaque control is fundamental to the prevention of gingivitis and in the maintenance of health following effective treatment. In chronic periodontitis, debridement of the root surfaces is the most effective routine approach for plaque control, although it is not possible to completely remove all of the attached microorganisms. In aggressive periodontitis, root planing may be supplemented with adjunctive systemic antimicrobial agents (see later). For caries, plaque control measures are particularly effective when combined with a reduction in the amount and frequency of sugar intake. It is difficult to alter established eating habits and to maintain a high degree of motivation for effective oral hygiene. Alternative preventive measures for caries and periodontal diseases are under development that require little cooperation from the public.

FISSURE SEALANTS

Occlusal pits and fissures are the most caries-prone areas of the human dentition. Strongly adherent, self-polymerizing and UV-light polymerizing plastic sealant materials have been applied to fissures as a barrier against microbial attack. The long-term retention of these materials in the mouth can be problematical.

FLUORIDE

It has been known for many decades that fluoride in the water supply can significantly reduce the incidence of caries. The caries benefit of fluoride was established from epidemiological surveys that showed a reduced caries incidence in certain geographical locations; the factor that correlated with protection was the natural fluoride content of the water supply. The optimum concentration for maximal protection against caries is approximately 1 part per million (1 ppm), but in some water supplies it occurs naturally at higher concentrations. Fluoride is also found in tea and in the bones of fish (especially soft-boned sardines and salmon). Excessive exposure to fluoride can cause fluorosis, which in extreme cases results in discolouration of teeth. Despite its proven value in decreasing caries incidence, the addition of fluoride to drinking water remains a controversial and emotive issue. Consequently, fluoride has been used to supplement other commodities (e.g. table salt, milk, toothpastes), so consumers can have a choice as to whether they want to gain further caries benefit. Fluoride can also be used in mouthwashes and gels for topical use, and in tablets for supplementation of the systemic effect, and has also been incorporated into topical varnishes and slow-release capsules. High concentrations of fluoride are used to treat caries-vulnerable groups, including xerostomic and disabled patients.

The precise mechanisms behind the anti-caries mechanisms of fluoride are still the subject of much debate. The original studies concluded that fluoride needed to be present pre-eruptively, so as to be incorporated into developing teeth. More recent evidence suggests that fluoride functions post-eruptively by favourably influencing the kinetics of de- and remineralization. Thus, fluoride can exert its effect on erupted teeth both topically (e.g. following the use of fluoridated toothpastes) and systemically after ingestion (e.g. via fluoridated water or milk). Low levels of fluoride appear in oral fluids (saliva, GCF) and interact with the surface of the enamel of erupted teeth to form fluorapatite. Fluorapatite is thermodynamically more stable than apatite and resists acid dissolution to a greater extent than hydroxyapatite.

Fluoride can also inhibit the metabolism of plaque bacteria (Ch. 4, Fig. 6.19) thereby affecting their competitiveness especially at low pH. Under acidic conditions, fluoride exists as HF, which is lipophilic and is able to easily cross bacterial membranes. The intracellular pH of bacteria is alkaline with respect to the extracellular pH; therefore, once inside the cell HF will dissociate and H^+ will acidify the cytoplasm and:

(1) inhibit various enzymes with pH optima near neutrality,

(2) reduce the transmembrane pH gradient, thereby affecting some uptake and secretion processes,

while F^- will:

(3) reduce glycolysis by direct inhibition of enolase,

(4) indirectly inhibit sugar transport by blocking the production of PEP for the PTS system, and

(5) inhibit the synthesis of intracellular storage (IPS) compounds, especially glycogen.

Dental plaque has been found to concentrate fluoride from ingested water. In areas where the concentration of fluoride in the water supply is low, dental plaque has been found to contain 5 to 10 ppm. In water supplies supplemented with 1 ppm fluoride, concentrations of up to 190 ppm have been found in dental plaque. Much of this fluoride is bound to organic components in plaque, but there is also evidence that it can be released when the pH falls, and be bioavailable to interfere with acid production by plaque bacteria. The sensitivity of oral bacteria to fluoride increases as the pH falls, so that concentrations of fluoride that are ineffective at resting pH values can be inhibitory at pH 5.0 or below. Mutans streptococci are particularly sensitive to low levels of fluoride at a moderately low environmental pH. Although surveys have failed to detect major changes in the qualitative and quantitative composition of plaque in humans residing in places with high or low natural levels of fluoride in the drinking water, fluoride is more likely to function prophylactically in these circumstances. Thus, mutans streptococci would be suppressed in plaque under conditions when they would otherwise be expected to flourish; the rate of change of pH in plaque following sugar metabolism would also be diminished.

Laboratory evidence supports this hypothesis; in a mixed culture system, *S. mutans* remained a minor component of plaque (<1% of the cultivable microflora) during glucose pulsing in the presence of 10 or 20 ppm sodium fluoride when, under similar circumstances but in the absence of fluoride, it had previously attained levels of around 20% of the microflora. Fluoride inhibited acid production from the glucose pulses so that the environmental pH did not fall as low or as fast. This influence on metabolism and pH will nullify the expected competitiveness that aciduric bacteria such as *S. mutans* and lactobacilli normally experience after sugar intake, relative to organisms associated with enamel health. Studies have shown that sufficient fluoride to affect the growth and metabolism of *S. mutans* can be released by acid attack from a fluoride-containing surface. Thus, fluoride can serve to stabilize the composition of the plaque microflora, a preventative mechanism which is consistent with the ecological plaque hypothesis. This antimicrobial effect can be enhanced by changing the counter-ion; thus, stannous fluoride is markedly more inhibitory to oral bacteria than sodium fluoride. Other antimicrobial agents will be discussed in the next section.

In the laboratory, mutans streptococci can eventually adapt to, and tolerate, even relatively high levels of fluoride. Concern has been expressed as to whether organisms might become resistant to fluoride due to the prolonged use of fluoride-containing toothpastes. Laboratory studies have shown that fluoride-tolerance reduces the acidogenicity and cariogenicity of mutans streptococci, so that even if adaptation occurs, there would be little increase in caries risk.

ANTIMICROBIAL AGENTS

For many individuals, it is difficult to maintain plaque at levels compatible with health by oral hygiene alone over prolonged periods. Consequently, the use of antimicrobial agents (not including antibiotics) to augment mechanical plaque control has been advocated for a number of years. These agents can be formulated into oral care products such as toothpastes and mouthrinses; they have been shown to reduce plaque, and some have anti-caries and anti-gingivitis benefits. The relatively short contact time between the inhibitor delivered from the product and the mouth dictates that it is essential that the agents bind effectively to oral surfaces, especially mucosal tissues (because of their large surface area); this property is termed **substantivity**. Once adsorbed, such inhibitors are released slowly from these 'reservoirs' back into the oral environment (especially saliva), from where they can be re-distributed around the mouth. In this way, effective agents can reduce the growth or metabolism of microorganisms for prolonged periods even at sub-MIC (sub-lethal) concentrations (Fig. 6.19). Some

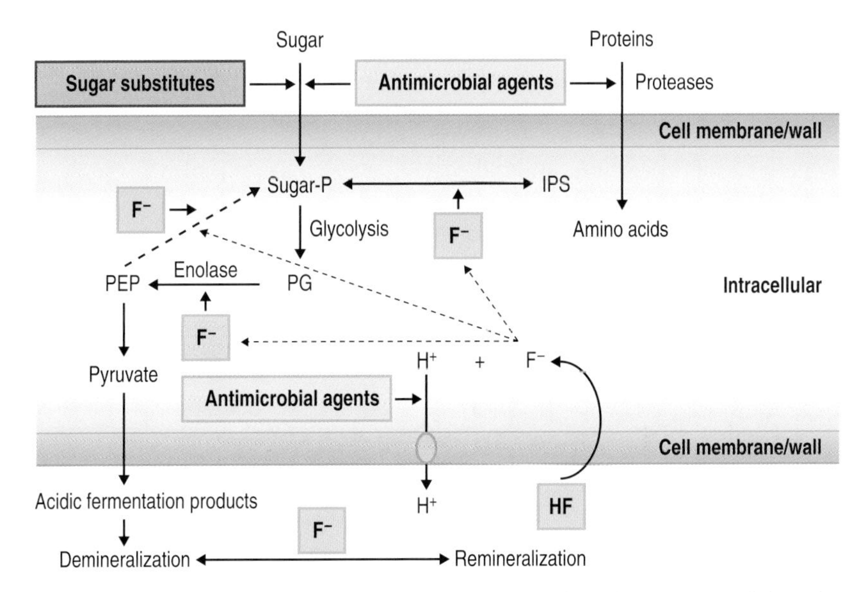

Fig. 6.19 The site of action of some classes of inhibitors used in dentistry. F = fluoride; IPS = intracellular polysaccharide; PG = phosphoglycerate; PEP = phosphoenolpyruvate

Table 6.9 Classes and examples of inhibitors used as antimicrobial agents in mouthwashes and toothpastes

Class of inhibitor	Examples
Bisbiguanide	Chlorhexidine, alexidine
Enzymes	Mutanase, glucanase; amyloglucosidase-glucose oxidase
'Essential oils'	Thymol, eucalyptol
Metal ions	Copper, zinc, stannous
Natural molecules	Plant extracts (apigenin, *tt*-farnesol)
Phenols	Triclosan
Quaternary ammonium compounds	Cetylpyridinium chloride
Surfactants	Sodium lauryl sulphate

products are anti-plaque rather than antimicrobial, e.g. they detach plaque without necessarily killing the microorganisms in the biofilm. Some examples of antimicrobial agents that have been successfully formulated into oral care products are listed in Table 6.9. Some agents that are used in mouthrinses cannot be formulated into toothpastes because of compatibility issues with other components of the dentifrice.

The most effective antimicrobial agent for oral use to date is chlorhexidine, which can be successfully formulated into a mouthrinse. This bisbiguanide has a broad spectrum of activity against yeasts, fungi, and a wide range of Gram positive and Gram negative bacteria. Chlorhexidine can reduce plaque, caries, and gingivitis in humans; it is not recommended for prolonged use because of side-effects such as staining of teeth and mucosal irritation. At high concentrations, chlorhexidine is bactericidal and acts as a detergent by damaging the cell membrane. Chlorhexidine is substantive, and is bound to oral surfaces from where it is released gradually into saliva over many hours at bacteriostatic concentrations. At these sublethal concentrations, chlorhexidine can still:

(1) abolish the activity of the PTS sugar transport system (Ch. 4) and thereby markedly inhibit acid production in streptococci;

(2) inhibit amino acid uptake and catabolism in some streptococci (e.g. *S. sanguinis*);

(3) inhibit a major protease (arg-gingipain) of *Porphyromonas gingivalis*, and

(4) affect various membrane functions, including the ATP-synthase and the maintenance of ion gradients in streptococci (Fig. 6.19).

Mutans streptococci are more sensitive to chlorhexidine than other oral streptococci, and this property has been exploited in those people at high risk of developing caries. Levels of mutans streptococci in the mouth have been reduced by the use of chlorhexidine mouthrinses while other oral streptococci, such as *S. sanguinis* (associated more with enamel health), were relatively unaffected. This approach has also been applied successfully to expectant mothers. The suppression of mutans streptococci in mothers reduced the transmission of these potentially cariogenic organisms to the baby and delayed the onset of caries. Chlorhexidine can be delivered either by gel (e.g. as a 1% gel in a custom-fitted vinyl applicator), as a mouthrinse, or as a varnish. Combinations of chlorhexidine with other agents such as fluoride or thymol in varnishes has resulted in additive or synergistic benefits, for example, in preventing caries in high risk patients such as those receiving radiation therapy for head and neck cancer. In these patients, the radiation therapy affects the salivary glands, and the reduced saliva flow is conducive to rampant caries.

Triclosan is the most commonly used antimicrobial agent in toothpastes. Triclosan has a broad spectrum of antimicrobial activity against yeasts and a wide range of Gram positive and Gram negative bacteria. However, under conditions of use in the mouth (i.e. high concentrations – short contact time; low concentrations – longer contact time), Triclosan has a more selective antimicrobial profile, and preferably inhibits the obligately anaerobic, Gram negative species that are prevalent in periodontal disease. Like chlorhexidine, Triclosan is substantive and multi-functional in its mode of action. At sub-MIC concentrations, it can inhibit acid production by streptococci and protease (arg-gingipain) activity by *P. gingivalis*. Triclosan can also reduce inflammation and the development of new aphthous ulcers in sufferers. The activity of Triclosan has been enhanced by combining it with either a copolymer to boost its oral retention, or with zinc citrate as a complementary antimicrobial agent. Zinc ions are also substantive and can inhibit sugar transport, acid production, and protease activity. There have been concerns raised over the widespread use of Triclosan. This compound has been found to accumulate in environmental samples, while repeated exposure to Triclosan has been linked with increased resistance of some microorganisms to important antibiotics.

Enzymes and essential oils have also been included in toothpastes. Examples include dextranases and glucanases (from fungi) to modify the plaque matrix and reduce plaque formation (Ch. 5), and glucose oxidase and amyloglucosidase to boost the activity of the salivary peroxidase (sialoperoxidase) system (Ch. 2). Essential oils (menthol, thymol, eucalyptol, etc) have been successfully formulated into a mouthwash and shown to penetrate plaque biofilms. Regular use of a mouthwash containing essential oils can reduce plaque and gingivitis over a six month period in clinical trials, and also reduce halitosis. The oils function by disrupting bacterial cell membranes and inhibiting key enzymes. Plant extracts with antiplaque and anti-metabolism activity have also been formulated into oral care products. New molecules have been discovered such as apigenin and *tt*-farnesol that can inhibit glucan synthesis and acid production by mutans streptococci; combinations of these new molecules with fluoride have additive anti-caries effects in rodent models. Inhibitors of mineralization, such as polyphosphonates, zinc salts, and pyrophosphates, can reduce calculus formation (Ch. 5).

Potentially, the regular, unsupervised use of antimicrobial agents from toothpastes and mouthrinses could lead to the disruption of the ecology of the oral microflora by either (a) perturbing the balance among the resident organisms, which might lead to the overgrowth by potentially more pathogenic species; or (b) the development of resistance. Guidelines are now laid down to ensure that manufacturers perform long-term clinical trials to confirm that these eventualities do not occur. The reason why oral care products containing antimicrobial agents are able to deliver clinical benefit without unduly disturbing the resident microflora of the mouth is probably due to the active agents functioning in a selective manner under the conditions of use (short contact time; increased tolerance of biofilms to inhibitors; Ch. 5) in the oral cavity (e.g. Triclosan preferentially inhibits anaerobes rather than the whole microflora).

In more advanced forms of periodontal disease, treatment requires professional plaque control which in some circumstances may require surgery so that clear access to the root surface is achieved. In extreme cases, not only is there a need to remove plaque and/or calculus, but also the outer surface layers of cementum (root planing), because of the possible penetration into cementum of cytotoxic or inflammatory products of subgingival bacteria, especially endotoxin (lipopolysaccharide, LPS). Even after thorough root planing to remove obvious deposits of plaque and calculus, residual bacteria may still be present, and sites can be re-populated rapidly leading to further loss of attachment in some pockets. Consequently, post-surgical control of microorganisms is sometimes necessary. This again can involve meticulous supragingival plaque control (to reduce the likelihood of subgingival colonization) or the use of antimicrobial agents, such as chlorhexidine, or even systemic antibiotics, such as tetracycline, amoxycillin or metronidazole. Antibiotics should only be used in special circumstances, such as some forms of aggressive periodontitis or in refractory periodontal disease, because of the global problems of antibiotic resistance. A potential strategy to treat periodontal pockets is to locally apply antimicrobial agents such as chlorhexidine, metronidazole and tetracycline. This can be by hollow fibres impregnated with the drug of choice, by direct irrigation of the pocket, or by inserting slow release materials. Mixed culture biofilms such as dental plaque are less susceptible to the action of antimicrobial agents than the same species grown singly in planktonic culture (Ch. 5; Table 5.4).

SUGAR SUBSTITUTES

Most humans enjoy and prefer to eat sweet substances. Unfortunately, many sweet foods are composed of mono- or disaccharides which are easily metabolized by plaque bacteria to acids and glucans, thereby predisposing teeth to dental caries. The use of inert (non-metabolizable) dietary sweeteners has been proposed to satisfy the human preference for sweet substances without causing caries. These sugar substitutes function by stimulating saliva flow in the absence of a significant acid challenge to enamel; indeed, the use of these agents can sometimes lead to the remineralization of enamel.

Artificial sweeteners are of two types: (a) the intense type many times sweeter than sucrose, and (b) the bulk agents which are usually not as sweet. The intense sweeteners include cyclamate, aspartame and saccharin, and are used in drinks. These sweeteners have some weak antimicrobial effects, with aspartame and saccharin being capable of inhibiting bacterial growth. The bulk agents, e.g. polyols such as sorbitol and xylitol, are not as sweet as sucrose, but cannot be metabolized by the majority of plaque bacteria and are used in the confectionery industry. Other polyols include mannitol, lactitol, Lycasin® (a mixture of sorbitol, mannitol, maltotriitol, and polysaccharide alcohols), and Palatinit® (a mixture of two 12-carbon polyols). Some of these polyols have been incorporated into sugar-free chewing gums; the use of these products three or more times a day can reduce the incidence of caries, by reducing the frequency of acid attack on the enamel (Fig. 2.3) and by stimulating saliva flow, thereby encouraging remineralization. Xylitol has been claimed to be superior to other sugar alcohols because of its effect on bacterial metabolism. Xylitol is transported into cells of mutans streptococci by the fructose-PTS (Fig. 4.10) where it enters a 'futile cycle' of phosphorylation, dephosphorylation and eventual expulsion. Xylitol interferes with sugar metabolism of mutans streptococci by consuming PEP and NAD^+ during the 'futile cycle' and competitively inhibiting glycolysis at the phosphofructokinase level. This futile cycle reduces the rate of growth and acid production (from exogenous sugars such as glucose) of cells, and leads to reduced levels of both mutans streptococci and caries in habitual users of xylitol-containing confectionery. The use of sugar substitutes is consistent with the 'ecological plaque hypothesis', since the prevention of periods of low pH in plaque during between meal periods would remove opportunities for the preferential growth of acid-tolerating bacteria.

FUTURE DIRECTIONS

Replacement therapy and probiotics

The possibility that antagonistic microorganisms could be exploited to control pathogens and prevent disease has been proposed for over 100 years, and is termed 'replacement therapy'. A major potential benefit of this approach is that it could provide life-long protection with minimal cost or compliance on behalf of the recipient once colonization by an 'effector' strain has been achieved. There are two main approaches: (a) pre-emptive colonization, where key ecological niches (functions) within plaque are filled by a harmless or beneficial organism before the undesirable strain has had a chance to colonize or become established. The initial colonizer becomes integrated into the ecosystem and subsequently excludes the pathogen. Low-virulence mutants of mutans streptococci have been produced that are deficient in GTF or intracellular polysaccharide production, or which lack lactate dehydrogenase activity, and which are designed to prevent subsequent colonization by 'wild-type' mutans streptococci. Similarly, genes encoding for alkali production are being cloned into acidogenic bacteria in order to reduce the acid challenge to enamel. An alternative approach is to (b) derive a more competitive strain that would displace a pre-existing organism from plaque. This strategy has the advantage that it is not dependent on treatment with the 'effector' strain at or before colonization by the undesirable organism. Examples of strains that have been designed for this role include *S. salivarius* (strain TOVE-R), which has been shown to displace *S. mutans* from the teeth of rats and to inhibit caries. This strategy is being evaluated in human trials using a strain of *S. mutans* that cannot make acid (lactate dehydrogenase has been replaced with alcohol dehydrogenase) and which produces a bacteriocin active against wild-type strains. Assurances over the safety of such 'effector' strains will be required by both the authorities and by the public.

Probiotics are live microorganisms which, when administered in adequate numbers, confer a health benefit on the host. Probiotics are proving popular with consumers in improving gastric health, and are now being considered for applications in oral care.

Active and passive vaccination

The oral cavity is provided with all of the components necessary to mount an effective immune response against microorganisms (Ch. 2). While the microbial aetiology of dental diseases is not totally specific, evidence implicates certain organisms as major causative bacteria in both caries and advanced periodontal disease. This has led to the proposal of using **active vaccination** to provide life-long protection against these diseases, with most progress being made on developing a caries vaccine.

A vaccine against dental caries using mutans streptococci (whole cell vaccines), or molecules derived from these bacteria (sub-unit vaccines), has been proposed for many decades. Early studies used crude whole cell preparations of *S. mutans* to protect animals. Although protection against caries and a reduction in the levels of mutans streptococci was achieved, concern was expressed over possible immunologically-mediated tissue damage in humans following exposure to streptococcal antigens (as occurs in, for example, rheumatic fever). Subsequent work has been directed towards characterizing the antigenic composition of mutans streptococci and selecting individual purified antigens that will confer protection but lack any potential for human tissue cross-reactivity. Three protein antigens have received most attention; these are (a) adhesins known as the Antigen I/II family (also referred to as antigen B, P1, SpaP, Pac, SpaA, Pag), (b) the glucosyltransferases (GTFs; Ch. 4), and (c) glucan-binding proteins. Early approaches used parenteral injection, but the main focus now is to develop strategies that engage the mucosal immune system by using oral or intra-nasal routes of vaccination. To this end, vaccines might be delivered with liposomes, mucosal adjuvants, or by bacterial vectors. Sub-unit vaccines have been shown to induce salivary secretory IgA and circulating IgG antibodies to antigens of mutans streptococci, and these are capable of reducing (a) colonization by these cariogenic bacteria, and (b) the number of caries lesions. Small scale human trials have confirmed the ability of putative vaccines to increase levels of specific sIgA antibodies to mutans streptococci in saliva and to delay their subsequent recolonization.

A major issue for the introduction of a caries vaccine will centre around the risk-benefit analyses. There have been no major field trials to assess their efficacy in humans even though potential vaccines against mutans streptococci have already been manufactured to standards that satisfy the legislative authorities. This is because the incidence of caries has fallen dramatically in most industrialized societies during the time of the development of these vaccines, probably as a result of fluoride, while the public acceptance of mass-vaccination programmes can be poor, even for serious medical infections. A major question facing health organisations is whether a vaccine is justified against a non-life threatening disease? It might be that vaccination could be considered of benefit to particular high-risk groups in the population.

Periodontal diseases represent an even more complex microbial challenge in terms of vaccination. The elevated levels of *P. gingivalis* in advanced forms of periodontitis have led some groups to investigate the feasibility of developing a vaccine against this organism. Pilot studies in animal models, using intact killed whole cells or proteases as the vaccine candidate, have shown reduced bone loss, although the microbial challenge consisted only of *P. gingivalis*. It remains to be determined whether such vaccines would have clinical benefit in a more realistic setting, involving a polymicrobial infection.

A development arising from the studies on vaccination is the concept of using pre-existing antibodies (**passive immunization**) to control putative pathogens. When the natural levels of mutans streptococci in the mouth were suppressed by chlorhexidine, the topical application to teeth of monoclonal antibodies directed against antigen I/II was shown to prevent subsequent recolonization by mutans streptococci in humans for up to 100 days, and protect against caries in primates. Similarly, bovine anti-mutans streptococci antibodies fed to germ-free rats significantly reduced colonization by *S. mutans* and *S. sobrinus*, as well as caries on buccal, sulcal and approximal surfaces; specific monoclonal antibodies also reduced colonization of rats by *S. sobrinus*. Transgenic plants have been genetically-engineered to produce a monoclonal secretory antibody with specificity for antigen I/II of mutans streptococci. The dimeric nature of this antibody enabled it to persist intact for longer periods in the mouth than the parent antibody. Application to human volunteers from whom indigenous mutans streptococci had been cleared, prevented recolonization by *S. mutans* for up to four months. Similar benefits have been reported following the use of monoclonal antibodies targeted against *P. gingivalis*. This approach has many advantages, not least being the reduction of any of the risks (however small) that are associated with active vaccination. Antibodies could be generated against a wider number of putative pathogens, and they could be applied by dental professionals at regular intervals as part of routine visits to the dentist. In the future, this could form the basis of a novel approach to maintaining dental plaque with a microbial composition that is compatible with oral health.

Photodynamic therapy, redox and anti-inflammatory agents

Other novel approaches to controlling pathogens in plaque may involve photodynamic therapy or redox agents. Periodontal pathogens, including *P. gingivalis, A actinomycetemcomitans* and *F. nucleatum*, and cariogenic bacteria, such as mutans streptococci, are susceptible to killing by low power laser light once cells have been treated with low concentrations of a photosensitiser dye such as toluidine blue. When activated, the dye liberates free radicals which are lethal to neighbouring cells. Photodynamic therapy works well on biofilms such as dental plaque; targeting of selected pathogens could be achieved by coupling the dye to an antibody that is specific for the pathogen. This approach is being used to treat infected root canals.

Agents that can alter the redox potential (degree of anaerobiosis; Ch. 2) of subgingival sites are being evaluated; these redox agents are designed to raise the Eh so that conditions will be less suitable for the proliferation of the obligate anaerobes that dominate in periodontal pockets. A new generation of anti-inflammatory agents are being developed (e.g. lipoxins, resolvins and docosatrienes) that could reduce bystander damage and reduce GCF flow thereby removing a key nutrient supply for periodontal pathogens.

SUMMARY

The mechanical removal of plaque by efficient oral hygiene can almost completely prevent plaque-mediated diseases. However, this level of oral care is difficult to maintain for long periods by many patients, and additional strategies need to be deployed. Many toothpastes and mouthwashes are supplemented with anti-plaque and antimicrobial agents (e.g. chlorhexidine, Triclosan, metal salts, essential oils, etc.), which even at sub-lethal concentrations can inhibit metabolic traits of plaque bacteria that are implicated in caries and periodontal diseases. The use of confectionery, drinks and chewing gums containing alternative sweeteners (e.g. polyols) that cannot be metabolized rapidly to acid can reduce the acidic challenge to teeth while stimulating saliva flow. Fluoride is the most effective strategy in reducing caries by promoting remineralization and reducing demineralization of teeth; fluoride can also reduce glycolysis and interfere with other key biochemical processes in cariogenic bacteria. New strategies are being developed including photodynamic therapy, replacement therapy, redox and anti-inflammatory agents, and vaccination (active and passive).

FURTHER READING – TREATMENT OF PLAQUE

Konopka K, Goslinski T 2007 Photodynamic therapy in dentistry. J Dent Res 86:694-707.

Marquis RE, Clock SA, Mota-Meira M 2003 Fluoride and organic weak acids as modulators of microbial physiology. FEMS Microbiol Revs 26:493-510.

Page RC 2000 Vaccination and periodontitis: myth or reality. J Int Acad Periodontol 2:31-43.

Persson GR 2005 Immune responses and vaccination against periodontal infections. J Clin Periodontol 32 Suppl 6:39-53.

Ribeiro LGM, Hashizume LN, Malz M 2007 The effect of different formulations of chlorhexidine in reducing levels of mutans streptococci in the oral cavity: A systematic review of the literature. J Dent 35:359-370.

Russell MW: Childers NK, Michalek SM, Smith DJ, Taubman MA 2004 A caries vaccine? The state of the science of immunization against dental caries. Caries Res 38:230-235.

Van Dyke TE 2007 Control of inflammation and periodontitis. Periodontology 2000 45:158-166.

CHAPTER SUMMARY

Distinct shifts in the balance of the microflora of dental plaque occur during the development of caries and periodontal diseases. Numerous cross-sectional and longitudinal surveys have found a strong association between the levels of mutans streptococci in plaque and the initiation of enamel caries. Increased proportions of lactobacilli are found in advanced lesions. However, the relationship between mutans streptococci and caries is not absolute, and other streptococci with relevant traits will also play a role. *Actinomyces* spp., mutans streptococci and lactobacilli are also implicated with root surface caries, while infected dentine has a complex microflora, with many anaerobic and proteolytic bacteria being detected.

The properties of cariogenic bacteria that correlate with their pathogenicity include the ability to rapidly metabolize sugars to acid, especially at low pH, and to survive and grow under the acidic conditions generated (i.e. cariogenic bacteria are acidogenic and aciduric). Additional properties include the ability to synthesize intracellular and extracellular polysaccharides. Strategies to control or prevent dental caries are based on (a) reducing levels of plaque in general, or specific cariogenic bacteria in particular, for example, by anti-plaque or antimicrobial agents,

(b) using fluoride to encourage remineralization and to strengthen the resistance of enamel to acid attack, and (c) reduce bacterial acid production by avoiding the frequent intake of fermentable carbohydrates in the diet, by replacing such carbohydrates with sugar substitutes, or by interfering with bacterial metabolism with fluoride or antimicrobial agents. Other strategies being developed for the future include (i) enhancing the colonization resistance property of plaque by replacement therapy, whereby harmless strains may exclude or suppress cariogenic species, and (ii) active or passive vaccination against mutans streptococci using sub-unit vaccines or specific antibodies, respectively.

Periodontal diseases are a group of disorders that affect the supporting tissues of the teeth but, as with caries, there is no single or unique pathogen. Many of the cultured bacteria from disease-affected sites are Gram negative and obligately anaerobic. Although the microflora in disease is diverse, certain species are recovered commonly at sites undergoing tissue breakdown; these include *Porphyromonas gingivalis, Prevotella intermedia, Aggregatibacter actinomycetemcomitans, Tannerella forsythia, Dialister pneumosintes, Fusobacterium nucleatum, Eubacterium* spp. and spirochaetes, although 50% of the organisms at these sites are unculturable, and their role in disease is still to be determined. Many of these species are highly proteolytic and can degrade host tissues and/or components of the host defences including key regulatory proteins of the inflammatory response. Bacterial invasion of tissues can occur, especially in some aggressive and necrotizing conditions such as NUG. Risk factors for periodontal diseases include abnormalities in the functioning of the host defences, smoking, and systemic disease such as diabetes mellitus. Organisms can evade or subvert the host defences by leukotoxin production or by the presence of a capsule; bacterial proteases can de-regulate the inflammatory response which can lead to by-stander damage to the host tissues. Periodontal diseases may also act as risk factors for more serious medical conditions, including pre-term, low birth weight babies and cardiovascular disease. Treatment and prevention of periodontal disease involves good oral hygiene and effective plaque control, which may be augmented by the use of antimicrobial agents.

Chapter | 7 |

Orofacial bacterial infections

As described in previous chapters, the mouth contains a rich and diverse microflora, only 50% of which can be cultivated. Dental plaque within a healthy mouth is a complex biofilm (Ch. 5), which has a commensal relationship with the host. However, plaque can become 'pathogenic' since it is involved in the two most prevalent human diseases, namely dental caries and periodontal disease (Ch. 6). Untreated, both of these conditions can progress into other forms of acute and chronic infection within the mouth and orofacial tissues (Fig 7.1). Small alterations in the local environment can produce microbial population changes that permit the development of opportunistic infections involving bacterial species that are usually regarded as non-pathogenic members of the oral microflora. On occasions, these infections can produce severe life-threatening situations.

Contemporary microbiological studies have revealed that the types of bacteria recovered from orofacial dental infections reflect the wide spectrum of facultative and strictly anaerobic bacteria that also are regarded as indigenous constituents of the host's oral microflora. Strict anaerobes comprise a major proportion of the microflora within acute suppurative infections. In addition, pathogenicity experiments in animals have implicated strictly anaerobic bacterial species, in particular Gram negative bacilli, as not only the predominant species but also the most likely pathogens, although the reasons for this are uncertain. One possibility is the occurrence of specific combinations of bacterial species since animal models have shown that *Prevotella* spp and *Fusobacterium* spp are more pathogenic when in combination with members of the anginosus group of streptococci than when inoculated subcutaneously separately (pathogenic synergism; Ch. 6). It has also been proposed that microaerophilic species produce an environment that favours the proliferation of strictly anaerobic species. The presence of an extracellular capsule on certain bacterial strains recovered from dentoalveolar abscesses has also been implicated as a potential pathogenic determinant since this may protect bacteria from phagocytosis or intracellular killing (Fig. 7.2). While found

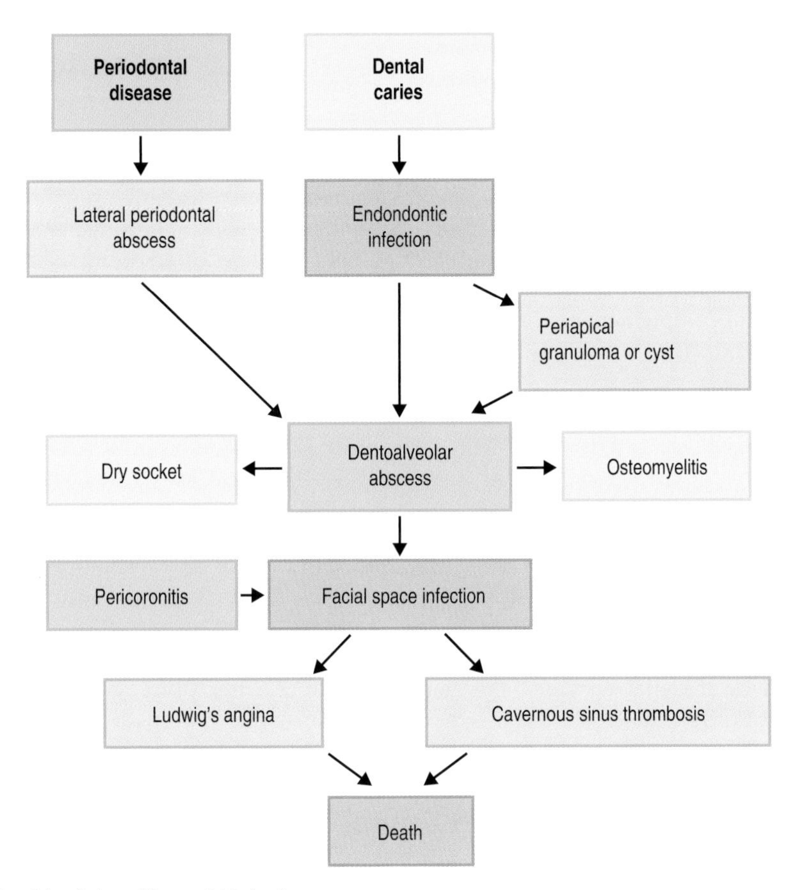

Fig. 7.1 Inter-relationship of dental bacterial infections.

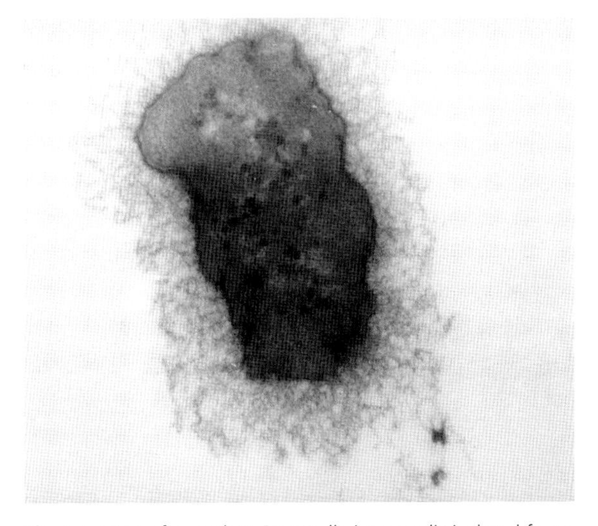

Fig. 7.2 TEM of capsulate *Prevotella intermedia* isolated from an acute dentoalveolar abscess.

on fresh clinical isolates, the capsule is lost after repeated subculture *in vitro*.

In an infection involving a diverse microbial community it is likely that environmental factors, such as availability of nutrients, local pH and the status of the immune defences, also play a major contributing role in determining the clinical outcome and whether or not an acute suppurative process develops. The primary source of nutrients is serum-derived proteins along with some host tissue components. Bacterial species within the infection may produce a range of complementary enzymes, in particular glycosidases and proteases, that permit progression of the infection (Ch. 4). *Prevotella oralis, P. intermedia* and *Porphyromonas endodontalis* have been identified as particularly effective in the degradation of serum proteins and immunoglobulins. These species also obtain essential growth elements such as iron and haemin from the catabolism of albumin, haptoglobin, haemopexin and transferrin. An example of the inter-relationship among the bacteria within the polymicrobial community is the degradation of proteins and peptides by *Prevotella* spp. for bacteria such as *F. nucleatum*, *Eubacterium* spp. and anaerobic streptococci. These consortia also produce metabolic substances, in particular hydrogen sulphide, indoles and amines, that inactivate host polymorphonuclear leukocytes and prevent complement action, in addition to acidic end products of metabolism that are cytotoxic.

Orofacial bacterial infections may present as either a localized abscess or diffuse cellulitis depending on the virulence of the bacteria, local anatomical structures and host defence mechanisms. On rare occasions, bacteria may enter the bloodstream to produce a potentially life-threatening septicaemia. An abscess is a localized collection of bacteria, inflammatory cells, tissue breakdown products, serum-derived proteins and other organic material. Tissue destruction is predominantly caused by bacterial enzymes although some damage is host-mediated. An abscess is hypertonic in relation to the immediate environment and pressure effects result in osteoclastic activity in surrounding bone. In dentoalveolar abscesses, perforation of bone permits spread of infection into the surrounding soft tissues. Subsequent inflammation in the soft tissue is termed cellulitis which is often accompanied by limited localized muscular movement (trismus). Bacterial metabolites, exotoxins and endotoxins along with host inflammatory substances then act on the temperature regulatory centre in the hypothalamus to raise the patient's temperature (pyrexia).

LABORATORY DIAGNOSIS

A major problem associated with the recovery of the causative microorganisms from specific orofacial infections is the high potential for sample contamination from microorganisms present in saliva. Contamination of a specimen with relatively rapid growing bacteria, such as streptococci or staphylococci, can potentially prevent the isolation of more slowly growing relevant species. As a basic principle the eventual microbiological report can only be as good as the quality of the specimen. In view of the likely presence of oxygen-sensitive bacteria in orofacial infections, all efforts must be made to ensure successful recovery of such strict anaerobes. Samples of pus should be obtained by aspiration to minimize the risk of contamination and protect oxygen-sensitive anaerobes from atmospheric oxygen (Fig. 7.3). If a swab is the only option for sampling, then this should be placed in appropriate transport medium. A microbiological specimen is a 'living' sample and as such must be transferred to the laboratory as rapidly as possible for processing to minimise the loss of viable bacteria.

On arrival at the laboratory a Gram stain of a smear of the sample can be used to confirm that the specimen is truly pus and not another substance, such as cyst fluid. The Gram stain of pus will reveal a large number of polymorphonuclear leukocytes and bacteria, probably a mixture of Gram positive and Gram negative bacteria (Fig. 7.4). The sample will routinely be plated onto non-selective blood-based media which will be incubated in an atmosphere of air plus 5% CO_2 and

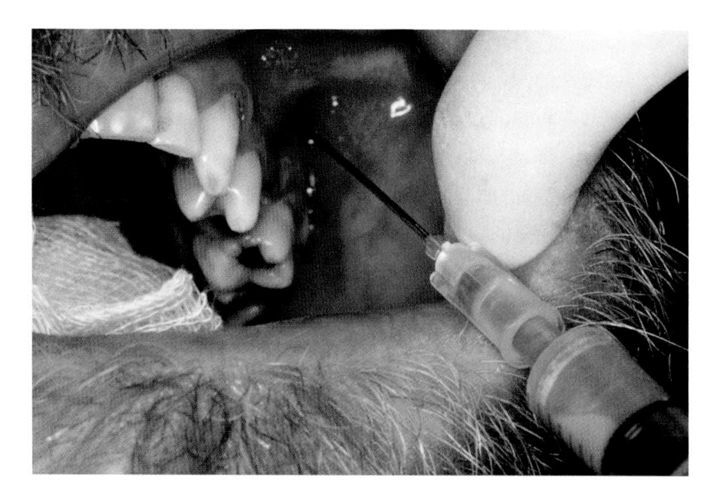

Fig. 7.3 Aspiration of pus from an acute dentoalveolar abscess.

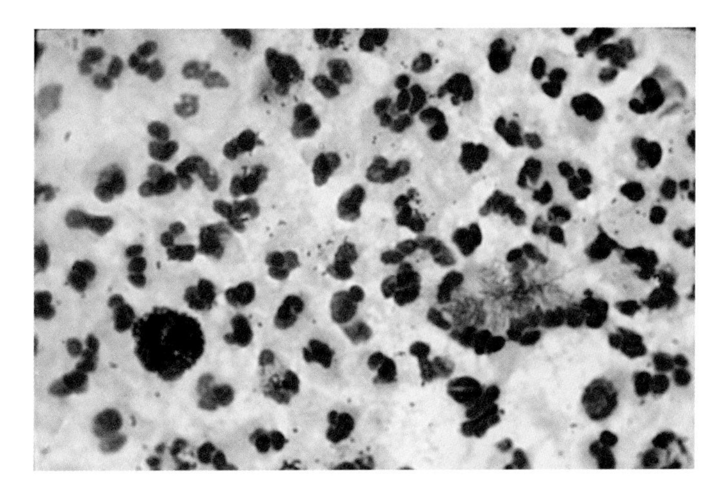

Fig. 7.4 Smear of pus obtained from acute dentoalveaolar abscess stained by Gram's method showing mixed infection.

anaerobically. Fastidious anaerobe agar is also used to ensure isolation of strict anaerobes. Plates are incubated at 37 °C and examined after 18–24 hours for primary growth before being returned to the incubator for prolonged incubation and re-examination on a daily basis up to 7 days. Representative colonies of any detected growth are subcultured for pure growth and determination of atmospheric requirements. Identification of bacteria within orofacial infections can take a number of days due to the slow-growing nature of many strict anaerobes. This factor limits the clinical benefit of sampling such infections. More recently, molecular-based techniques have been developed to provide rapid identification and detection of specific bacterial species in dental infections (Chs 3 and 4). Rapid identification methods will improve the clinical usefulness of microbiology when managing severe dental infections.

Culture methods fail to recover the full diversity of microorganisms within orofacial infections (Ch. 3). Molecular studies, in which DNA has been extracted from pus obtained from acute dentoalveolar abscesses and 16S rDNA has been amplified using universal primers, have revealed that unculturable species account for a high percentage of the microflora in the sample when compared to results of culture. Similar findings have recently been reported for endodontic infections. These observations should be taken into account when considering the microbiological aspects of the individual infections described below since it is likely that unculturable and novel bacterial species have an aetiological role in all dental infections but their exact role is not fully understood at the present time.

ANTIMICROBIAL SUSCEPTIBILITY

The global emergence of antibiotic resistance is of great concern, and bacteria recovered from orofacial infections are now being found to have reduced in vitro antimicrobial susceptibility to penicillins and other antibiotics. Historically, isolates from acute suppurative dental infections rarely demonstrated resistance to penicillin but this is no longer the case. The incidence of resistance to penicillin has increased dramatically in Gram negative strictly anaerobic bacilli, in particular *Prevotella* spp, due to the production of beta-lactamases. Studies in the UK have revealed that the incidence of penicillin resistance in acute dentoalveolar infections rose from 3% of isolates in 1986 to 23% of isolates in 1995. Similar incidences of penicillin resistance have now also been reported in the USA (33%), Sweden (38%) and Japan (39%).

Susceptibility testing is traditionally performed using a disc diffusion method on solid agar media. This technique allows a basic assessment of susceptibility. Calculation of the minimum inhibitory concentration (MIC) requires more labour intensive broth or agar dilution methods. In recent years, the development of a simple disc diffusion method called the E-test has permitted direct reading of antimicrobial MIC from an agar plate (Fig. 7.5).

Molecular techniques have been developed that permit rapid detection of penicillin-resistance genes in pus specimens. These techniques may prove to be helpful in clinical management if they become more widely available in the future. The presence of

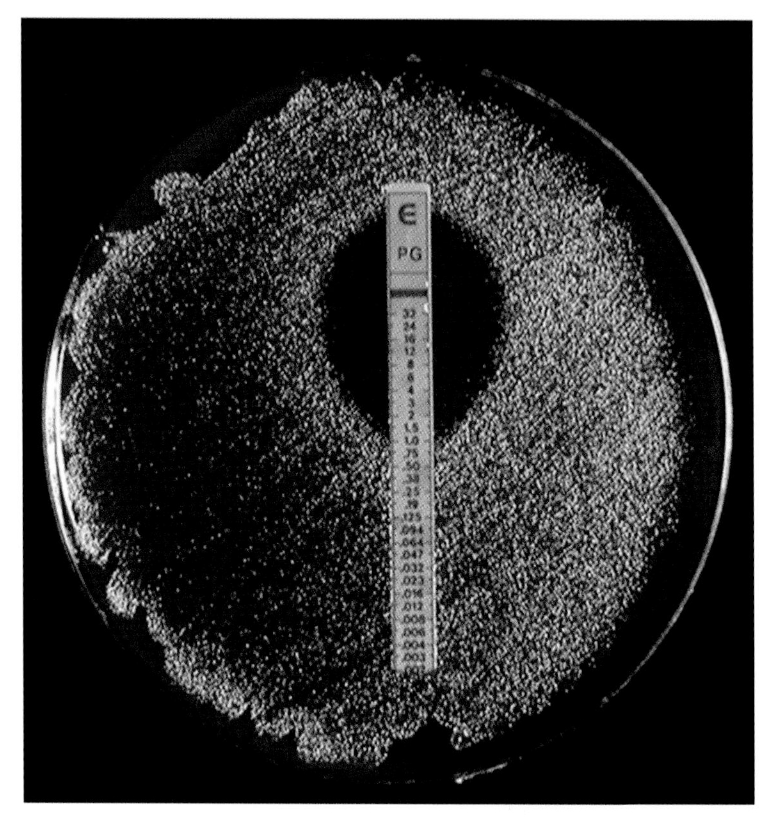

Fig. 7.5 Incubated plate of a *Prevotella* species demonstrating susceptibility to penicillin using the E-test.

penicillin-resistant bacteria has been reported to be responsible for treatment failures in head and neck infections of dental origin. The production of beta-lactamases not only plays a direct pathogenic role by destroying the drug but also indirectly 'shields' non-beta-lactamase producing, penicillin-sensitive bacteria within the infection. The widespread use of penicillin has contributed to this problem, because it has been shown that the administration of penicillin leads to the emergence of beta-lactamase-producing bacteria, especially Gram negative bacilli, in sites such as the oropharynx. Increased resistance to other antibiotics prescribed for dental infections does not appear to have been reported. Of specific interest is the extremely low incidence of resistance to clindamycin, even in countries such as Germany and Japan, where this agent is frequently used to treat acute dental infections.

PRINCIPLES OF MANAGEMENT

The actual treatment for an individual patient will be dependent on the specific circumstances. The basic principle consists of drainage of pus, if present, and removal of the source of infection, usually by pulp extirpation or extraction of the affected tooth. Consideration should be given for the need for antimicrobial therapy. Undoubtedly, in the past, antibiotics have been prescribed frequently either inappropriately or unnecessarily. Such habits have contributed to the emergence of penicillin resistance in bacterial species encountered in the mouth. Despite this, if required, members of the pencillin group (amoxicillin, phenoxymethylpenicillin), given orally, remain the antibiotic therapy of first choice. Erythromycin and metronidazole are suitable alternative agents for patients with hypersensitivity to penicillins. Standard dosages usually are used for dental outpatients, although increased dosages and combination therapy have been recommended for severe infections. The concept of a complete course of antibiotics is obsolete and patients should take the drug for as short a time as possible, in practical terms until symptoms have resolved. A short course of two 3g administrations of amoxicillin 12 hours apart has been found to be effective for acute dentoalveolar abscesses.

The range of other antimicrobial agents that have been suggested for the treatment of dentoalveolar infections include ornidazole, cephalosporin, azithromycin, spiramycin, amoxicillin-clavulanate and clindamycin.

ENDODONTIC INFECTION

The presence of microorganisms in root canals immediately prior to and during endodontic treatment has been studied extensively in recent years. Different sampling techniques and identification methods have been used and this, in part, probably explains the wide spectrum of bacteria recovered. Overall the microflora encountered is similar in nature to that found in acute dentoalveolar abscesses. In recent years, cloning and sequencing techniques coupled with denaturing high performance liquid chromatography have revealed that root canals typically contain between 7–20 different species, in particular *Olsenella profusa*, *P. gingivalis*, *Dialister* spp. and anaerobic streptococci. *E. faecalis* has received special attention since it had been proposed that it was specifically associated with endodontic failures. However, molecular studies have revealed that this bacterial species is frequently present in necrotic pulps prior to treatment as well as following failed endodontic therapy. Phylogenic analysis of bacterial and archaeal 16S rRNA has detected a *Methanobrevibacter oralis*-like species along with *Treponema denticola*. Furthermore, animal studies have implicated *Treponema denticola* as being the cause of disseminating infection from the root canal to distant organs. In addition to the identification of bacteria, studies have quantified the presence of endotoxins within root canals; higher levels of lipopolysaccharide were found in teeth with clinical symptoms compared to asymptomatic teeth. These contemporary studies indicate a complex polymicrobial community within endodontic infections and substantiate the link between oral disease and systemic conditions.

DENTOALVEOLAR INFECTION

The term dentoalveolar infection can be used to describe pyogenic (pus-forming) conditions that affect the teeth and supporting structures, and includes lateral periodontal abscess and acute dentoalveolar (periapical) abscess.

Lateral periodontal abscess

The lateral periodontal abscess can be differentiated from the dentoalveolar abscess by the fact that the tooth that it is associated with has a vital pulp. The periodontal abscess develops as a result of blockage, occasionally due to the presence of foreign material such as fish bone or toothbrush bristle, in an established periodontal pocket. Clinically, the abscess develops rapidly producing localized swelling and erythema. Pus is likely to discharge from the gingival margin. Obtaining a 'true sample' without contamination of the specimen is almost impossible. Not surprisingly, studies have reported the presence of those bacterial species also associated with subgingival plaque, in particular, *Porphyromonas* spp., *Prevotella* spp., *Fusobacterium* spp., haemolytic streptococci, *Actinomyces* spp., *Capnocytophaga* spp. and spirochaetes. The abscess should be treated by drainage and irrigation with an antiseptic mouthwash, such as 0.2% chlorhexidine. An assessment should be made in relation to the long-term prognosis of the tooth, since on many occasions there is advanced periodontal disease and loss of supporting bone which are indications for extraction. Antibiotic therapy is rarely required.

Acute dentoalveolar abscess

Acute dentoalveolar abscess is the most frequently occurring orofacial bacterial infection. This condition represents the onset of a suppurative process at the apex of the root of a tooth with necrotic pulp. Pulp death usually occurs due to invasion of bacteria from advanced dental caries. However, occasionally the pulp may have become necrotic due to loss of its blood supply as a result of trauma to the apical vessels, such as may occur during a blow to the tooth. The majority of acute dentoalveolar abscesses are preceded by a period of chronic infection and development of periapical granulation tissue that may persist for many months or years. Evidence of a long-standing inflammatory process at the apices of the roots is seen radiographically as an area of radiolucency at that site on radiographs (Fig. 7.6). Interestingly, microscopic examination of periapical granuloma, obtained in the absence of acute symptoms, has revealed the presence of low numbers of bacteria in the tissues, often within macrophages. Bacteria probably gain access to the apical tissue by one of three routes: direct spread from the pulp chamber, through the periodontal

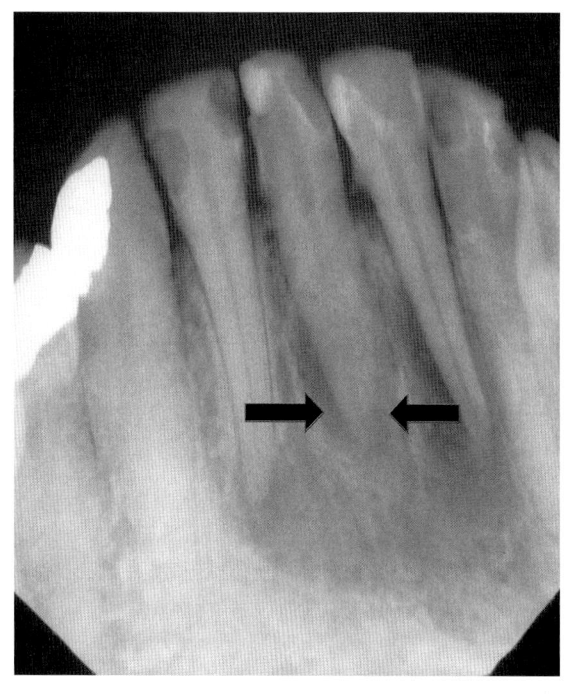

Fig. 7.6 Intra-oral radiograph showing periapical radiolucency due to bone loss associated with dentoalveolar infection (arrows).

membrane on the root surface or by seeding from local blood vessels (anachoresis). The mechanisms that cause a chronic asymptomatic lesion to change into an acute suppurative process are unknown, but the occurrence of specific combinations of bacteria or the sudden provision of nutrients via local tissue damage is involved. The onset of acute inflammation produces the characteristic symptom of severe pain. Other signs and symptoms will depend on the individual case. However, clinical examination often reveals a carious or discoloured tooth that is tender to touch with localized swelling, erythema and trismus (Fig. 7.7). The onset of raised body temperature and malaise are a response to circulating inflammatory cytokines, interleukins and tumour necrosis factor, in response to bacterial endotoxins.

Investigations using culture and molecular methods have confirmed the polymicrobial nature of this infection, which usually involves five or six bacterial species. The most frequently recovered facultatively anaerobic isolates are streptococci, in particular members of the anginosus group of streptococci, *Actinomyces* spp., while the predominant strictly anaerobic isolates are anaerobic streptococci, *Veillonella, Prevotella, Porphyromonas* and *Fusobacterium* spp. Quantitative studies have revealed the viable microbial flora of acute dentolveolar abscess to be between 10^6–10^8 colony forming units (cfu)/ml of pus. The number and proportions of strictly anaerobic species encountered in dentoalveolar abscesses are greater than the number of facultatively anaerobic species. Strict anaerobes are not only the predominant species, often accounting for four or more of the six or seven species encountered within the mixed microflora, but they also comprise 80–90% of the overall

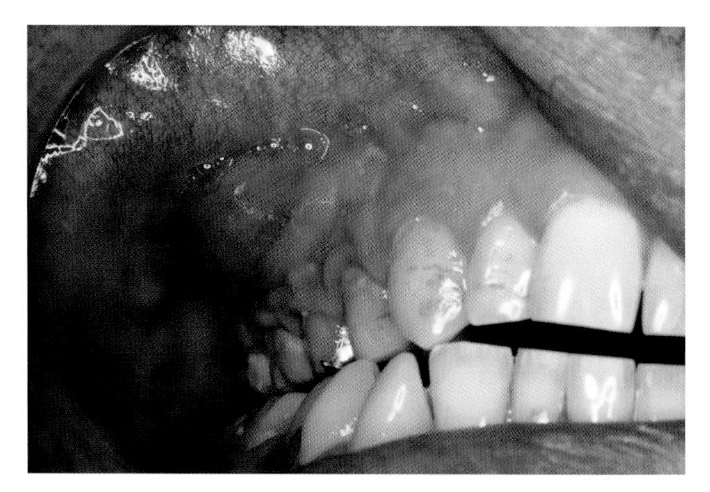

Fig. 7.7 Dentoalveolar abscess presenting as a fluctuant swelling in the buccal sulcus.

cultivable microflora. Molecular approaches often detect species that are difficult to grow by traditional culture techniques, and some novel species have been found.

The majority of cases of dentoalveolar abscess can be managed successfully by establishing surgical drainage alone. This should involve aspiration of pus from the abscess in situations where a microbiology service is available for culture prior to incision of the soft tissues, extirpation of the pulp or removal of the tooth. However, occasions do arise when adequate drainage cannot be achieved, or the patient has clinical signs of systemic upset. In these circumstances, it may be necessary to provide antimicrobial therapy. Selection of antimicrobial therapy is based on published susceptibilities rather than identification of the causative organisms and determination of antimicrobial susceptibility in a specific patient. A pus specimen from an individual patient cannot be processed fast enough by traditional methods to be of value in making treatment decisions since information is rarely available to the clinician within the first 48 hours. Agents in the penicillin group, principally amoxicillin and phenoxymethylpenicillin, are still the antimicrobials of choice in the treatment of acute dental infections while metronidazole or erythromycin should be used as an alternative agent for patients with hypersensitivity to penicillins. Clindamycin is used as the antibiotic of first choice in some parts of the world.

Immediate referral to a specialist is required when a patient presents with symptoms of cellulitis, difficulty in swallowing, tachycardia, hypotension, raised temperature, lethargy or dehydration. Specialist care may also become necessary when standard outpatient treatment fails to result in symptomatic improvement. Infection may spread into a number of tissue spaces and this is influenced by the local anatomy, in particular, muscle attachment and their relationship to the position of the apices of the tooth involved (Fig. 7.8, A and B). Spread into the facial spaces of the neck may lead to difficulty in swallowing. Hospitalization permits the provision of intravenous antibiotics and fluids. There is also the ability to secure the airway with a tracheostomy, if required. Rarely, infection from dentoalveolar infection in the maxilla may spread into the facial air sinuses via the facial vein and cause cavernous sinus thrombosis, a condition that is associated with high mortality.

LUDWIG'S ANGINA

An inadequately treated dentoalveolar infection can progress to cause widespread swelling of the tissue spaces (submental, sublingual and submandibular) in the head and neck with the spread of infection though fascial spaces to the mediastinum, a situation referred to as Ludwig's angina.

The tissues of the neck become markedly swollen and tense leading to difficulty in breathing. Hence, the use of the term 'angina', which literally means choking. Death from Ludwig's angina still occurs, especially in developing countries, due to late intervention or treatment failure. Airway management, involving intubation or tracheostomy, is usually required. The bacterial species most frequently encountered in Ludwig's angina include *Prevotella* spp., *Porphyromonas* spp., *Fusobacterium* spp. and anaerobic streptococci. Occasionally, staphylococci, enterobacteria and coliforms have been recovered in cases of Ludwig's angina. Awareness of the potential presence of these bacterial species is important to ensure appropriate antibiotic therapy. Initial treatment must include broad spectrum antibiotic therapy, such as a combination of ceftriaxone and metronidazole, delivered intravenously.

OSTEOMYELITIS

Osteomyelitis is defined as inflammation of the medullary bone within the maxilla or mandible with possible extension into the adjacent cortical bone and overlying periosteum. This condition may be acute or chronic and can be extremely difficult to treat effectively. It is perhaps surprising that there are not more cases of osteomyelitis in the jaws following tooth extraction when the potential for members of the oral microflora to gain access to the underlying bone is considered. The good blood supply to the jaws is probably responsible for such a small number of cases. This concept is supported by the observation that the rare cases of osteomyelitis that do occur are often seen in situations where vascularity is reduced, such as that following radiotherapy (see Ch. 11). In recent years, osteomyelitis has been observed in patients taking bisphosphonates for the treatment of osteoporosis or breast cancer. Treatment is based on local debridement and topical antiseptic on exposed areas. Clindamycin is a recommended antibiotic due to its ability to achieve therapeutic levels within bone.

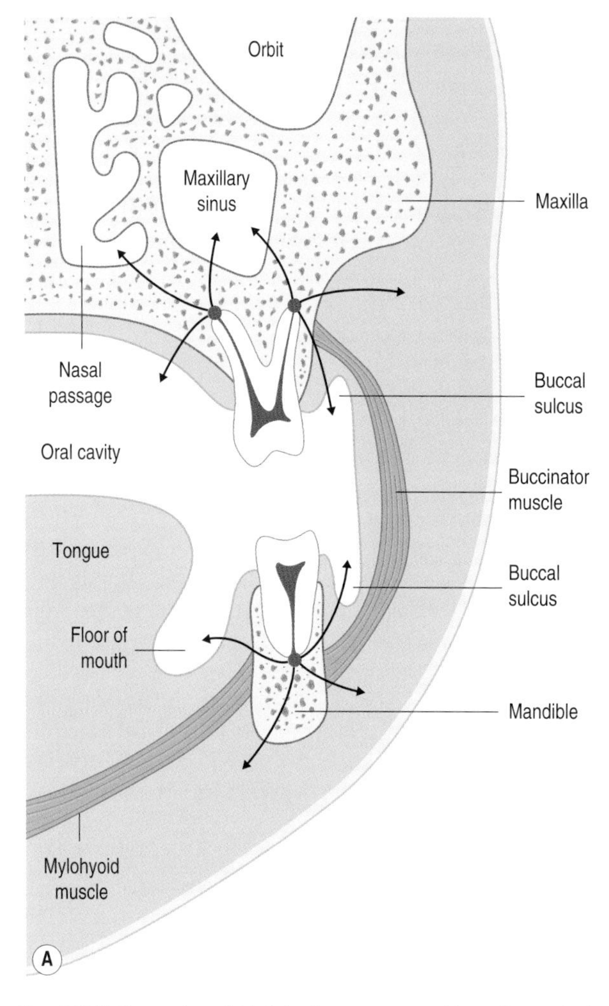

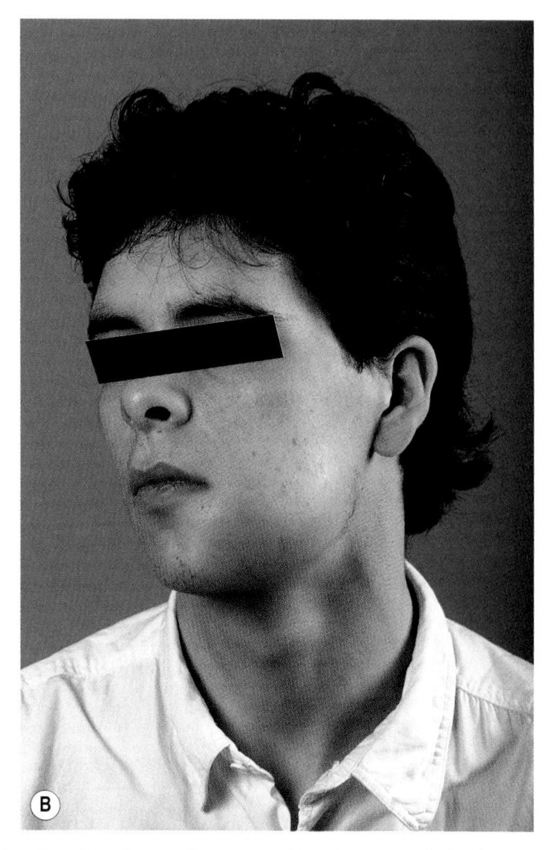

Fig. 7.8 Pathways by which infection may spread from the periapical region. Muscle attachments and local anatomy (A) influence whether the swelling presents intra-oral or extra-orally. (B) Extra-oral fluctuant swelling due to abscess on a lower second molar.

DRY SOCKET

This extremely painful condition, which is a localized form of alveolar osteitis, occurs after approximately 3% of routine extractions and 20% of surgical extractions. Examination will reveal an empty socket at the site of extraction in the preceding 2–3 days (Fig. 7.9). The aetiology is not fully understood but involves fibrinolysis of the blood clot, which may occur due to opportunistic infection by strict anaerobes. However, the causative role of bacteria has not been conclusively established. Clinically, there is a pronounced halitosis

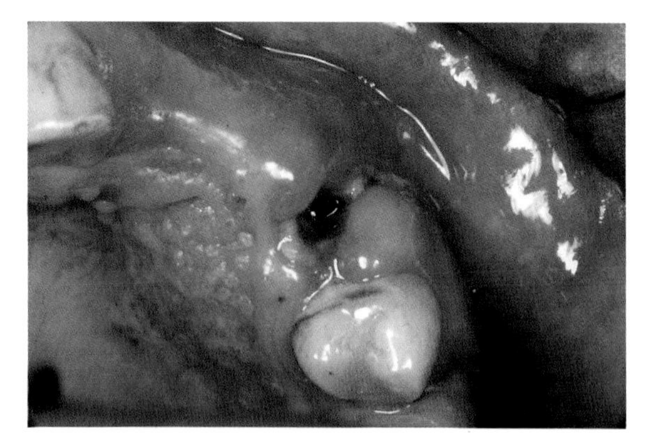

Fig. 7.9 Dry socket following extraction of an upper first premolar.

which has implicated the presence of strict anaerobes and led to the use of metronidazole in treatment.

PERI-IMPLANTITIS

Peri-implantitis is an emerging form of periodontitis that is a direct consequence of the increasing use of dental implants. Peri-implant disease refers to the general category of pathological changes that can occur in the hard and soft tissues surrounding an implant. The integration of an implant can be jeopardized by the presence of inflammatory changes that causes loss of the supportive bone (Fig. 7.10). However, most peri-implant disease is plaque-induced and the spectrum of bacterial species recovered in dentate patients is comparable to that encountered in adult periodontitis, namely *A. actinomycetemcomitans, P. gingivalis, P. intermedia* and *F. nucleatum* (Ch. 6). Interestingly, but perhaps not surprisingly, the microflora encountered on healthy stable implants in edentulous individuals is similar to that found on the mucosa and includes Gram positive facultative streptococci.

Peri-implantitis has been shown to respond to local mechanical and chemical means of reducing the microflora in the immediate vicinity of the implant. However, consideration has to be given to the possibility of causing physical damage to the surface of the implant. Irrigation with an antiseptic, such as 0.2% chlorhexidine, has been found to be beneficial. Alternatively, the provision of systemic antimicrobial therapy, such as amoxicillin, metronidazole, ornidazole or tetracycline, has also been recommended.

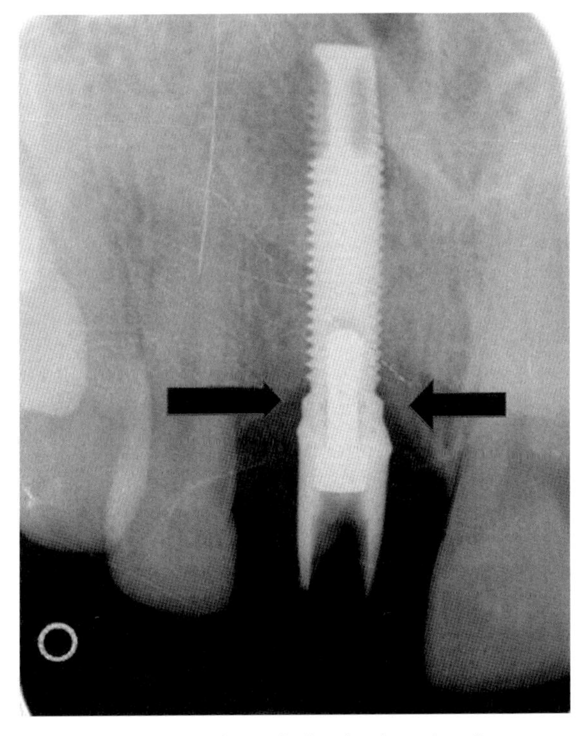

Fig. 7.10 Intra-oral radiograph showing bone loss due to peri-implantitis around a single tooth implant (arrows).

PERICORONITIS

Inflammation of the soft tissues covering or immediately adjacent to the crown of a partially erupted tooth can cause extreme pain, particularly when the opposing teeth cause additional trauma (Fig. 7.11). This condition occurs fairly frequently in relation to erupting lower third molar teeth in young adults, and is due to infection in the space between the tooth and overlying soft tissue. Strict anaerobes, in particular *P. intermedia*, anaerobic streptococci and *Fusobacterium* spp, are often present, and more contemporary studies have also isolated *Aggregatibacter* (formerly *Actinobacillus) actinomycetecomitans* and *Tannerella forsythia*. Treatment is local irrigation, but if the opposing tooth is non-functional then it should be extracted. In severe cases it may be necessary to prescribe metronidazole or amoxicillin.

BACTERIAL SIALADENITIS

Inflammation of the salivary glands is termed sialadenitis and this may arise due to either bacterial or viral infection. Historically, suppurative sialadenitis was regarded as an infection principally caused by *Staphylococcus aureus* and the condition was a recognised post-operative complication in hospitalized patients undergoing general surgery. However, this post-operative parotitis is now rare due to a better understanding of maintaining fluid balance and the reduced likelihood of *S. aureus* colonization of the mouth due to improved oral hygiene measures. Sialadentitis within the parotid gland is usually due to the presence of underlying xerostomia, due to Sjögren's syndrome or previous radiotherapy, while sialadenitis in the submandibular gland is most frequently secondary to blockage of the duct by salivary stone. The clinical presentation involves painful swelling of the infected gland and discharge of pus from the duct orifice (Fig. 7.12).

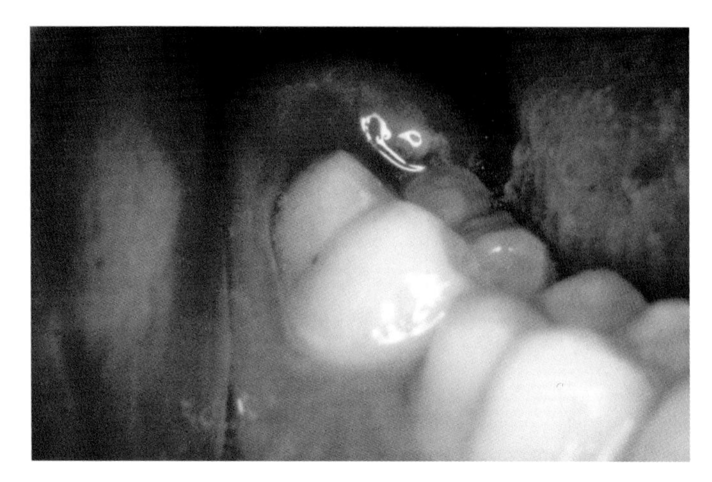

Fig. 7.11 Localized inflammation leading to pericoronitis over a lower right third molar tooth.

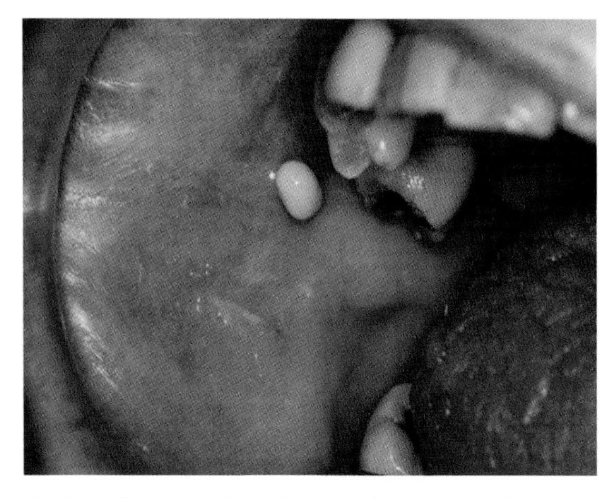

Fig. 7.12 Discharge of pus from the right parotid salivary gland duct.

Knowledge of the microbiology of suppurative sialadenitis has become clearer due to the use of improved sampling techniques. Ideally, pus should be collected by aspiration of the duct orifice in order to minimize the risk of sample contamination from the oral microflora. If a swab technique is used, then great care should be taken to avoid sample contamination from the adjacent oral mucosa. Rarely, pus may also spread extra-orally and a sample can be obtained by external aspiration. Quantitative microbiological studies of suppurative parotitis have revealed a viable flora of 10^6–10^8 cfu/ml involving a wide spectrum of bacterial species, such as alpha-haemolytic streptococci, *Haemophilus* spp., *Eikenella corrodens, Prevotella* spp. and strictly anaerobic Gram positive cocci. On rare occasions, *Mycobacterium tuberculosis* and atypical mycobacteria are encountered in parotitis.

Antimicrobial therapy should be prescribed with amoxicillin the agent of choice and erythromycin used in patients with a hypersensitivity to the penicillins. If microbiological investigation reveals the presence of strict anaerobes then the use of metronidazole could be considered.

Recurrent parotitis of childhood is a relatively rare condition in which sufferers develop a purulent discharge from one of the parotid glands about two or three times a year. The microbiology of the infection is similar to that encountered in other forms of suppurative sialadenitis. It has been suggested that patients would benefit from long-term antibiotic therapy, although most patients are managed adequately with the provision of amoxicillin or erythromycin as and when acute symptoms develop.

ANGULAR CHEILITIS

This condition represents an area of inflammation that is localized to the angles of the mouth (Fig. 7.13). Angular cheilitis is usually bilateral, although only one side of the mouth may be affected on occasions. The inflammatory changes are associated with the presence of *Staphylococcus* aureus, including methicillin resistant *Staphylococcus aureus* (MRSA), or *Candida* spp., either alone or in combination. Streptococci are also recovered from approximately a third of cases. As a generalization, staphylococci

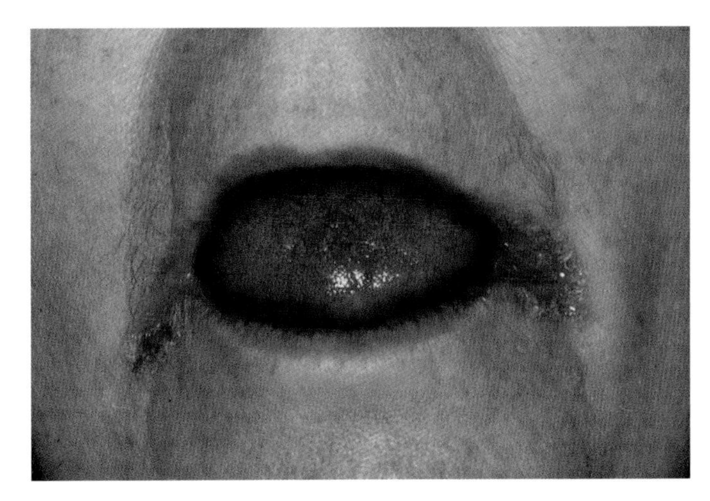

Fig. 7.13 Angular cheilitis presenting as erythema at both angles of the mouth.

are usually encountered in dentate individuals while candida are found in patients with dentures or an orthodontic appliance. The reservoir of staphylococcal infection is often the anterior part of the nose while the mouth is the source of the candida. Treatment should involve not only the angles but also the appropriate reservoir of infection. In the case of staphylococci, fusidic acid cream can be prescribed, with one tube for the angles and a separate tube for the nose. Miconazole cream is also useful in cases where there is uncertainty about the microoganism that may be present since this agent has activity against candida and Gram positive cocci. An antifungal agent should be given in cases involving candida (Ch. 9).

CERVICOFACIAL ACTINOMYCOSIS

Actinomycosis is an example of an opportunistic infection caused by members of the *Actinomyces* genus. Although a range of *Actinomyces* species are encountered in plaque, dentinal caries and dentoalveolar abscess (Chs. 3, 5 and 6), cervicofacial actinomycosis, which characteristically presents as a submandibular swelling, is associated with *A. israelii* in 90% of cases. Occasionally, *A. bovis* or *A. naeslundii* may be isolated either alone or in combination with *A. actinomycetemcomitans*, *Haemophilus* spp., *Propionibacterium* spp. or *Prevotella* spp., any of which may account for up to 25% of the microflora. It has been proposed that the aetiology involves the introduction of these bacterial species into the deeper tissues following trauma or extraction of a tooth. The characteristic swelling at the angle of the mandible, which may be either localized or diffuse, progresses slowly until multiple sinuses develop within an indurated overlying skin (Fig. 7.14). Pus expressed from the sinuses is thick and yellow with granular particles consisting of calcified aggregates

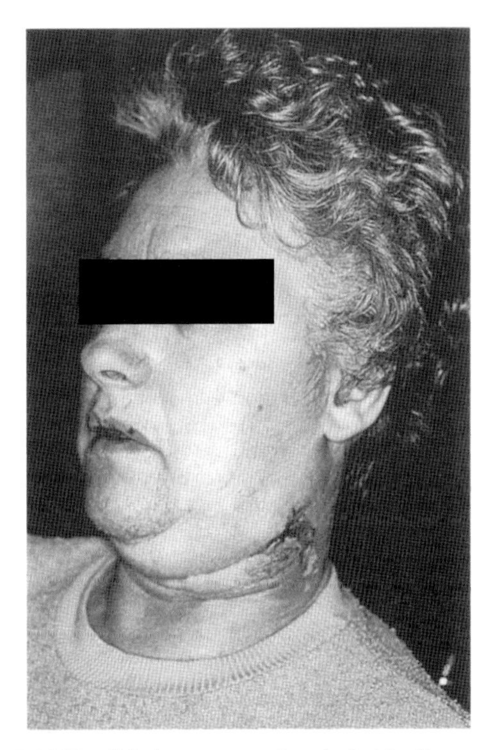

Fig. 7.14 The clinical appearance of cervicofacial actinomycosis.

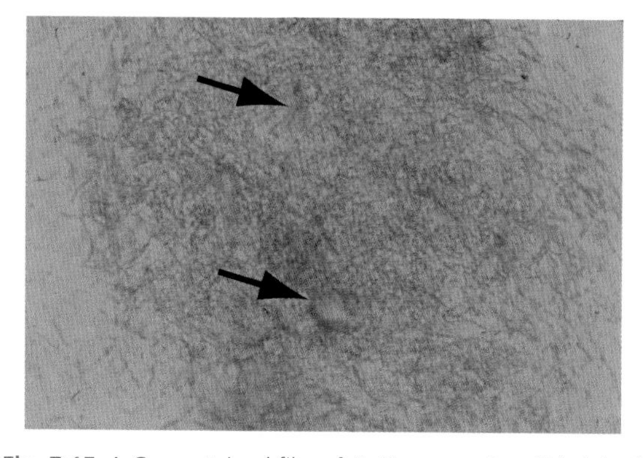

Fig. 7.15 A Gram-stained film of *Actinomyces israelii* (original magnification ×100). Note the branching filaments and the tendency to form granular masses (arrows).

of *Actinomyces* filaments that are referred to as 'sulphur granules'. Diagnosis is based on Gram staining of these granules combined with an eosin counter stain that produces a clubbing effect on the peripheral filaments (Fig. 7.15). Cultures should be incubated anaerobically for up to 14 days; colonies of *A. israelii* on blood agar are sometimes described as being shaped like 'molar teeth'. Although the submandibular region is by far the most frequently affected area, cases of actinomycosis have also been reported in the maxillary antrum, tongue and major salivary glands. This infection induces a granulomatous reaction in the surrounding tissues which results in multiple pus-filled pockets within the tissues. This particular aspect of actinomycosis has implications for treatment since it is essential to break these pockets down surgically to allow drainage. Amoxicillin is the antibiotic of choice although erythromycin or clindamycin should be used if the patient is hypersensitive to penicillins. Therapy may have to be prolonged (4–6 weeks) due to failure to achieve adequate drug levels in the granulation tissue.

STAPHYLOCOCCAL LYMPHADENITIS

Infections in the head and neck region can cause enlargement and pain in the regional lymph nodes. While this is a general observation in a number of infections, there is a specific condition in which a patient, usually a child, develops a localized painful swelling of the facial lymph node. This is due to infection involving a *Staphylococcus* spp which has spread from colonization within the nose. Flucloxacillin should be used systemically to treat the lymphadenitis and topical fusidic acid should be applied to the anterior part of the nose to eliminate the source of infection.

FACIAL LACERATIONS

Superficial lacerations involving the face, neck and scalp have the potential to become infected with members of the commensal skin microflora, such as *Staphylococcus epidermidis* and *Propionbacterium acnes*. Soft tissue wounds should be treated within 24 hours by thorough cleaning prior to suturing. Infection in lacerations is rare and there is seldom a need to prescribe antibiotics. If infection develops in a wound, a swab should be taken and sent for culture. In these circumstances an antibiotic with known activity against staphylococci, such as flucloxacillin, can be provided empirically. Wounds that cannot be closed by sutures or adhesive strips, and/or which may become infected, benefit from applications of a topical agent such as 2% mupirocin ointment or 2% fusidic acid cream, which may be applied two or three times daily. There is interest in the use of semi-occlusive wound dressings to improve wound healing and reduce scarring, which is of particular aesthetic importance in the management of facial wounds.

CHAPTER SUMMARY

Orofacial bacterial infections are usually opportunistic polymicrobial conditions involving those species that are also regarded as members of the host commensal microflora, particularly strict anaerobes. Wherever possible, samples should be obtained by aspiration in order to minimize the risk of contamination from saliva and other oral surfaces. Specimens need to be transported to the laboratory promptly for processing. The use of molecular microbiological techniques has revealed that many unculturable bacterial species are often present. The reason why these microorganisms become pathogenic is uncertain but synergistic relationships between some species are likely to be involved. The formation of such consortia is likely to protect infecting microorganisms from the host defences. Antibiotic resistance is relatively rare in dental infections although reduced susceptibility to penicillins due to beta-lactamase production, particularly by Gram negative strictly anaerobic bacilli, is being encountered increasingly. Treatment of such infections should be based on local measures to drain and clear infection. Antibiotic therapy is rarely required and should only be given if symptoms of systemic involvement are present.

FURTHER READING

Kuriyama T, Absi EG, Williams DW, Lewis MAO 2005 An outcome audit of the treatment of acute dentoalveolar infection: impact of penicillin resistance. Brit Den J 199:759-763.

Kuriyama T, Karasawa T, Nakagawa K et al 2001 Incidence of β-lactamase production and antimicrobial susceptibility of anaerobic gram-negative rods isolated from pus specimens in orofacial odontogenic infections. Oral Micobiol Immunol16:10-15.

Mitchell DA 2006 An introduction to oral and maxillofacial surgery. Oxford University Press, Oxford.

Munson MA, Pitt-Ford T, Chong B et al 2002 Molecular and cultural analysis of the microflora associated with endodontic infections. J Dent Res 81:761-766.

Sakamoto M, Rôças IN, Siqueria JF, Benno Y 2006 Molecular analysis of bacteria in asymptomatic and symptomatic endodontic infections. Oral Microbiol Immunol 21: 112-122.

Stefanopoulos PK, Kolotronis AE 2004 The clinical significance of anaerobic bacteria in acute orofacial infection. Oral Surg Oral Med Oral Pathol, Oral Radiol Endod 98:398-408.

Chapter 8

Antimicrobial prophylaxis

ANTIMICROBIAL AGENTS

Antimicrobial agents are compounds which inhibit the growth, or kill microorganisms. Some of the early antimicrobial agents were derived from microorganisms and were called antibiotics. Nowadays antimicrobial agents are compounds which are synthesized to target certain specific functions in the microbial cell and are not derived from microorganisms; they are, therefore, not termed antibiotics but are referred to as antimicrobial agents.

Antimicrobial agents can be used for either treatment or prevention of infectious disease but must be used properly and accurately. The empirical overuse of antibiotics has been accompanied by an enormous increase in the emergence of microbial resistance; this has made some antimicrobials useless for the treatment of some common diseases. The use of antimicrobials in the prevention of disease is called prophylaxis and is controversial. In many cases the use of prophylactic antimicrobials in oral surgery is a matter of clinical habit rather than based on sound evidence-based clinical science. There are four occasions when prophylactic antimicrobials are indicated and these are:

- When the risk of post-operative infection is high.
- When wounds are contaminated with soil or dirt (e.g. after road traffic accidents) and there is a risk of infection (e.g. *Clostridium tetani*).
- Where the consequences of infection are serious or life threatening.
- When a person's defences against infection are compromised (see Ch. 11).

This chapter will concentrate on the first and third indications for prophylactic antimicrobials where oral operations are concerned.

WHEN DOES POST-OPERATIVE INFECTION OCCUR?

The majority of post-operative infections occur at the time of surgery. Secondary infection can occur following surgery (e.g. if a wound is disturbed or sutures are lost), but this is not usual. In a series of animal experiments in the 1960s it was demonstrated that post-operative infections are usually infected at the time of surgery. The source of the post-operative infection can either be endogenous or exogenous. Endogenous infections are derived from the patient's own microflora and are introduced at the time of the operation; they then proliferate and an infection results. The commonest time when endogenous post-operative infection occurs is when the surgery is done on a site already infected with the person's own microflora. Ideally surgery should not be done on areas that are not infected, but this is not always possible. Exogenous wound infections arise from microorganisms being introduced into the mouth from a source outside the oral cavity, and are usually caused by poor aseptic technique or by non-sterile instruments. Exogenous wound infections can often be prevented by careful preparation of the operation site with judicious use of antiseptics.

There are two types of post-operative infection: immediate or late. Immediate post-operative infections occur in the first 2–3 days following the operation. Late infections can occur weeks or months after the operation and are due to microorganisms remaining quiescent within the site and then being reactivated. Late infections of this kind are particularly associated with implants or surgically-placed prostheses and are often called latent infections.

HOW DOES PRE-SURGICAL ANTIMICROBIAL PROPHYLAXIS WORK?

The mechanism of antimicrobial prophylaxis is still controversial. Most antimicrobial agents work best on actively dividing microorganisms which does not usually apply to most immediate wound infections. Successful antimicrobial prophylaxis does appear to suppress microbial growth. A number of other mechanisms could explain how prophylactic antimicrobials work and include:

- Antimicrobials attaching to the surface of the microorganisms and forming complexes that increase phagocytosis.
- Antimicrobial/microorganism complexes increasing opsonization.
- Antimicrobial/microorganism complexes increasing complement activation by either the classical or alternative pathways.
- Antimicrobials preventing microorganisms from directly attaching to prostheses by blocking binding sites.

The above explanations all have some experimental evidence to support them, but it is all derived from *in vitro* experiments. The lack of any direct experimental evidence of the mechanism has led many people to question whether antimicrobial prophylaxis is necessary at all, especially with oral surgical operations where the incidence of post-operative infection is very low.

PRE- OR POST-OPERATIVE ANTIMICROBIALS OR BOTH?

Despite the evidence that infection occurs at the time of operation many clinicians still give courses of antimicrobial prophylaxis at times that are inappropriate and will miss the critical time when antimicrobial protection is required. For example, a common time to give antimicrobials is if an extraction cannot be achieved by simple forceps action and a surgical operation is necessary. Often it is many hours after the operation by the time the antimicrobials are dispensed. All the available clinical evidence has shown that giving antimicrobials some time after the operation has no effect on the outcome. There are now a large number of double-blind clinical trials that have shown that only an antimicrobial given before the operation, in sufficient time for serum and tissue concentrations to be maximal, will have a prophylactic effect on post-surgical infection.

One important factor to consider when selecting the antimicrobial agent is that it should be able to penetrate the tissues concerned and in particular bone. Clindamycin, the cephalosporins and metronidazole all penetrate bone well, but amoxicillin does not and is not licensed for use in this tissue.

The macrolides also do not have good bone penetration. Amoxicillin is by far the most commonly given prophylactic antimicrobial and to reach appropriate prophylactic concentrations in bone, for example, it is necessary to give high doses. This is not the case with clindamycin, the cephalosporins and metronidazole where standard adult doses give high and prophylactic concentrations in bone. Most antimicrobial agents that penetrate bone do so rapidly in the oral skeletal structures usually attaining maximal concentrations within one hour.

ANTIMICROBIAL PROPHYLAXIS FOR ORAL SURGERY

One branch of surgery where the chances of post-operative infection could be high is oral surgery, as this is inevitably done in sites where many millions of potential infectious agents could be present. In practice, the rates of post-operative infection in oral surgery are extremely low. Most simple soft-tissue surgery within the oral cavity does not require any antimicrobial prophylaxis. The current consensus of opinion is that the rate of post-operative infectious complications is so low that antimicrobial prophylaxis cannot be justified and would not affect the outcome. For example, in simple periodontal surgery, where numerous potential pathogens are present (Ch. 6), the elimination of pocket stagnation does not require antimicrobial prophylaxis, although it is often given. Antimicrobials given before deep root planing or extensive scaling probably have some effect on healing, but the difference between those given prophylaxis and those without is not statistically significant.

THIRD MOLAR SURGERY

The use of prophylactic antimicrobials for the removal of third molars has always been controversial. Until quite recently, third molars were removed whether they gave symptoms or not. The extraction of unerupted third molars often involves the removal of bone and, as a consequence, pain, swelling and trismus (restriction of mouth opening) can occur. Post-operative infection is rare following third molar surgery, but the swelling associated with this procedure is often mistaken for infection. It is a common practice to give antimicrobial agents before and after third molar surgery and there is a strong cadre of surgeons who still perpetuate this practice. There have been nine double-blind randomized trials of a variety of prophylactic antimicrobial agents given before and after third molar surgery. All of these trials have come to the same conclusion that antimicrobial agents have no statistically significant effect on swelling, pain, trismus or post-operative infection. One trial also measured the effect of prophylactic antimicrobials on C-reactive protein and alpha-1 trypsin serum levels which could be indicators of inflammation or infection. The antimicrobials were found to have no effect on the serum concentrations of these markers. This evidence would strongly support the contention that antimicrobials should not be given prophylactically for third molar removal.

JOINT REPLACEMENTS

The replacement of joints such as hips and knees with artificial prostheses is now common orthopaedic practice. Some orthopaedic surgeons believe that the bacteria that enter the bloodstream following dental procedures can pose a threat of early or late infections in the prosthesis. The consequences of infection in an orthopaedic prosthesis can be extremely serious. An infected hip prosthesis would require another surgical replacement operation and has an approximately 25% chance of being successful. This means that a person with an infected hip has only a 25% chance of being able to satisfactorily walk again. Some orthopaedic surgeons insist that persons with implanted prostheses have prophylactic antimicrobials before all dental treatment. The prophylactic antimicrobial recommended is usually amoxicillin which is ironic, because this probably does not penetrate joints, has no proven prophylactic action in this site and is not licensed for this purpose. A risk assessment and review of the literature reveals a paucity of proven cases where infected joint replacement prostheses have been linked with dental treatment. The use of prophylactic antimicrobials for dental patients with implanted orthopaedic prostheses, therefore, is not recommended or justified scientifically.

DENTAL IMPLANTS

The pioneering work of Bränemark devised techniques for the placement of dental implants that integrated with bone. The use of such implants has revolutionised prosthetic dentistry and many thousands of dental implants are placed successfully each year. The surgical placement of dental implants is an elective operation done under aseptic conditions and, therefore, should not require antimicrobial use, but many surgeons around the world insist that they are given before and after implant placement. There have now been at least nine substantial double-blind placebo controlled randomized trials on the use of prophylactic antimicrobials and implant placement.

One review of these trials called the use of prophylactic antimicrobials for the placement of implants 'at best equivocal, but probably not of use'. It would again appear that the use of antimicrobial agents for the placement of implants is not justified.

ORAL SURGERY WHERE THE CONSEQUENCES OF POST-OPERATIVE INFECTION ARE POTENTIALLY SERIOUS

One potential post-operative infection following dental procedures that could be serious and life-threatening is infective endocarditis. The link between this infection and dentistry is highly controversial, as is the use of antimicrobial prophylaxis to prevent this condition. It is pertinent first to review what causes infective endocarditis and its consequences.

Infective endocarditis

Infective endocarditis is an infection of the endothelium (lining) of the heart. If the blood flow through the heart is disrupted either by congenital, or acquired disease then it can clot. This is due to the flow being slowed where there is eddy or whirling of the flow. One common cause of slowing of blood flow is narrowing of the valve exits, where the blood is pumped from a narrow area into a larger area (the so called Venturi effect). Again the blood is slowed and clots form deposits on the undersides of the valves. These clots are often called 'vegetations,' because they resemble vegetationous growths. If bacteria enter the blood stream (bacteraemia) and enter the heart they can attach to these vegetations and start to grow. They grow extremely slowly on these vegetations often taking between 12 and 18 hours to double in number and form biofilms (Fig. 8.1; Ch. 5). Eventually they can cause inflammation of the heart lining (called the endothelium) and infective endocarditis can ensue. One source of the infective agents has been postulated to be streptococci from the mouth which are released into the blood stream during dental procedures.

Infective endocarditis is an extremely dangerous condition, but fortunately it is rare with only 1000 patients developing the disease in the UK each year. Even when prolonged intravenous antibiotics are given promptly to kill the infecting agent, endocarditis still has a high mortality rate of between 25–40%. The disease is quite difficult to diagnose from its initial signs and symptoms which are influenza-like symptoms, night sweats and lassitude which gradually progress. The diagnosis is usually made on the basis of a culture of blood which yields the infective

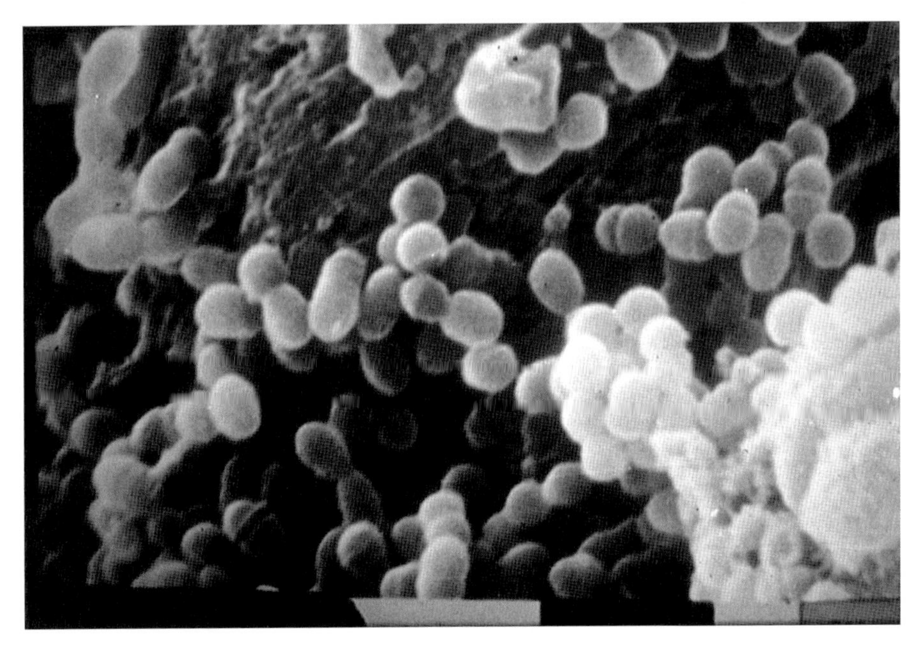

Fig. 8.1 SEM showing streptococci colonizing a heart valve from a case of fatal endocarditis.

agents. If the patient recovers, the heart valves may need replacement and the vegetations need removal. This requires open-heart surgery which carries a significant mortality risk. Replacement of the heart valves unfortunately means that the patient may have a 25% chance of getting infective endocarditis again. During the period when the patient has infective endocarditis small portions of the vegetations may break off and block peripheral blood vessels; this is particularly serious if it is in the brain.

The microorganisms which cause infective endocarditis are listed in Table 8.1. The principal bacteria that cause this disease are now staphylococci (probably derived from the skin), but until recently oral streptococci were the main cause. The rise in the number of people developing infective endocarditis due to staphylococci is probably due to the use of unsterile needles by intravenous drug addicts.

Oral streptococci have long been associated in the development of infective endocarditis. This is because many dental procedures such as scaling, extractions and gingival manipulations have been shown to release oral bacteria, and in particular streptococci, into the bloodstream (i.e. cause a bacteraemia). The principal oral streptococci associated with infective endocarditis are *Streptococcus sanguinis*, but *S. gordonii* and *S. oralis* are also frequently isolated. Although these bacteria are readily found in the mouths of patients with infective endocarditis (Ch. 4), they can also be recovered from elsewhere in the body, for example, on the genitalia and in the upper respiratory tract. It is, therefore, by no means certain that the mouth is always the portal of entry for these bacteria on their way to the heart.

Table 8.1 Microorganisms isolated from cases of human infective endocarditis

Microorganism	% Isolation Frequency
Staphylococci	44
Oral streptococci*	36
Enterococci	12
Aggregatibacter (Actinobacillus) actinomycetemcomitans	3
Coxiella burnettii	2
Candida spp	1
Other microorganisms including viruses	2

*Most common species isolated are *S. sanguinis* and *S. oralis*

The exact mechanism by which oral streptococci cause infective endocarditis is still a matter of debate. Undoubtedly oral streptococci enter the blood stream and circulate to the heart and attach to the vegetations, but this is probably not the main route of infection. It has been postulated that on entering the blood stream oral streptococci are 'shocked' by the change in their environment. This 'shock' may cause the exposure on their cell surface of specific adhesins (Ch. 4). These adhesins are not normally exposed on the surface of the streptococci that possess them and because of this have been given the term cryptitopes. At least two specific adhesins have been identified: a rhamnose-rich glycoprotein with a collagen-like domain and another protein which has not been fully characterized. The rhamnose-rich protein binds the oral streptococci to platelets and induces their aggregation, for this reason it is often given the acronym PAAP (platelet aggregating protein). It is the complexes of platelets and streptococci which bind to the vegetations on the heart and cause infective endocarditis. Not all strains of oral streptococci possess PAAP, but its presence is probably not essential for the pathogenesis of infective endocarditis, as other oral streptococcal strains without this factor can cause the disease. In addition to PAAP, the presence of glucan-forming enzymes, the glucosyltransferases (Ch. 4), have been implicated in the adherence of oral streptococci to vegetations, but it is not clear if this is an essential requirement for infective endocarditis to occur.

Antimicrobial prophylaxis against infective endocarditis

The prevention of infective endocarditis is of paramount importance as the disease is so serious and potentially life threatening. One possible preventative method is to give antimicrobials before certain types of dental treatment with the intention of preventing the infection. Animal studies, particularly in the rabbit, have been used to simulate the disease. If large doses of antimicrobials are given before the susceptible rabbit is inoculated then 90% of the animals can be protected against infective endocarditis. The protection is not 100% effective in animals and this is also true for humans where infective endocarditis is not completely prevented by administration of prophylactic antimicrobials. There is also some doubt in humans as to the exact dose of antimicrobial agent required, for example, 3 g amoxicillin (given orally) is used in the UK while in the USA the dose is 2 g.

There are over 44 inter-related conditions that can be associated with a susceptibility to infective endocarditis but some of these are rare. Thus there is confusion as to which patients should receive antimicrobial prophylaxis. Also there is doubt as to whether antimicrobial prophylaxis works at all, as the animal studies do not completely simulate human infective endocarditis. For this reason, expert groups have met around the world and issued guidelines as to which patients should receive antimicrobial prophylaxis and for which types of dental treatment.

There have also been large numbers of authorities that are questioning whether antimicrobial prophylaxis should be given at all before dental treatment for patients susceptible to infective endocarditis.

The largest review summating all the evidence has been done by the National Institute for Clinical Excellence (NICE) in the UK in 2008. Using all the data they had available from studies around the world they concluded that there were four groups of patients that are particularly susceptible to infective endocarditis: these were those with acquired valvular damage, structural congenital heart disease, valve replacements and cardiomyopathy. These four groups alone could justify antimicrobial prophylaxis. NICE also looked at the effects of antimicrobial prophylaxis on bacteraemias and concluded that the effect was impossible to measure. NICE therefore recommended from March 2008 that no further antimicrobial prophylaxis should be given before any dental treatment in any group of patients susceptible to infective endocarditis in the UK.

CHAPTER SUMMARY

Antimicrobial prophylaxis is not justified for patients who have received hip replacements, before implant placement, minor oral surgery or third molar removal. The UK has also recommended that antimicrobial prophylaxis is not given before dental treatment for patients susceptible to infective endocarditis. In situations where antibiotics are appropriate, they should be selected carefully and should penetrate the target tissues.

FURTHER READING

Esposito MP, Coulthard R, Oliver P, Thomsen P 2004 Antibiotics to prevent complications in implant treatment. Cochrane Data Base System Review CDOO4152.

Ford I, Douglas CWI 1997 The role of platelets in infective endocarditis. Platelets 8: 285-294.

Infective endocarditis. The NICE recommendations. National Institute for Clinical Research, 2008.

Martin MV, Kanatas AN, Hardy P 2005 Antibiotic prophylaxis and third molar surgery. Br Dent J 198: 327-330.

Petersen LJ 1990 Antibiotic prophylaxis against wound infections in oral and maxillofacial surgery. J Oral Maxillofac Surg 48:617-620.

Chapter 9

Oral fungal infections

Candida species are fungi that are frequently encountered in the mouth of healthy individuals and as such can be considered to be normal residents of the oral microflora. The actual incidence of oral candidal carriage is estimated to be between 35 and 55% of healthy individuals, depending on the population group studied. Other fungi, such as *Saccharomyces* spp., *Geotrichum* spp. and *Cryptococcus* spp. are also encountered (Table 9.1), but their occurrences are rare and these are not generally implicated with oral infection. While *Candida* species are normally harmless commensals, when conditions in the mouth alter to one that favours proliferation of *Candida*, a shift to a pathogenic state can occur. As such, *Candida* infection is invariably an opportunistic one dependent upon some form of underlying host predisposition. Infection with *Candida* is described in the literature as a candidosis (candidoses, pl) or candidiasis (candidiases, pl). Both terms are widely used, although candidosis is often preferred due to its consistent use of the 'osis' stem with the terminology for other fungal infections. The term *Candida* originates from the Latin word *candid*, meaning white.

PATHOGENIC *CANDIDA* SPECIES

The genus *Candida* contains over 200 different species that are ubiquitously distributed. However, only a few of these have been implicated in human infection. The most prevalent *Candida* species recovered from the human mouth, in both commensal state and cases of oral candidosis, is *Candida albicans*. It is estimated that this species accounts for over 80% of all oral yeast isolates. In terms of oral prevalence, *C. albicans* is followed by *C. glabrata, C. krusei, C. tropicalis, C. guilliermondii,*

Table 9.1 Fungal species recovered from the human mouth.	
***Candida* species**	**Other fungal species (rare)**
Candida albicans	*Paracoccidioides brasiliensis*
Candida glabrata	*Aspergillus* spp.
Candida tropicalis	*Cryptococcus neoformans*
Candida krusei	*Histoplasma capsulatum*
Candida lusitaniae	*Mucor* spp.
Candida dubliniensis	*Saccharomyces* spp.
Candida kefyr	*Geotrichum* spp.
Candida guilliermondii	*Rhizopus* spp.
Candida parapsilosis	

C. kefyr and *C. parapsilosis*. In more recent years there has been a greater recognition of the importance of the non-*albicans Candida* species in human disease. *Candida glabrata* and *C. krusei* are species that have received attention due to their enhanced resistance to certain antifungal agents. *Candida dubliniensis* is a recently identified pathogenic species, first described in 1995 when it was co-isolated with *C. albicans* from cases of oral candidosis in HIV-infected individuals.

CANDIDA VIRULENCE FACTORS

The transition of *Candida* from a harmless commensal to a pathogenic organism is complex and may relate to subtle environmental changes that lead to the expression of a range of virulence factors (Table 9.2). It is likely that it is the combined effect of both host and candidal factors that ultimately contribute to the development of oral candidosis.

Adherence

One of the key virulence factors of *Candida* spp. is the ability to adhere to host surfaces. In the oral cavity, this allows the organism to avoid removal through the effects of salivary flow and swallowing. Adherence can be to oral epithelial tissue or to biomaterials of prosthetic devices such as dentures, that have been introduced into the mouth. Attachment to such oral surfaces can be specific or non-specific, the latter involving electrostatic or hydrophobic interactions, together with the simple physical entrapment of the microorganism at specific locations in the mouth.

The cell surface molecules on *Candida* that are involved in its specific adherence are described as adhesins (Ch. 4). The host cell component that these adhesins interact with, are referred to as receptors. A wide range of adhesins have been identified

Table 9.2 Putative virulence factors associated with *Candida albicans*.	
Virulence factor	**Effect**
Adherence	**Promotes retention in the mouth**
• Relative cell surface hydrophobicity	• Non-specific adherence process
• Expression of cell surface adhesin molecules	• Facilitates specific adherence mechanisms
Evasion of host defences	**Promotes retention in the mouth**
• High frequency phenotypic switching	• Antigenic modification through frequent cell surface changes
• Hyphal development	• Reduces likelihood of phagocytosis; allows phagocytosed yeast to escape phagocyte
• Secreted aspartyl proteinase production	• Secretory IgA destruction
• Binding of complement molecules	• Antigenic masking
Invasion and destruction of host tissue	**Enhances pathogenicity**
• Hyphal development	• Promotes invasion of oral epithelium
• Secreted aspartyl proteinase production	• Host cell and extracellular matrix damage
• Phospholipase production	• Damage to host cells

for *C. albicans* and include mannoproteins, fibrillar adhesins that bind to fucosyl receptors and proteins that bind to complement receptors on host cells. Candidal adherence is a complex and multifactorial process, dependent on both host and candidal characteristics.

Morphology

Candida have the ability to grow in several morphological states including budding yeast cells, pseudohyphae (elongated chains of yeast cells), and also true filamentous hyphae (Fig. 9.1). Pseudohyphae and hyphae are distinguishable as the former contains constrictions at the septa of the filaments. Once attached to host surfaces the ability of *Candida* and in particular *C. albicans* to switch from its yeast morphology to a filamentous form may promote penetration of the epithelium and increase resistance of cells to phagocytosis by host immune cells.

Candida glabrata is notable for its inability to form filaments while other non-albicans *Candida* species can develop pseudohyphae. True hyphal development is an attribute reserved for *C. albicans* and the closely related *C. dubliniensis*. A number of genes have been shown to positively control hyphal production in *C. albicans* including *HGC1* which encodes for a cytoplasmic protein (hyphae-specific G1 cyclin) without which the hyphal morphology will not occur. Studies examining mutants of *C. albicans* unable to express *HGC1* show that non-filamentous strains are less virulent.

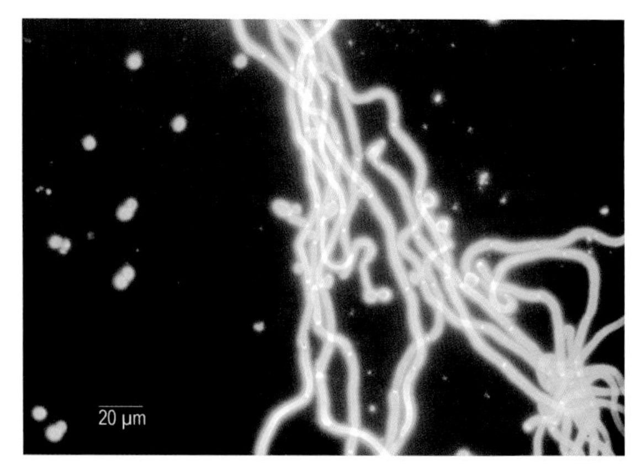

Fig. 9.1 Fluorescent microscopy image of *Candida albicans* as a mixture of yeast and filamentous growth forms.

Phenotypic switching

The candidal phenomenon of high frequency switching is related to cell morphology and reflected *in vitro* as reversible changes in colony morphology induced by exposure to various environmental stimuli. Switching has multiple effects on the *Candida* cells and is associated with altered gene expression which affects surface antigenicity, adhesiveness, drug susceptibility, and resistance to phagocytosis by polymorphonuclear leukocytes. A high switching mode is a strain-dependent trait and can clearly influence strain virulence.

Hydrolytic enzymes

Destruction of host tissues by *Candida* may be facilitated by the release of hydrolytic enzymes into the local environment and secreted aspartyl proteinases (SAPs) and phospholipases are the enzymes most frequently implicated with *C. albicans*.

Secreted aspartyl proteinases (SAPs)

At present, 10 different genes have been identified that encode for candidal SAPs. Expression of these genes can be induced under different conditions and three (*SAP4*, *SAP5* and *SAP6*) appear to be expressed during hyphal development. All SAPs exhibit a number of common characteristics including an activity restricted to a largely acidic environment and inhibition by pepstatin A (a hexa-peptide originally isolated from *Actinomycete* species). The exact role of these enzymes in virulence remains unclear, however their ability to degrade host extracellular matrix proteins would be an obvious pathogenic factor as would the destruction of host proteins involved in defence against infection.

Phospholipases (PLs)

In addition to SAPs, enzymes categorized as phospholipases (PLs) are often considered to be factors in *Candida* pathogenicity. Phospholipases are enzymes that hydrolyse phospholipids into fatty acids. Four classes of phospholipases (A, B, C, and D) have been defined depending upon the type of ester bond cleaved. The production of all classes of phospholipase has been described for *Candida* species and their production could contribute to host cell membrane damage which could promote cell lysis or expose receptors to facilitate adherence.

SUMMARY

Several *Candida* species are recognized as important opportunistic pathogens of humans and the ability to cause disease is dependent upon the delicate balance that exists between the host defence processes and the expression of virulence factors by the infecting *Candida*. No single predominant virulence factor for *Candida* is recognized although there are a number of factors that have been implicated in promoting the infection process. These include attributes involved in the adhesion of *Candida* to oral surfaces (e.g. relative cell surface hydrophobicity and the presence of specific adhesin molecules), the ability to resist host immune defence mechanisms (e.g. high frequency phenotypic switching and morphological transition) and the release of hydrolytic enzymes (e.g. secreted aspartyl proteinases and phospholipases) that can induce damage to host cells.

Table 9.3 Host related factors associated with oral candidosis.

Suggested host factor
Local host factors
• Denture wearing
• Steroid inhaler use
• Reduced salivary flow
• Carbohydrate rich diet
Systemic host factors
• Extremes of age
• Endocrine disorders *e.g.* diabetes
• Immunosuppression
• Receipt of broad spectrum antibiotics
• Nutritional deficiencies

ORAL CANDIDOSIS

Candidosis is a 'disease of the diseased' which highlights the importance of host-related factors on the development of oral candidosis. This is most clearly exemplified by the high incidence of oral candidosis in Human Immunodeficiency Virus (HIV)-positive individuals and Acquired Immunodeficiency Syndrome (AIDS) sufferers. However, transition from healthy oral carriage to a diseased state can be triggered by less extreme changes within the oral environment and numerous other factors have been implicated (Table 9.3).

Oral candidosis is not a single entity, and four distinct primary oral candidoses are frequently described, based on their clinical presentation (Fig.9.2).

Pseudomembranous candidosis

Pseudomembranous candidosis (Fig. 9.2A) is characterized by the presence of white plaque-like lesions on the oral mucosa and has traditionally been most frequently found in the mouths of neonates and in the elderly. Pseudomembranes occur on the surface of the labial and buccal mucosa, hard and soft palate, and tongue. The lesions can be removed by gentle scraping to reveal the underlying erythematous mucosa and this is a diagnostic clinical feature of the infection. When viewed by light microscopy, the removed pseudomembranes are seen to consist of desquamated epithelial cells and fungal elements. Pseudomembranous candidosis is often described as 'oral thrush' and is generally regarded as an acute infection resulting from an underlying host predisposition. Management and correction of any host related factor generally results in resolution of the condition. However, in recent years and with the advent of HIV infection and the increasing incidence of AIDS, a more chronic variant of pseudomembranous candidosis has been reported that can persist for several months if not years. Furthermore, in such immunocompromised individuals, progression of the oral infection to an oesophageal involvement is often evident and this can lead to added complications such as difficulties in swallowing and chest pain. The increasing prevalence of steroid inhaler use, particularly in young adults as part of the management of asthma, has been associated with frequent cases of pseudomembranous candidosis in the soft palate.

Acute erythematous candidosis

Acute erythematous candidosis (Fig. 9.2B) is characterized by the presence of painful reddened patches on the oral mucosa, typically on the dorsum of the

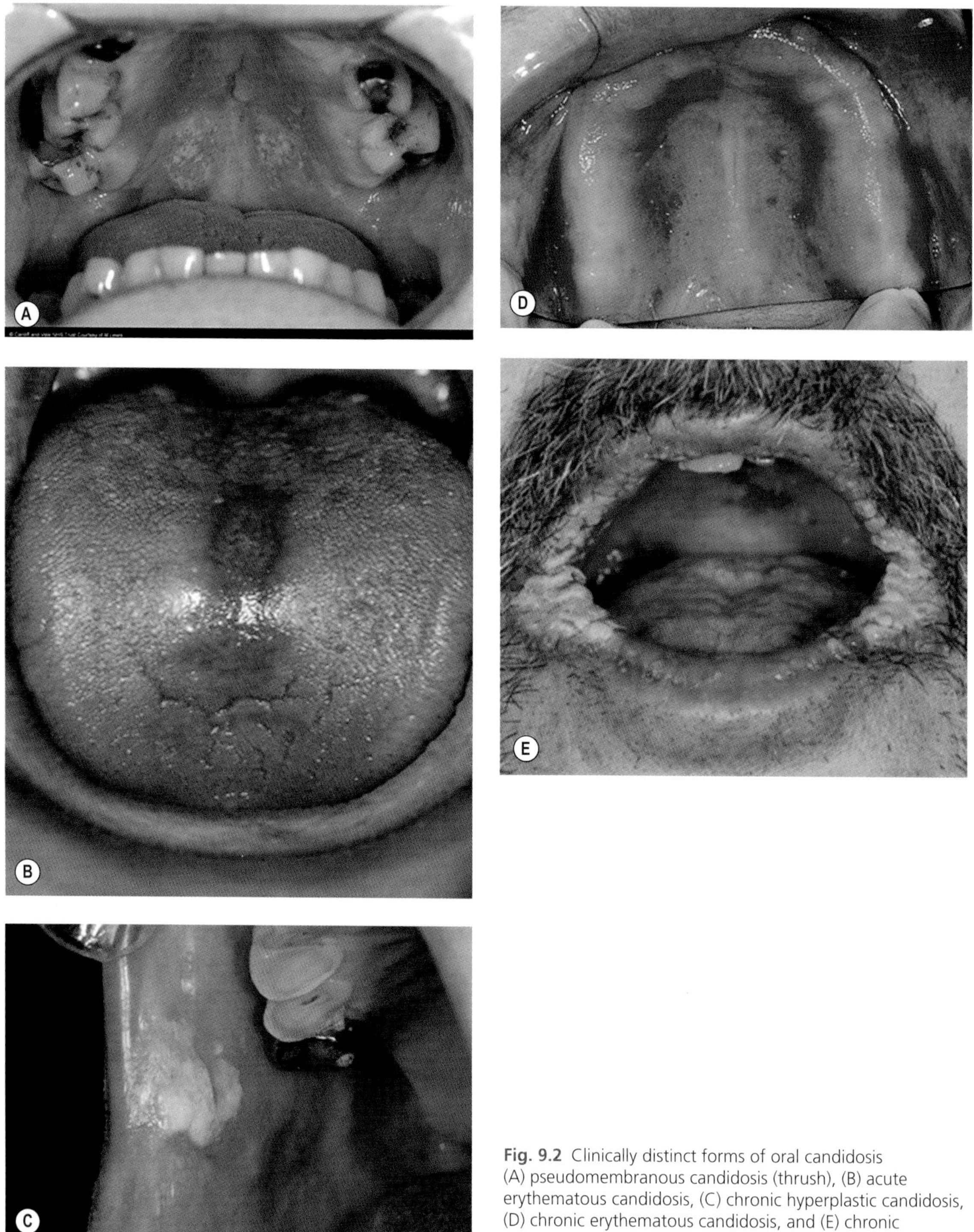

Fig. 9.2 Clinically distinct forms of oral candidosis (A) pseudomembranous candidosis (thrush), (B) acute erythematous candidosis, (C) chronic hyperplastic candidosis, (D) chronic erythematous candidosis, and (E) chronic mucocutaneous candidosis.

tongue. The condition is most frequently associated with the administration of a broad spectrum antibiotic, particularly if the patient also uses a steroid inhaler. It is believed that the antibiotic decreases the bacterial community within the oral microflora, allowing *Candida* numbers to increase. Cessation of antibiotic treatment will generally result in resolution of the lesion. The relationship between antibiotic therapy and this form of oral candidosis has resulted in the use of an alternative description, namely, 'antibiotic sore mouth'.

Chronic hyperplastic candidosis

Chronic hyperplastic candidosis (CHC; Fig. 9.2C) is a relatively rare form of oral candidosis with its highest prevalence seen in middle aged men who are tobacco smokers. The condition is generally asymptomatic and if left untreated some cases (5–10%) go on to exhibit dysplasia and subsequent development of oral cancer at the lesional site. Unlike other forms of oral candidosis, CHC is characterized by the invasion of the oral epithelium by hyphal forms of *Candida*. The condition can occur at any site on the oral mucosa but is most frequently encountered as bilateral white patches in the buccal commissure regions. The lesions cannot be removed by gentle scraping without bleeding and two lesional types have been described based on clinical appearance. Homogeneous lesions are smooth and white which contrasts with heterogeneous lesions where areas of erythema can be seen giving a nodular or speckled appearance to the infected site. Some studies suggest that it is the heterogeneous form of the lesion that is more prone to malignant transformation.

Chronic erythematous candidosis

The most frequently encountered form of oral candidosis is chronic erythematous or '*Candida* associated denture stomatitis' (Fig. 9.2D). As its name implies, this infection presents as reddening of the mucosa beneath the fitting surface of a denture. Up to 65% of denture wearers have clinical signs of this condition, although the sufferer is usually unaware of infection. This condition can develop under any acrylic denture or intra-oral appliance, but is almost invariably seen in the palate rather than on the mandibular mucosa. Inadequate oral hygiene or the presence of a poorly fitting denture are both strongly associated with chronic erythematous candidosis.

Other secondary forms of oral candidosis

In addition to the primary forms of oral candidosis described above, other *Candida*-associated lesions are recognized and include conditions such as angular cheilitis, median rhomboid glossitis, and chronic mucocutaneous candidosis.

Angular cheilitis

Angular cheilitis characteristically presents as erythematous lesions at the corners of the mouth (Fig. 7.13). The condition is frequently associated with another form of oral candidosis, typically chronic erythematous candidosis. While *Candida* can be recovered from the lesional sites, the exact role of this organism in the infection can be difficult to ascertain as frequently bacterial species such as *Staphylococcus aureus* or streptococci are also present.

Median rhomboid glossitis

Median rhomboid glossitis is seen as a symmetrical shaped area in the midline of the dorsum of the tongue. The condition is chronic and represents atrophy of the filiform papillae. Recovery of *Candida* from this area is high, and the condition would appear to be strongly associated with both smoking and the use of inhaled steroids.

Chronic mucocutaneous candidosis

Chronic mucocutaneous candidosis (CMC) is a condition that comprises a group of candidal infections largely confined to the skin, mucous membranes (Figure 9.2E) and nails of an individual. A number of relatively rare congenital conditions are associated with CMC and the key predisposing factor would appear to centre on an impaired cellular immunity against *Candida*.

It remains unclear as to why individuals present with these different infections, which are all seemingly caused by the same fungus. Host determinants are important with the different infections varying in prevalence amongst distinct patient groups. What is also evident is that *C. albicans* is an extremely heterogeneous species whose strains differ markedly, both phenotypically and genotypically. Thus, candidal strain variation could be a factor in determining which type of infection develops, whether the host actually manages to clear the colonizing strain or whether the strain is retained as a commensal. It is highly conceivable that strain variation could promote pathogenesis through elevated expression of virulence determinants and by affecting the nature of the hosts' immune response.

SUMMARY

Oral candidosis is not a single disease presentation and four clinically distinct forms are often described. These include the acute infections of pseudomembranous candidosis and acute erythematous candidosis with chronic infections represented by chronic erythematous candidosis and chronic hyperplastic candidosis. In more recent years and with the advent of the AIDS epidemic, chronic forms of pseudomembranous candidosis are more frequently encountered. Each infection has a distinct clinical presentation and associated host predisposing factors. The role of the infecting organism in determining the type of infection that occurs remains unclear.

HOST RESPONSE TO ORAL CANDIDOSIS

Appropriate host immunity is essential in the prevention of oral candidosis. Innate immunity is first encountered in the oral cavity in the form of antimicrobial peptides (AMPs), also referred to as host defence peptides (HDPs; Ch. 2) found in saliva or released by oral epithelial cells. Release of these molecules from epithelial cells is believed to be triggered when *Candida* binds to a particular group of receptors on epithelial cell surfaces. These receptors are often referred to as pattern-recognition receptors, and toll-like receptors (TLRs) are a major class of these. In humans, TLR2 and TLR4 are responsible for recognising fungal pathogens resulting in activation of intracellular pathways leading to cytokine production, activation of the innate immune response and release of AMPs.

Examples of AMPs include lactoferrin, α- and β- defensins, histatins, lysozyme, secretory immunoglobulin A, mucins, sialoperoxidase and transferrin (Ch. 2). The main function of these molecules is to either kill the colonising *Candida* or limit its adherence to oral surfaces. Histatins are largely specific to the mouth and have an anti-candidal activity. Reduced histatin levels have been linked with elevated *Candida* colonization of the oral mucosa.

Also of importance in early host defence is the phagocytotic clearing of *C. albicans* by polymorphonuclear cells (PMNs) and monocytes. Stimulation of macrophages may arise through direct contact with a range of candidal cell-wall component molecules. After phagocytosis, killing of *C. albicans* is believed to involve reactive oxygen and nitrogen intermediates. The phagocyte-dependent protection of the host can be promoted or impaired by the release of cytokines by T-helper (Th) cells. The importance of an appropriate Th response in protecting against oral candidosis is best exemplified by the high incidence of oral candidosis in HIV-positive individuals in whom a decline in T-cell activity occurs. The type of Th response generated can be influenced by the effect of the infecting organism on antigen-presenting cells (APCs) such as dentritic cells (DCs) that perform a sentinel role within the oral mucosa. After contact with *Candida*, or its products, DCs migrate into the draining lymph node where they mature and direct $CD4^+$ T cells to develop into either Th1 or Th2 cells through *Candida* antigen presentation and cytokine production. A Th1 type response is considered to be protective, while a Th2 response is believed to lead to *Candida*-related pathology.

Evidence suggests that the environment of initial DC stimulation may be important in ultimately determining the type of Th response. Studies in mice indicate that early release of proinflammatory cytokines such as interferon-γ (IFN-γ) and tumour necrosis factor-α (TNF-α) by macrophages, and interleukin-12 (IL-12) by DCs are important in directing Th cell maturation towards the Th1 type. In contrast, release of IL-4 and IL-10 would appear important for Th2 cell development. Different *C. albicans* strains could influence this process by stimulating tissues to produce particular cytokine profiles, or affecting the DC phenotype and thus the influence of DCs on naive Th cell maturation. There is evidence suggesting that the latter occurs with the different morphological forms of *C. albicans*, as DCs have been shown to discriminate between yeast and hyphal forms of *C. albicans*, which respectively promote Th1 and Th2 responses. Recent studies have also proposed a role for regulatory T cells ($CD4^+CD25^+$ T lymphocytes; Treg) in the immune response to *C. albicans* with the possibility that 1L-10 and transforming growth factor β (TGFβ)-mediated responses stimulate the production of Treg cells which suppress the normally protective Th1 responses.

Antibody driven (humoral immunity) protection against oral candidosis is first encountered by the action of secretory IgA which is considered to be an important inhibitor of the adhesion of *Candida* (and indeed other oral microbes) to oral surfaces. Serum antibodies probably constitute a secondary defence line and become important once either tissue penetration or systemic infection occurs.

SUMMARY

Host defence against oral candidosis initially involves a complex combination of non-specific antimicrobial molecules found in saliva and gingival crevicular fluid, the phagocytic clearing activity of polymorphonuclear and monocytic cells, and classical cell mediated defence mechanisms. In the event of tissue penetration, antibody based protection will become more prominent. A deficiency in the functioning of any of these defence mechanisms has the effect of predisposing an individual to *Candida* infection.

DIAGNOSIS OF ORAL CANDIDOSIS

Diagnosis of oral candidosis can often be made on the nature of the clinical presenting features although microbiological specimens should be taken if possible in order to both identify and quantify any *Candida* that may be present and provide isolates for antifungal sensitivity testing. Identification of infecting strains is important since the emergence of species with reduced sensitivity to frequently administered antifungals is becoming increasingly evident.

Isolation of *Candida* from the oral cavity

Oral samples can be obtained by a variety of methods (Table 9.4) with the most common approaches being swab, imprint culture, oral rinse and culture of whole saliva. Each method has its merits as well as its drawbacks and the most appropriate method is largely governed by the presentation of the lesion. Where an accessible and defined lesion is evident, a direct sampling approach such as the use of a swab or an imprint is often preferred as this will provide information of the organisms present at the lesion itself. In cases where there are no obvious lesions or in instances where the lesion is difficult to access, an indirect sample based on culturing saliva specimens or an oral rinse is more acceptable.

In the case of chronic hyperplastic candidosis, a biopsy of the lesion is necessary for subsequent detection of invading *Candida* by histological staining using either the periodic acid Schiff or Gomori's methenamine silver stains.

Quantitative estimation of fungal load at the lesion has been justified as a means of differentiating between commensal carriage and pathogenic existence of oral *Candida*, with higher loads considered likely in the latter. On this basis, the imprint culture and the oral rinse offer advantages over the other approaches.

Table 9.4 Methods of recovering *Candida* from the oral cavity.

Isolation method	Advantages	Disadvantages
Culture of whole saliva	Sensitive; viable organisms isolated	Problems may occur with collection of sample; not site specific
Concentrated oral rinse	Quantitative; viable cells isolated	Some patients have difficulty in using rinse; not site specific
Swab	Simple to use; viable cells isolated; site specific	Difficult to standardise
Smear	Simple to use; not reliant on culture	Viable cells not determined; species identity not readily confirmed
Imprint culture	Quantitative; viable cells isolated; site specific	Some sites difficult to sample
Biopsy	Essential for chronic hyperplastic candidosis	Invasive; not appropriate for other forms of candidosis

Oral samples for detection of *Candida* are generally cultured on Sabouraud Dextrose Agar (SDA) which will support the growth of all oral *Candida* species with the added benefit of suppressing bacterial growth due to its relatively low pH. Occasionally microbiologists will incorporate antibiotics into SDA to further increase its selectivity. In recent years, other differential media e.g. CHROMagar® *Candida* (Fig. 9.3), have been developed that allow identification of certain *Candida* species based on colony appearance and colour following primary culture. The advantage of such media is that the presence of multiple *Candida* species in a single infection can be determined which can be important in selecting subsequent treatment options.

Presumptive identification of yeasts based on primary culture media can be confirmed through a variety of supplemental tests traditionally based on morphological and physiological characteristics of the isolates. As previously mentioned, *C. albicans* and *C. dubliniensis* are the only species that produce true hyphal growth and this trait can be exploited for identification through the use of the 'germ-tube test'. In this test, the organism is subcultured in horse serum at 37°C for 2–4 hours, after which time the culture is examined by light microscopy for the presence of germ-tubes (Fig. 9.4).

Candida albicans and *C. dubliniensis* can also be identified from other species based on their ability to produce morphological features known as chlamydospores. Chlamydospores are refractile, spherical structures generated at the termini of hyphae following culture of isolates on a nutritionally poor medium such as cornmeal agar. Isolates are inoculated in a cross-hatch pattern on the agar and overlaid with a sterile coverslip. Agars are incubated for 24–48 hours at 37°C and then examined microscopically for chlamydospore presence (Fig. 9.5).

Biochemical identification of *Candida* species is largely based on carbohydrate utilization and a range of commercial systems are now available to facilitate such tests. Isolate identification is determined by the profile of carbohydrates that can be utilized by the test organism. Traditional testing would have involved culture of test isolates on a basal agar lacking a carbon source. Carbohydrate solutions would then be placed within wells of the seeded agar or upon filter paper discs located on the agar surface. Growth in the vicinity of the carbon source would indicate utilization. Commercial systems such as the API 32C system are based on the same principle but test carbohydrates are housed in plastic wells located on a test strip. Growth in each well is read by changes in turbidity or colour changes in certain kit systems. Numerical codes obtained from the test results are used to identify the test organism based on database comparison.

Increasingly, molecular-based identification methods are used within diagnostic laboratories and there are a number of reports using species-specific polymerase chain reaction (PCR) approaches for *Candida*

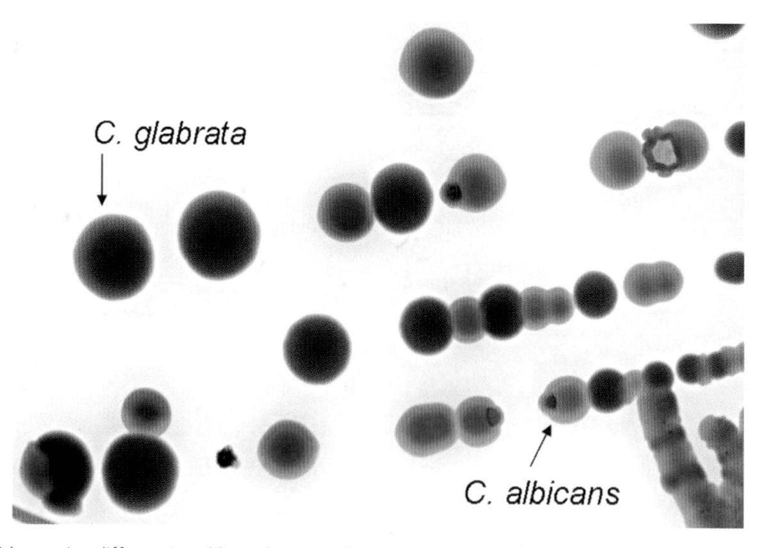

Fig. 9.3 Mixed *Candida* species differentiated by culture on CHROMagar® *Candida*. *Candida albicans* appear as green colonies, non *C. albicans* species frequently present with purple or alternative colouration.

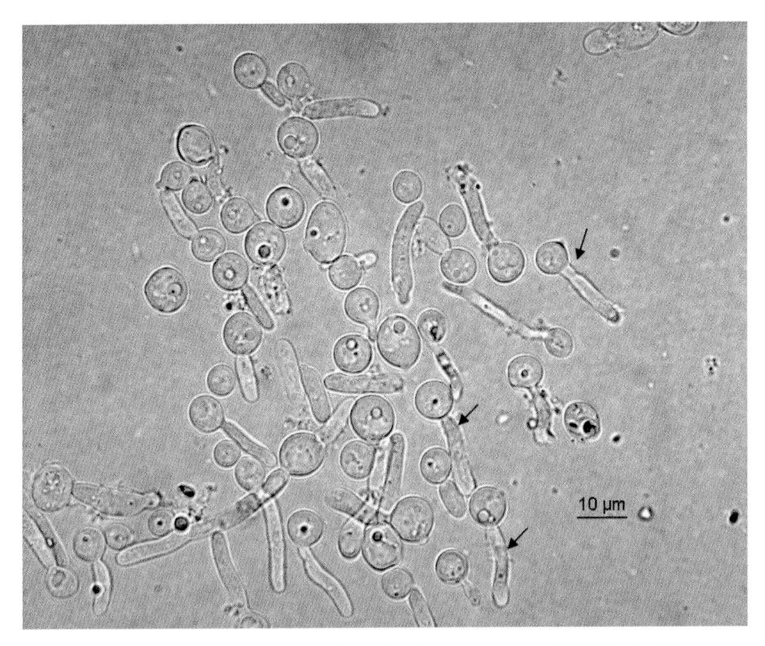

Fig. 9.4 Germ tube production (arrowed) by *C. albicans* cultured in horse serum at 37°C for 2–4 hours.

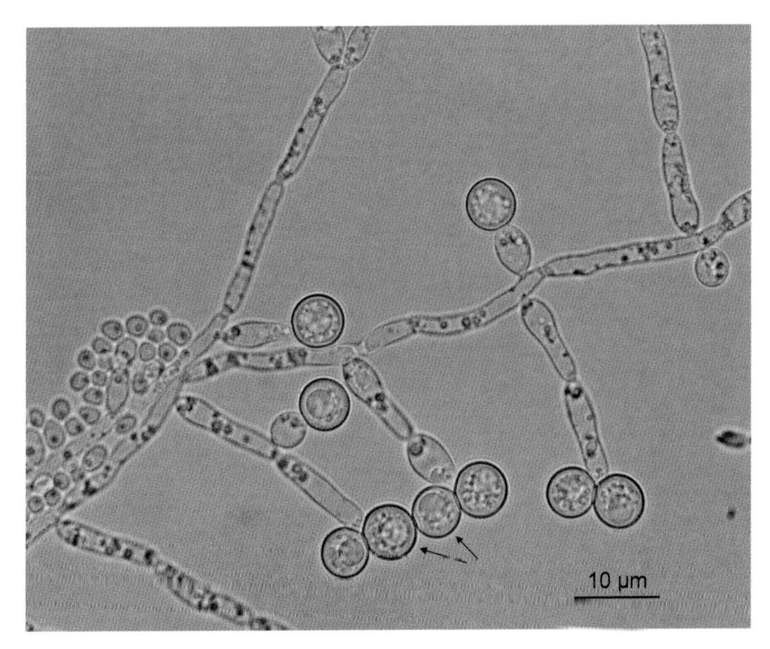

Fig. 9.5 Chlamydospores (arrowed) produced by *Candida albicans* on cornmeal tween 20 agar.

identification. Several target genes have been reported for *Candida* species discrimination, although those most frequently amplified are the sequences of the ribosomal RNA operon. Identification can be obtained based on PCR product sizes obtained following gel electrophoresis resolution, or PCR product sequence variation determined either by direct sequencing or through the use of restriction fragment analysis following cutting of PCR sequences with restriction endonucleases. Molecular-based technology can also be used to identify strains of *Candida* species although the use of techniques such as Pulsed

Field Gel Electrophoresis (PFGE), Random Amplified Polymorphic DNA (RAPD) analysis and REP (repeat sequence amplification) PCR are largely reserved for epidemiological investigations in research of oral candidosis.

SUMMARY

In recent years greater emphasis has been placed on the reliable identification of *Candida* species from human clinical samples. Key to this has been the recognition that a range of different species are associated with human infection and, importantly, may vary in both pathogenic potential and susceptibility to administered antifungal agents. Since *Candida* are frequent components of the resident microflora in health, appropriate sampling methods are required to assist in ascertaining the exact location of the organisms in the mouth together with their number. There are a wide variety of phenotypic methods available for identifying isolated *Candida* including the use of differential agar media, morphological culture tests and biochemical screening panels. These methods have recently been supplemented with more sophisticated molecular tests involving analysis of the DNA of isolated organisms.

MANAGEMENT OF ORAL CANDIDOSIS

In view of the fact that oral candidosis is an opportunistic infection, identification and elimination of any underlying host predisposing factor (Table 9.3) is the key to patient management. Consideration of the patient's medical history is highly significant in developing a management regime for a sufferer of oral candidosis. Predisposing factors need to be identified and resolved wherever possible. Such goals are achievable in many instances, for example, improving the oral hygiene in denture wearers who have chronic erythematous candidosis is paramount to management of this condition. Cessation of smoking for sufferers of CHC or median rhomboid glossitis should also be targeted together with educating asthmatics who use steroid inhalers about the importance of rinsing their mouths after administration of the inhaler. Haematological tests may reveal inadequate levels of vitamins and minerals and such situations can be readily addressed through management of diet and/or the use of supplements. Undiagnosed or poorly controlled diabetes is a recognised predisposing factor to oral candidosis and therefore assessment of blood glucose may be required.

In some cases, however, the predisposing factors cannot be resolved, such as with individuals who are immunosuppressed through the receipt of an immunosuppressant drug required for the treatment of a cancer, or to avoid organ rejection following transplant surgery.

ANTIFUNGAL INTERVENTION

In comparison with antibiotics, the development of antifungal agents has been relatively slow. This can be attributed to several factors including the inherent problems in developing an effective agent that acts upon a eukaryotic fungal cell type without toxicity to eukaryotic host cells. In addition, it is only relatively recently that diagnostic procedures have highlighted the significant role of fungi in disease and their increasing occurrence, largely due to medical interventions leading to host susceptibility.

The classification of antifungal drugs is currently based on their target of activity (Table 9.5) and the use of these agents often varies with the type of oral candidosis and condition of the patient (Table 9.6). Resistance to antifungal drugs is an increasingly recognized phenomenon and can be defined clinically as the persistence of signs and symptoms of the infection despite adequate delivery of a normally appropriate and tolerable level of the drug. Depending on the drug and the yeast species, the mechanism of antifungal resistance can either be intrinsic (present without previous exposure to the antifungal) or inherent, where resistance develops in a previously susceptible organism following exposure.

Polyene antifungals

Polyene antifungals are fungicidal due to their ability to interact with the ergosterol component within the fungal cell membrane to generate pores within the membranes causing cell leakage and loss of cytoplasmic content. The principal polyene antifungals are amphotericin B and nystatin and these agents are generally regarded to have the broadest spectrum of antifungal activity. These agents are frequently used topically and can be administered in a variety of oral formulations in the treatment of oral candidosis including suspensions, lozenges and pastilles. Polyenes are very poorly

Table 9.5 Antifungals used in the management of candidosis.

Antifungal	Mode of action	Administration
Polyenes	Disruption of fungal cell membrane	
• Nystatin		topical
• Amphotericin		topical
Azoles	Inhibition of ergosterol synthesis	
• fluconazole		systemic
• miconazole		topical
• ketoconazole		topical/systemic
• clotrimazole		topical
• itraconazole		systemic
• voriconazole		systemic
• posaconazole		systemic
5-flucytosine	Inhibition of DNA and protein synthesis	systemic, often in combined therapy with amphotericin
Echinocandins	Inhibition of ß 1, 3 D-glucan synthesis	intravenous
• caspofungin		
• micofungin		
• anidulafungin		

Table 9.6 Recommended antifungal therapy for primary forms of oral candidosis.

	PMC	AEC	CEC	CHC
Topical delivery				
Nystatin			Yes	
Amphotericin			Yes	
Miconazole			Yes	
Clotrimazole			Yes	
Systemic delivery				
Ketoconazole	Yes	Yes		Yes
Fluconazole	Yes	Yes		Yes
Itraconazole	Yes	Yes		Yes

PMC, pseudomembranous candidosis; AEC, acute erythematous candidosis;
CEC, chronic erythematous candidosis; CHC, chronic hyperplastic candidosis,
Nystatin is available as both an ointment and oral suspension
Amphotericin is available as a lozenge
Miconazole is available as an oral gel and cream
Clotrimazole is available as a cream and pessary
Other antifungals are available and these may be more frequently used in hospitalized patients

absorbed through the gut and as such their use is relatively limited. In cases of serious invasive *Candida* infections, intravenous administration of amphotericin B is often the preferred treatment option for hospitalized patients.

Azole antifungals

Azole antifungals inhibit the biosynthesis of ergosterol by interference with the fungal enzyme, lanosterol demethylase. A key function of this enzyme is to convert lanosterol to ergosterol and inhibition leads to a depletion of the sterol in the fungal cell membrane. Azole antifungals have a fungistatic rather than fungicidal activity against *Candida* species and, consequently, it is important to simultaneously address underlying host conditions during azole therapy to provide the best chance of disease resolution. The two azole agents that have been used most frequently to treat oral candidosis are fluconazole and itraconazole. The major benefit of the drugs is that they can be given orally and are well absorbed from the gut. Fluconazole is especially effective since it is secreted in saliva and the salivary levels are almost equal to those achieved in the blood. In contrast, itraconazole is a lipid based drug that achieves excellent tissue levels. Emergence of *Candida* resistance against the azoles has been described and can be either inherent or acquired. Several mechanisms of azole resistance are known and include (a) overproduction or an alteration in the demethylase enzyme targeted by azoles; (b) removal of the azole drug from the cytoplasm via multidrug transporters; or (c) compensation by other sterol synthesis enzymes involved in membrane synthesis.

5-Flucytosine (5-FC)

The antifungal 5-FC was originally synthesized in 1957 when the drug was used as a cytosine analogue treatment in leukaemic patients. Several years later the antifungal properties of 5-FC became evident. The drug enters the fungal cell through a cytosine permease and is then converted by the fungus into 5-fluorouracil. This nucleoside analogue becomes incorporated into RNA molecules and that serves to interfere with the synthesis of DNA and the manufacture of proteins within the fungal cell. Human cells are not affected due to the lack of cytosine permease in the cell membrane.

Future strategies for anti-candidal therapy

In recent years, several new antifungals have been developed that act upon cell wall targets. The synthesis of β1,3 D-glucan is one such target as this represents a key component in the fungal cell wall. The basis of the activity is through interference with the enzyme β1,3 D-glucan synthetase. The antifungals demonstrating this mechanism of action are referred to as the echinocandins and three such drugs (caspofungin, micofungin, and anidulafungin) demonstrate activity against *Candida* species. Another cell wall component that offers an attractive antifungal target is chitin which is a polysaccharide absent from host cells but which is an essential component of fungal cell walls where it offers structural support. Nikkomycins represent a class of drug that inhibits the enzyme chitin synthase and while good activity is evident against certain fungal species which have cell walls rich in chitin e.g. *Histoplasma capsulatum* and *Blastomyces* species, current drug forms appear to have limited or modest action against *Candida* species. A number of studies do however indicate synergistic activity of nikkomycin with azole drugs against *Candida*.

SUMMARY

Management of oral candidosis has to involve the identification and control of any host factor that may be predisposing to the infection. In addition, a range of antifungal agents are available to directly combat the infecting *Candida*. The variety and number of these agents is low when compared with traditional antibiotics against bacteria which is in part due to the difficulty in developing an antifungal agent that is effective against its targeted organism and is devoid of toxic effects against host cells. Suitable antifungal strategies include either directly targeting the ergosterol component in the fungal cell membrane (polyene antifungals) or the enzymes involved in its biosynthesis (azole antifungals). More recently, constituents of the fungal cell wall such as chitin (target site of nikkomycin antifungals) and glucan (echinocandin group antifungals) have received attention, although the use of these agents is currently limited with regard to oral candidosis.

CHAPTER SUMMARY

Several species of the fungal genus *Candida*, are frequently encountered as harmless members of the normal oral microflora of humans. In instances where debilitation of the host occurs, these organisms can cause infection which may manifest in several forms of oral candidosis, each with distinct clinical presentations.

Candida albicans is the species most frequently isolated from the oral cavity and while it also represents the principal species associated with oral candidosis, several other species have more recently also been shown to cause oral infection.

Candida albicans expresses a number of putative virulence factors that contribute to its pathogenicity. The ability to switch from a yeast morphology to a filamentous hyphal one has been linked with both protection against host immune defences and the invasion of the oral epithelium by the organism. In addition, a number of hydrolytic enzymes including secreted aspartyl proteinases and phospholipases are implicated in causing damage to host cells and host defence molecules. The expression of these virulence factors alone is probably not sufficient to cause infection and needs to be coupled with a lowering of host defence mechanisms in order for there to be subsequent infection.

In recent years, significant advances have been made in developing methods aimed at identifying *Candida* species. These advances correlate with the increasing incidence of all forms of candidosis as the proportion of debilitated and immunosuppresed people has increased. The reasons for such increases in human candidoses have largely been attributed to the wider use of invasive surgical procedures, immunosuppressive therapies and the spread of HIV and AIDS infection.

An important aspect of patient management of oral candidosis is to address any underlying host predisposing factor. This may take the form of advising patients on aspects of their oral hygiene or denture cleansing, administration of appropriate therapeutics or correcting any nutritional deficiencies. In many cases, however, antifungal therapy will have to be used, particularly when any underlying host factors cannot be identified or modulated.

It is not surprising that there has also been much emphasis in recent years on the development of antifungal agents used in the management of candidosis. Such development has again been, in part, a response to the increasing incidence of candidosis and is also a reflection of the increasing detection of non-*Candida albicans Candida* species in human infection. Such species, while often considered to be inherently less pathogenic than *C. albicans*, frequently exhibit greater resistance to certain antifungal agents.

FURTHER READING

Additional resources on the clinical aspects of oral candidosis include the works of Samaranayake & MacFarlane (1990), Oral candidosis, Wright, London, United Kingdom; and the reference book of Odds (1988), *Candida* and candidosis: a review and bibliography, Bailliere Tindale, London, United Kingdom. More specific references on aspects covered in this Chapter are listed below.

Ellepola ANB, Samaranayake LP 2000 Antimycotic agents in oral candidosis: an overview: 1. Clinical variants. Dent Update 27:111–116.

Ellepola AN, Samaranayake LP 2000 Antimycotic agents in oral candidosis: an overview: 2. Treatment of oral candidosis. Dent Update 27:165-70, 172-174.

Fidel PL Jr 2002 Immunity to *Candida*. Oral Dis 8 Suppl 2:69-75.

Li L, Redding S, Dongari-Bagtzoglou A 2007 *Candida glabrata*: an emerging oral opportunistic pathogen. J Dent Res 86:204-215.

Naglik J, Albrecht A, Bader O, Hube B 2004 *Candida albicans* proteinases and host/pathogen interactions. Cell Microbiol 6:915-926.

Sitheeque MA, Samaranayake LP 2003 Chronic hyperplastic candidosis/ candidiasis (candidal leukoplakia). Crit Rev Oral Biol Med 14:253-267.

Soysa NS, Samaranayake LP, Ellepola ANB 2008 Antimicrobials as a contributory factor in oral candidosis – a brief overview. Oral Dis 14:138-143.

Williams DW, Lewis MA 2000 Isolation and identification of *Candida* from the oral cavity. Oral Dis. 6:3-11.

Chapter 10

Orofacial viral infections

It has been estimated that 90% of adults harbour viruses that have been acquired as a result of infection during earlier life. Many viruses have the property of latency and may reside in the tissues asymptomatically for the remainder of the patient's life. The oral tissues are a frequent site for symptomatic primary infection and also reactivation of latent viruses. The presence of these viruses often becomes apparent at times when the host immune defence is compromised. This may range from short episodes of localized symptoms in otherwise healthy individuals to widespread prolonged problems in HIV positive patients.

Viruses, which are some of the smallest microorganisms (100–300 nm), consist of a core (genome) containing either DNA or RNA surrounded by a protein shell (capsid) (Fig. 10.1), can cause a range of important human diseases. Certain viruses also possess an outer lipoprotein coat derived from infected host cells. Viruses are obligate intracellular parasites in that they require the protein synthesizing apparatus (ribosomes) of the host cell. Viral replication is a complex process but comprises a number of recognized steps including, adsorption/penetration into the host cell, uncoating, transcription, synthesis of viral components, assembly and finally, release of new virions (Fig. 10.2).

ANTIVIRAL AGENTS

Knowledge of the different steps in viral replication has been the principle basis for the development of the antiviral drugs that are presently available. Relatively few antiviral agents have been developed when compared to the number of antibacterial drugs that are available. The intracellular nature of infection and the ability of viruses to establish latent forms have contributed to the difficulty in designing effective antiviral drugs.

The development of aciclovir was a milestone in antiviral therapy, representing the first true specific antiviral agent, recognized by the award of the Nobel Prize for Medicine. Aciclovir is a nucleoside analogue drug that has activity against members of the herpes group of viruses, in particular herpes simplex

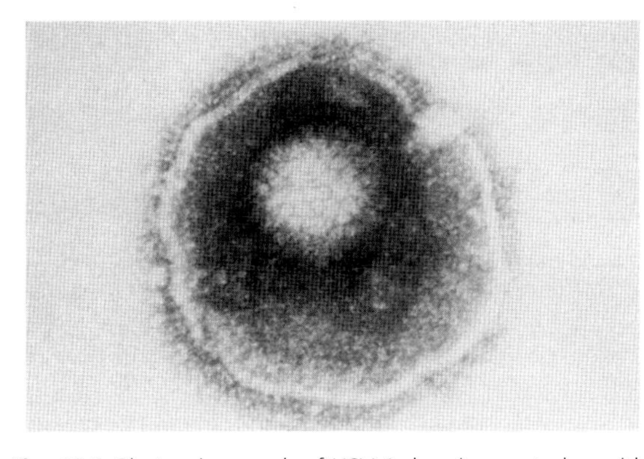

Fig. 10.1 Photomicrograph of HSV-1 showing central capsid and surrounding envelope (original magnification ×100,000).

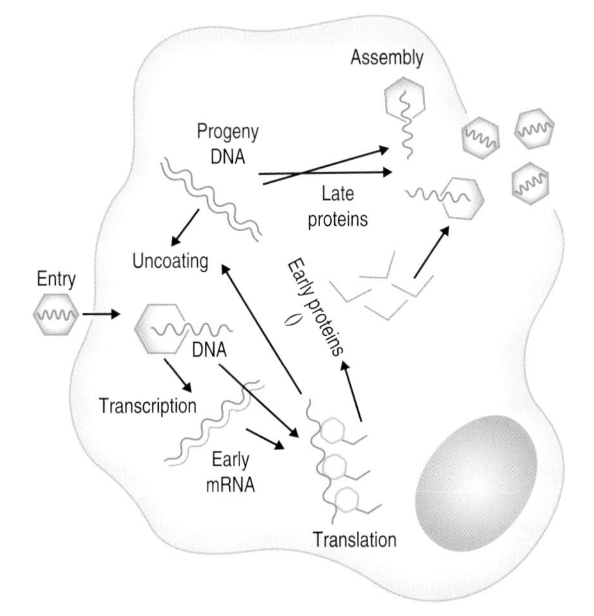

Fig. 10.2 Stages of viral infection and replication within a host cell.

virus type 1 (HSV-1) and herpes simplex virus type 2 (HSV-2). Viral enzymes, within HSV-infected cells, phosphorylate aciclovir to monophosphate and the agent becomes cell bound. Subsequent further phosphorylation to aciclovir triphosphate produces an analogue to deoxyguanosine triphosphate that inhibits viral DNA synthesis and prevents further viral replication.

Since aciclovir acts by blocking viral replication, a decision to provide the drug should be made at an early stage, preferably within 48 hours of the onset of acute symptoms in herpes simplex or varicella zoster infections. Antiviral therapy started later than this time is unlikely to produce any significant clinical benefit, and therefore is not justified unless the patient is otherwise medically compromised.

Aciclovir may be applied topically or given systemically in severe infection. Other antiviral agents used for orofacial herpes simplex and varicella zoster infections include valaciclovir (which is given systemically and has a longer intracellular half-life than aciclovir), penciclovir (available only in topical form) and famciclovir (the oral pro-drug of penciclovir). These agents act essentially in the same way as aciclovir. Docosanol, an agent that alters the cell membrane to prevent viral entry, is also available for topical application for orofacial herpes simplex infections. Ganciclovir and foscarnet are two other antiviral agents that are used in specialist units for treatment of infections due to cytomegalovirus.

LABORATORY DIAGNOSIS

A variety of laboratory methods have been developed for the detection, isolation and identification of viruses within clinical samples (Table 10.1). These techniques involve microscopy, culture, serology and nucleic acid amplification. However, the most appropriate method of sampling depends on the nature of the suspected infection.

Electron microscopy can be used to provide a provisional identification based on the morphological appearance of viral particles but this approach has low specificity and requires additional tests. Routine light microscopy can be used in conjunction with immunofluoresence and monoclonal antibodies to detect the presence of specific viruses (Fig. 10.3). This is a relatively rapid method giving a result within 30 minutes but the technique is not widely available.

Viruses can be grown in tissue culture usually involving baby hamster or monkey kidney fibroblasts. A swab of the lesion should be placed in viral transport medium, which contains at least two antibiotics, usually penicillin and streptomycin, to prevent bacterial growth, combined with an antifungal, such as amphotericin, to eliminate any fungal contamination. The transport medium should also contain serum and a buffer to maintain virus viability. The specimen should be sent to the laboratory promptly although it will not be processed for 24 hours to allow the antimicrobials mentioned above time to have an effect. The first stage of processing is inoculation into a

Table 10.1 Special investigations used in the diagnosis of orofacial viral infection.

Investigation	For	Against
Electron microscopy of vesicular fluid	Easy sample Rapid result	Insensitive Not specific
Light microscopy of lesional smear	Easy sample of smear Widely available Rapid result	Not specific
Light microscopy of lesional smear with immunofluorescence	Easy sample Rapid result Specific	Not routinely available
Culture of swab of lesion	Easy sample Can be specific Widely available	Result may not be available for up to 10 days
Antibody titre in venous blood	Requires paired venous samples	Two haematological samples required. Result not available for at least two weeks
PCR amplification of vesicular fluid or swab of lesion	Easy sample Rapid result	Not widely available

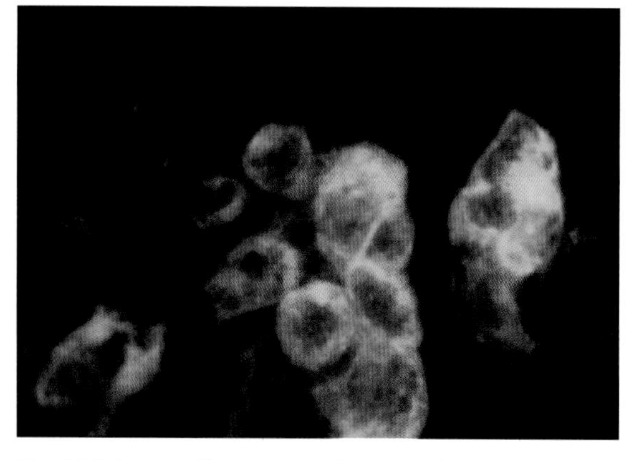

Fig. 10.3 Immunofluorescence of a smear showing presence of HSV-1.

monolayer of tissue culture. The presence of virus is determined in the laboratory by detection of a cytopathic effect, which is seen as the development of multinucleate giant cells (Fig. 10.4). This may take up to 10 days although the cytopathic effect occurs more rapidly in the presence of high numbers of virus particles.

Alternatively, diagnosis may be confirmed retrospectively by the detection of a four-fold rise in antibody titre between acute and convalescent sera taken from the patient. However, this technique has limited clinical benefit in diagnosis due to the prolonged time involved in obtaining a result. Molecular methods are being used increasingly to detect virus DNA or mRNA and in the future it is likely that these will provide a rapid diagnosis.

HERPES VIRUSES

The name herpes comes from the Greek word 'herpein' which means to creep (chronic, recurrent). While more than 100 herpes viruses have been isolated in nature, only eight herpes viruses have been described in humans and these are classified according to their biological properties into three subfamilies: Alphaherpesvirinae, Betaherpesvirinae and Gammaherpesvirinae (Table 10.2), all of which may be encountered in orofacial tissues.

Herpes simplex type 1 (HSV-1)

Primary infection

Primary infection with HSV-1 usually occurs during the first few years of life and serum markers of infection with the virus are found almost universally in the population in the Western world by 15 years of age. Oral clinical symptoms are characterized by the development of generalized oral discomfort and widespread gingivostomatitis. These features are relatively mild and often mistakenly diagnosed as an episode of 'teething' in young children. However, it has been estimated that clinical changes are severe

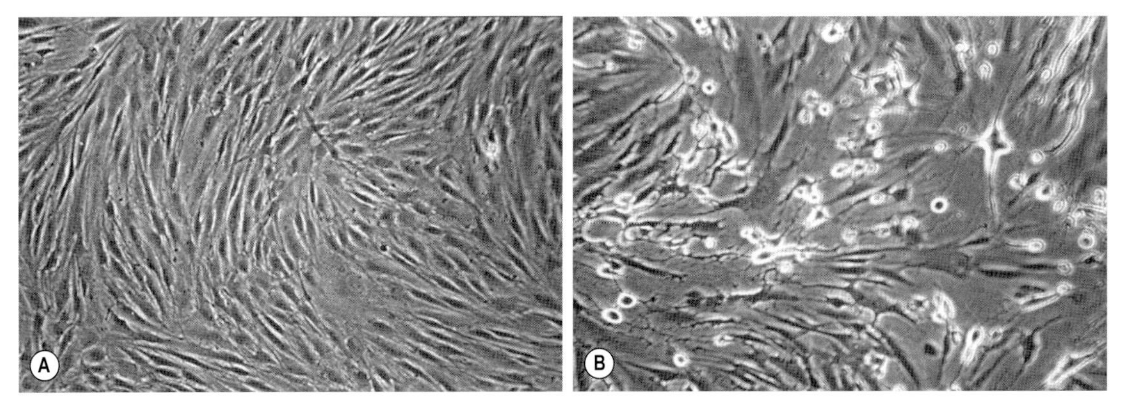

Fig. 10.4 (A) Monolayer of baby hamster kidney fibroblasts inoculated with swab specimen at day 1. (B) Same monolayer at day 7 showing cytopathic effect as destruction of architecture and development of multinucleate cells.

Table 10.2 Nomenclature of human herpes viruses (*Herpesviridae*).

Name	Trivial name	Acronym
Alphaherpesvirinae		
Human herpesvirus 1	Herpes simplex virus 1	HSV-1
Human herpesvirus 2	Herpes simplex virus 2	HSV-2
Human herpesvirus 3	Varicella zoster virus	VZV
Betaherpesvirinae		
Human herpesvirus 5	Cytomegalovirus	HCMV
Human herpesvirus 6		HHV-6
Gammaherpesvirinae		
Human herpesvirus 4	Epstein-Barr virus	EBV
Human herpesvirus 7		HHV-7
Human herpesvirus 8	Kaposi's sarcoma herpesvirus	HHV-8

in up to 10% of cases and manifest as blood-crusted lips (Fig. 10.5), gingival swelling, multiple oral ulcers, lymphadenopathy and pyrexia. Regardless of the severity of the primary infection, all signs and symptoms resolve within 10 days. The signs and symptoms of primary herpetic gingivitis are often sufficiently characteristic that a diagnosis can be made on the findings of clinical presentation alone. However, diagnosis of HSV-1 infection is most easily made by isolation of the virus. Large numbers of virus are present not only on the ulcerated mucosa but also within the saliva.

Treatment is supportive although a decision must be made on the need to provide the patient with antiviral therapy. The agent of choice is aciclovir, preferably as a suspension, since the tablet form is difficult to swallow in the presence of widespread oral ulceration. Aciclovir (200 mg) should be given five times daily for 5 days. Children under the age of 2 years should receive a half-dose, while those over 2 years of age should receive the adult dose. Regardless of the use of an antiviral agent, HSV-1 is not eliminated from the body following resolution of the acute symptoms and the virus remains within the tissues in a latent form, and can reactivate.

Secondary infection

Up to 40% of HSV-1 positive individuals suffer from recurrent episodes of secondary infection.

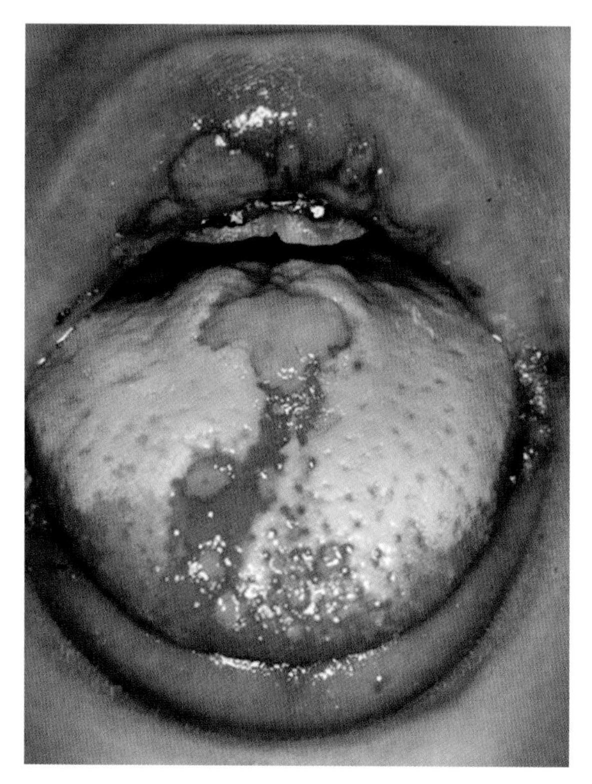

Fig. 10.5 Blood encrusted lips and oral ulceration of primary HSV-1 infection.

Reactivation of latent HSV-1 is related to either a breakdown in local immunosurveillance or an alteration in local inflammatory mediators. Traditionally, it has been thought that reactivated HSV-1 migrates from the trigeminal ganglion to the peripheral tissues of the lips or face. While this is true, it is becoming increasingly apparent that HSV also resides more locally in neural and other tissues.

Reactivation of HSV-1 characteristically produces herpes labialis, known more commonly as a cold sore or fever blister (Fig. 10.6). The symptoms of herpes labialis characteristically begin with a tingle or burning sensation (prodrome) in a localized region of the lips at the vermillion border. However, approximately 25% of episodes have no prodromal stage and the lesion initiates as vesicles. Within 48 hours the vesicles rupture to leave an erosion, which subsequently crusts over and eventually heals within 7–10 days. The clinical appearance is so characteristic that diagnosis is based on this alone. However, if necessary, the presence of HSV can be confirmed by isolation of virus in tissue culture or the use of immunofluorescence on a smear of the lesion. Factors that predispose to the development of herpes labialis in susceptible individuals include sunlight, trauma, stress, fever, menstruation and immunosuppression. A sunscreen applied to the lips can also be effective in reducing the frequency of sunlight-induced recurrences. The topical application of aciclovir or penciclovir can reduce the duration of the outbreak. Individuals with severe or frequent recurrences can benefit from the prophylactic use of systemic aciclovir (200 mg two or three times daily).

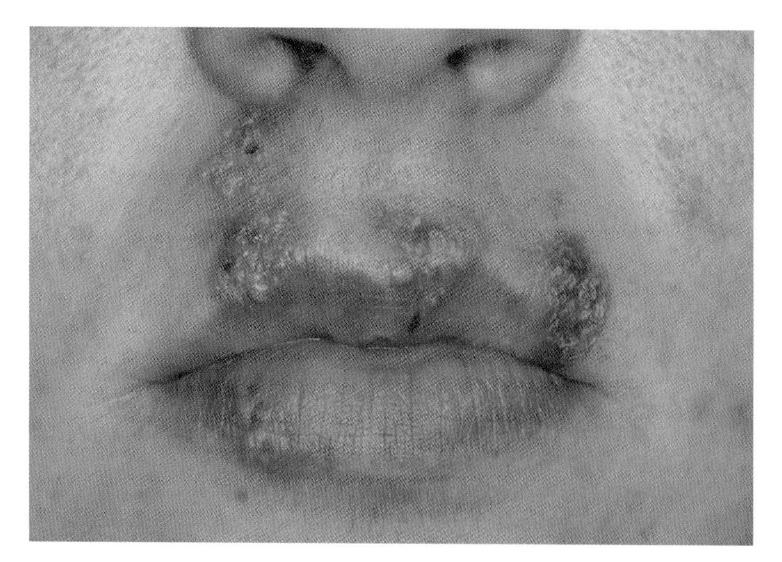

Fig. 10.6 Recurrent herpes labialis (cold sore) due to reactivation of HSV-1.

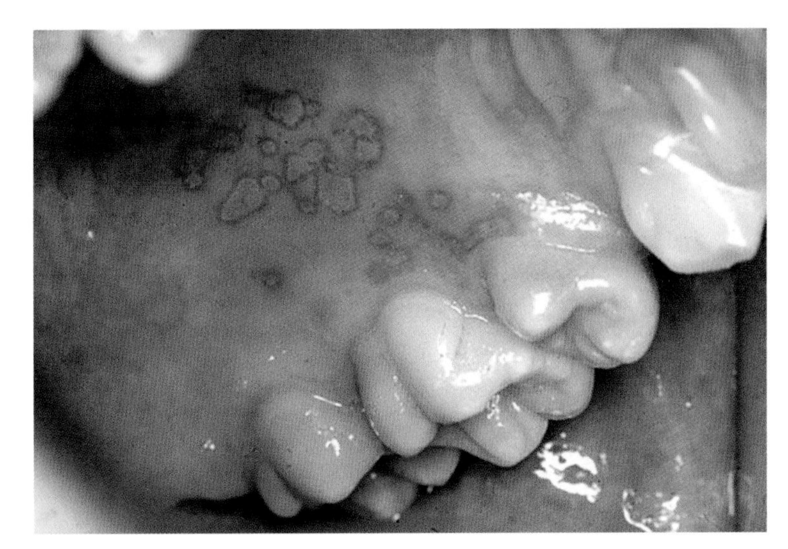

Fig. 10.7 Localized cluster of ulcers in the palate due to reactivation of HSV-1.

Reactivation of HSV-1 can also produce recurrent intra-oral ulceration. In a similar way to herpes labialis, the patient with an intra-oral lesion is usually aware of prodromal tingling. The mucosa of the hard palate (Fig. 10.7) is the site most frequently involved. It is also recognised that HSV-1 is asymptomatic and shed periodically in the saliva of up to 70% of the population at least once a month. Such shedding represents a risk of spread of the virus and in part explains the widespread nature of HSV-1 in the community. Reactivation of HSV-1 has also been implicated as an aetiological factor in periodontal disease and erythema multiforme.

Herpes simplex type 2 (HSV-2)

It has traditionally been taught that HSV-2 is only encountered in the genital region. However, it is becoming increasingly apparent that on rare occasions HSV-2 can cause oral lesions clinically identical to those of secondary HSV-1 infection. This observation is probably due more to the frequent transmission of virus as a result of direct contact during orogenital sexual practices but may, in part, also reflect the more widespread use of typing methods for suspected orofacial herpetic infections. The presence of HSV-2 can be confirmed by viral culture or, if available, direct immunofluoresence on a smear. Aciclovir is the agent of first choice for treatment of HSV-2 infection. While at present HSV-2 is associated with an increased risk of cervical cancer, a similar association has not been shown for oral cancer.

Varicella zoster virus (VZV)

Primary infection

Varicella zoster virus (VZV), the third member of the herpes group of viruses, spreads by droplet infection and the primary infection occurs most frequently in childhood causing chickenpox. The skin rash of chickenpox appears 2–3 weeks after infection and may occasionally be accompanied by the development of vesicles in the palate and faucial region, which rapidly rupture to produce small ulcers (2–4 mm). The diagnosis is made from the history and characteristic appearance of the cutaneous lesions. Culture of the virus is difficult and, therefore, if a microbiological diagnosis is required this needs to employ electron microscopy, immunofluorescence or serology. Treatment is supportive although aciclovir in high dose, valaciclovir or famciclovir may be used if the patient is immunocompromised.

Secondary infection

Reactivation of latent VZV in sensory nerve ganglia produces the clinical condition of herpes zoster, which is more commonly described as shingles. Herpes zoster is characterized by the onset of a unilateral area of severe pain which is accompanied within a few days by the development of vesiculobullous lesions (Fig. 10.8). The trigeminal nerve is affected in about 15% of cases of herpes zoster and involvement is limited to one division of the nerve. Although the diagnosis can

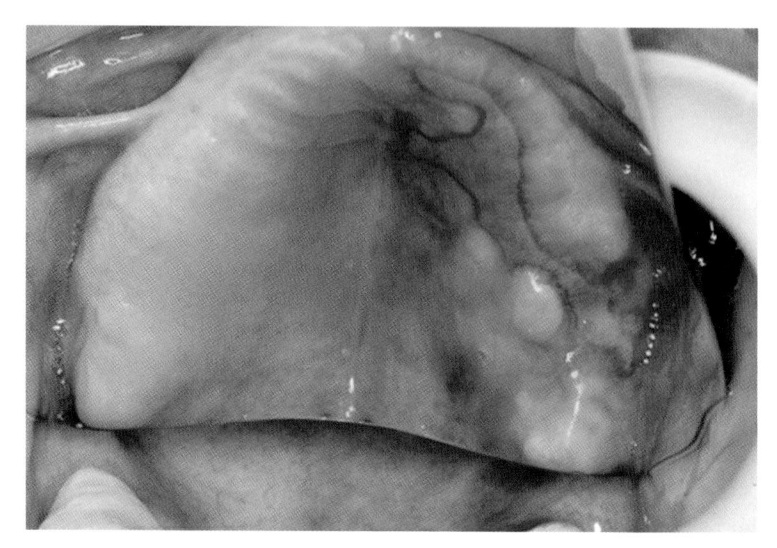

Fig. 10.8 Unilateral ulceration in the palate due to reactivation of HZV (shingles).

be made on the basis of clinical presentation alone, confirmation of herpes zoster can be made by isolation of VZV in cell culture or immunofluorescence on a smear. Antiviral treatment should be instituted as early as possible, preferably within the first 48 hours of symptoms, and should constitute either famciclovir 250 mg every 8 hours (or 750 mg once daily) for 10 days, or valaciclovir 1 g every 8 hours for 10 days. Post-herpetic neuralgia may be a subsequent problem in these patients, and this is why it is recommended that antiviral therapy should be provided for at least 10 days to reduce the likelihood of this extremely painful condition.

Epstein–Barr virus (EBV)

The fourth member of the herpes group is Epstein–Barr virus (EBV), named after the two virologists who first observed it. EBV has been subsequently associated with a number of infections that affect the orofacial region, including infectious mononucleosis, Burkitt's lymphoma, oral hairy leukoplakia, nasopharyngeal carcinoma and post-transplant lymphoproliferative disease. The virus is prevalent in the population with approximately 70% of adults carrying the virus by the age of 30 years. Like HSV, this virus is also periodically and asymptomatically shed in the saliva.

Infectious mononucleosis

Infectious mononucleosis, also known as glandular fever, is an acute infectious disease that is spread most frequently during kissing. The onset of a painful throat and submandibular lymphadenopathy is accompanied by fine petechial haemorrhages in the hard and soft palate. A white pseudomembrane may develop on the tonsils. Diagnosis is supported by demonstration of a lymphocytosis and atypical mononuclear cells (Downey cells) in a blood film or, alternatively, by detection of heterophile antibodies ('Monospot test'), EBV specific antibody using immunofluorescence methods or EBV DNA by PCR.

Hairy leukoplakia

Hairy leukoplakia was first described in the mouths of gay men with AIDS in California, and has subsequently become recognized as a specific oral manifestation of HIV infection or immunosuppression. Characteristically, hairy leukoplakia presents as a corrugated white lesion on the lateral border of the tongue, although it has also been described on the dorsum of the tongue and the buccal mucosa. EBV has been demonstrated in lesional tissue by *in situ* hybridization with appropriate DNA probes. Although the exact role of EBV in hairy leukoplakia is still uncertain, temporary clinical resolution of the condition can occur following provision of high doses of aciclovir. Imprint cultures of hairy leukoplakia often yield candidal species, but it is likely that this represents opportunistic secondary infection.

Burkitt's lymphoma and nasopharyngeal carcinoma

EBV is regarded as an oncogenic virus and is associated with Burkitt's lymphoma, an aggressive tumour of the jaws seen in areas where malaria is also prevalent, and nasopharyngeal carcinoma, especially in China and South-East Asia.

Human cytomegalovirus (HCMV)

While HCMV, the fifth herpes group virus, is widespread in the community it has only rarely been associated with the presence of oral symptoms similar to those seen in infectious mononucleosis. It can be detected by direct immunofluoresence. HCMV is a potential pathogen in the developing foetus and immunodeficient individuals. Ganciclovir and foscarnet are two antiviral agents used in management of serious HCMV infection.

Human herpes virus 6 (HHV-6)

Human herpes virus 6 is found in latent form in lymphoid tissue but is also asymptomatically shed in the saliva of most adults. The virus is implicated in infectious mononucleosis-like symptoms and skin rashes (roseola infantum). It has also been suggested that HHV 6 is the cause of erythematous papules in the soft palate and uvula (Nagayama's spots) seen in these children.

Human herpes virus 7 (HHV-7)

Human herpes virus 7 has been found in saliva but its role in human disease is unknown at present.

Human herpes virus 8 (HHV-8)

Human herpes virus 8 has been encountered in all forms of Kaposi's sarcoma and is believed to be the aetiological agent of this condition. Kaposi's sarcoma is a proliferation of endothelial cells producing a mass, particularly in association with HIV infection but occasionally in other immunosuppressed patients. Small lesions can be excised, treated with low-dose radiotherapy or by the injection of chemotherapeutic drugs, such as vinblastine. Larger lesions may require the use of systemic chemotherapy. HHV-8 has also been associated with sarcoidosis.

COXSACKIE VIRUSES

The coxsackie viruses are enteroviruses that affect the gut and are named after the village in New York where they were first detected. Several subspecies of type A and type B are now recognized and some may cause orofacial infection. These viruses are highly infectious and are widespread in the community due to transmission by the faecal–oral route or by nasal/pharyngeal secretions.

Hand, foot and mouth disease

Hand, foot and mouth disease is usually caused by Coxsackie virus subspecies A16, but may also be due to infection with types A4, A5, A9 and A10. As the name of the condition implies, the distribution of lesions involves macular and vesicular eruptions on the hands, feet and mucosa of the pharynx, soft palate, buccal sulcus or tongue. The cutaneous lesions of hand, foot and mouth disease are transient, lasting only 1–3 days, and are unlikely to cause any significant symptoms. The diagnosis of hand, foot and mouth disease is usually made on the basis of the characteristic clinical signs. Viral culture for coxsackie infections is not widely available, and therefore if confirmatory diagnosis is required this has to be based on demonstration of an increase in convalescent antibody levels. Antimicrobial treatment is rarely required.

Herpangina

Herpangina is due to infection by either Coxsackie virus subspecies A2, A4, A5, A6 or A8. This condition occurs predominantly in children, and presents as sudden onset of fever and sore throat with subsequent development of papular, vesicular lesions on the oral mucosa and pharyngeal mucosa. Severity of symptoms is variable, but clinical resolution usually occurs within 7-10 days, even in the absence of treatment. The diagnosis of herpangina is usually made on the basis of the characteristic clinical signs and symptoms. Viral culture for Coxsackie infections is not widely available and, therefore, if required, confirmatory diagnosis is based on demonstration of an increase in convalescent antibody levels. Treatment consists of bed rest and the use of an antiseptic mouthwash, such as 0.2% chlorhexidine gluconate two or three times daily. Patients should be encouraged to maintain adequate fluid intake.

HUMAN PAPILLOMA VIRUSES (HPV)

More than 80 serological types of human papilloma virus have been described, some of which have been encountered in benign conditions while others have been implicated in the aetiology of cancer at various body sites.

Verruca vulgaris

HPV types 2 and 4 are frequently encountered in mucosal warts (Fig. 10.9). Development of orofacial lesions may be associated with transmission from warts on the hands. Alternatively, the oral lesions may arise from orogenital contact, where HPV types 6, 11 and 16 are more prevalent. The labial and lingual mucosa are the most common sites for oral warts which present as small localized growths. The clinical appearance is characteristic but most lesions are removed and, therefore, histopathological findings can confirm the diagnosis. Histologically, the structure of the lesion is similar to papilloma but there are large clear cells (koliocytes) in the prickle cell layer. Immunostaining may be used to detect presence of papilloma virus. Excision is usually curative and recurrence is uncommon except in immunocompromised individuals.

In recent years, there has been increasing interest in the potential role of HPV 16 in the aetiology of oropharyngeal carcinoma as a result of oral sexual practices. Further evidence of the involvement of HPV 16 in this situation would support vaccination against this virus. The recognised association of this virus in cervical cancer has led to the proposal that all females are vaccinated against HPV 16 at the age of 12 years.

Focal epithelial hyperplasia (Heck's disease)

Heck's disease is a benign condition first described in Native Americans and the Inuit but also now seen in other populations. An infectious aetiology due to human papilloma viruses (HPV types 13 and 32) has been shown by both epidemiological and molecular studies. The lesions appear as discrete or clustered, smooth-topped pink papules most frequently on the buccal mucosa, labial mucosa, tongue and gingivae. The diagnosis is made on ultrastructural studies that show 50 nm viral particles of the HPV within biopsy material.

PARAMYXOVIRUSES

The paramyxoviruses are enveloped RNA viruses that comprise four groups: parainfluenza virus, mumps virus, measles virus and respiratory syncytical virus.

Mumps

Mumps (endemic parotitis) is traditionally associated with painful swelling of the major salivary glands. Diagnosis can usually be made on the basis

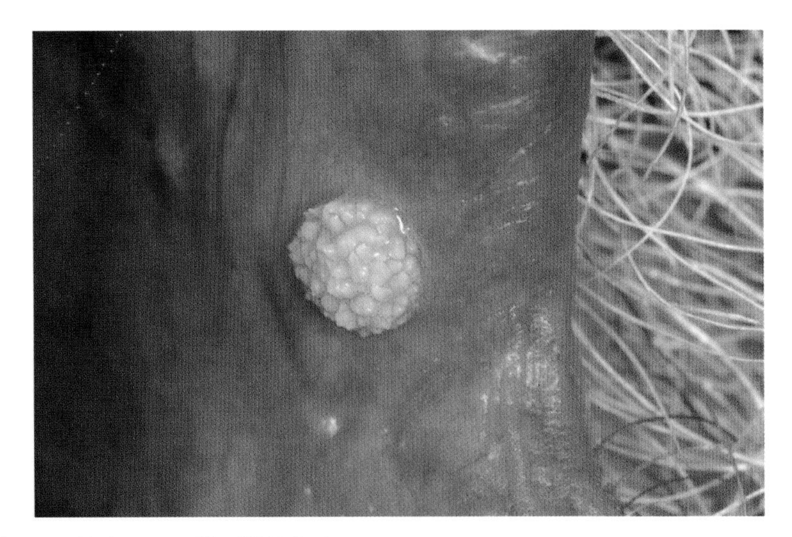

Fig. 10.9 Localized mucosal lesion caused by HPV infection.

of clinical symptoms; mumps can be differentiated from suppurative sialadenitis by the absence of a purulent discharge from the salivary duct orifice. However, if there is doubt then serological investigation to demonstrate the presence of specific IgM antibody can be used. In addition, a sample of saliva, collected by cannulation of the parotid duct, can be examined by electron microscopy or tissue culture to demonstrate the presence of virus. Treatment is supportive and it should be remembered that antibiotic therapy is not required.

Measles

Measles, a common disease of childhood, is spread by droplet infection and is highly infectious. The MMR (mumps, measles and rubella) vaccine provides immunity but in areas of low uptake or non-availability of the vaccine, measles still presents a serious illness due to potentially life threatening bronchopneumonia or encephalomyelitis. In Saharan Africa, the virus has also been implicated in gross destruction of the orofacial tissues (noma) in malnourished individuals (Ch. 6). In more typical milder cases, the characteristic skin rash and fever may be accompanied by transient small discrete macules in the buccal mucosa (Koplik's spots).

CHAPTER SUMMARY

Viruses within the herpes group, which contains eight distinct viruses, are encountered frequently in the orofacial tissues. Evidence of infection with herpes simplex type 1 (HSV-1), which causes primary herpetic gingivostomatitis, is found in the majority (80–90%) of the adult population and subsequent reactivation of latent HSV-1 produces herpes labialis (cold sores) in approximately a third of these at some time in their life. Other members of the herpes group, coxsackie A viruses, human papilloma viruses and paramyxoviruses can cause a range of signs and symptoms within the orofacial tisues, particularly in immunocompromised individuals. A relatively small number of antiviral agents are available although aciclovir and penciclovir do prevent replication of herpes viruses and are used frequently.

FURTHER READING

Arduino PG, Porter SR 2008 Herpes simplex virus type 1 infection: overview on relevant clinico-pathological features. J Oral Pathol Med 37:107-121.

Campsi G, Panzarella V, Giuliana M, Lajolo C et al 2007 Human papilloma virus: its identity and controversial role in oral oncogenesis, premalignant lesions and malignant lesions. Int J Oncol 30:813-823.

Cappuyns I, Gugerli P, Mombelli A 2005 Viruses in periodontal disease – a review. Oral Dis 11:219-229.

Dockrell H, Roitt IM, Zuckerman M et al 2007 Mims' medical microbiology (Trauma Manual) 4th edn. Mosby, London.

Lewis MAO 2004 Herpes simplex virus: an occupational hazard in dentistry. Int Den J 54:103-111.

Porter SR, Di Alberti L, Kumar N 1998 Human herpes virus 8. Oral Oncol 34:5-14.

Woo SB, Challacombe SJ 2007 Management of recurrent oral herpes simplex infections. Oral Surg Oral Med Oral Pathol Oral Radiol Endod 103:S12.e1-18.

Scully C, Samaranyake L 1992 Clinical virology in oral medicine and dentistry. Cambridge University Press, Cambridge.

Chapter 11

Oral implications of infection in compromised patients

The term 'medically compromised' is often misused. The definition of a medically compromised patient is one who by virtue of their medical condition, or its treatment, is susceptible to infection and other serious complications. Conditions which cause patients to be medically compromised can either be congenital or acquired. Medical compromise can be due to a whole variety of factors, some of which are illustrated in Table 11.1. The term 'immunocompromised' refers specifically to congenital or acquired alterations of the immune system, which may render an individual susceptible to infection. The number of immunocompromised individuals is increasing rapidly, mostly because of the AIDS pandemic, but also through intervention therapy (drugs which deliberately modify the immune system). A good example of the latter is deliberate suppression of the immune system with drugs to prevent rejection during and following solid organ transplantation. The oral microflora in immunocompromised patients is changed either by colonization with exogenous microorganisms which are not normally found in the mouth, or by the occurrence of opportunistic infection. It used to be believed that any person who was immunocompromised had to be given prophylactic antibiotics to prevent infection after surgery. This is not necessary unless there is a proven degree of impairment of immune defences which renders them susceptible to infection. The extent to which an immunocompromised patient is susceptible to infection can be measured by a variety of blood tests to assess the function of their immune system. These include simple tests on the number and proportion of their immunological cells (predominantly white cells), their function, or their degree of abnormality. Only where there is a proven loss of functional protective immunity is there a necessity to give prophylactic antimicrobials before surgery (Ch. 8).

Table 11.1 Orofacial infections that may occur in medically compromised patients

Disorder	Example	Orofacial infection
Endocrine disorders	Diabetes mellitus	Oral fungal infections
Respiratory disorders	Asthma	Oral fungal infections
Neurological disorders	Epilepsy	Gingival hyperplasia and periodontal disease
Neoplastic disease	Oral carcinoma	Dental caries and mucositis following radiotherapy
Chronic infection	Tuberculosis	Oral tuberculosis
Immunological disorders	HIV and AIDS	Oral viral and fungal infections
Haematinic deficiencies	Anaemia	Angular cheilitis and oral fungal infections

The status of the teeth and oral soft tissues is often a reflection of systemic health. Thus, opportunistic orofacial infection may be the presenting initial feature of systemic disease. In this chapter, the types of orofacial infection that are seen in medically compromised patients as a result of the presence of underlying disease or as a result treatment will be considered.

OSTEORADIONECROSIS

Cancer in the oral region is treated usually by surgery, radiotherapy, chemotherapy or a combination of all three. Radiotherapy destroys the rapidly dividing cancer cells, but it also destroys surrounding bone. This bone is highly susceptible to secondary radiation as it absorbs a great deal of energy. Bone is affected by radiation in three ways; there is a decrease in the number of cells (hypocellularity) and reduction in blood vessels (hypovascularity) and, as a consequence, less oxygen in the tissue (hypoxia). As the bone heals after irradiation, fibrous tissue is generated instead of bone, especially in the mandible. The effects of radiation therapy are not transitory and the hypovascularity increases with time. A simple operation on tissues which have been irradiated, such as a tooth extraction, can result in spontaneous death of the surrounding bone (necrosis). Death of the bone after irradiation can be progressive and is called osteoradionecrosis and has been associated with oral ulceration caused by ill-fitting dentures, scaling of the teeth, facial bone fractures and root canal therapy. In the past, the radiation therapy was not so highly focussed (collimated) on the malignant tissue and the surrounding normal structures were also often affected. In these conditions, the incidence of osteoradionecrosis in oral bone varied from 17–37%. With careful collimation, shielding of surrounding tissues, use of small but effective repeated radiation doses (fractionation), the incidence of osteoradionecrosis has been reduced to 2–5%.

Osteoradionecrosis is likely to arise due to a combination of radiation, trauma and infection. However, extensive animal studies support a view that the microorganisms are contaminants and cause secondary infection of pre-existing necrosis. Interestingly, molecular techniques applied to necrotic tissue obtained from cases of osteoradionecrosis have detected a predominantly anaerobic microflora, including *Porphyromonas* spp. and *Prevotella* spp.. Osteoradionecrosis is a difficult condition to treat despite the provision of an antibacterial agent, such as metronidazole or clindamycin, combined with surgery.

POST-IRRADIATION MUCOSITIS

Another of the consequences of irradiation of the oral region is non-specific inflammation of the oral mucosa, often called mucositis (Fig 11.1). This can be extensive and cause considerable pain with difficulties in feeding. Symptoms may be severe enough to influence the patient to abandon the radiation treatment. At first it was thought that radiation mucositis was due to infection by *Candida* spp., and other yeasts. However, provision of antifungal therapy has no effect, suggesting that yeasts are not causing the condition. More extensive sampling of the mucosa has shown that the microflora associated with mucositis is mainly composed of Gram

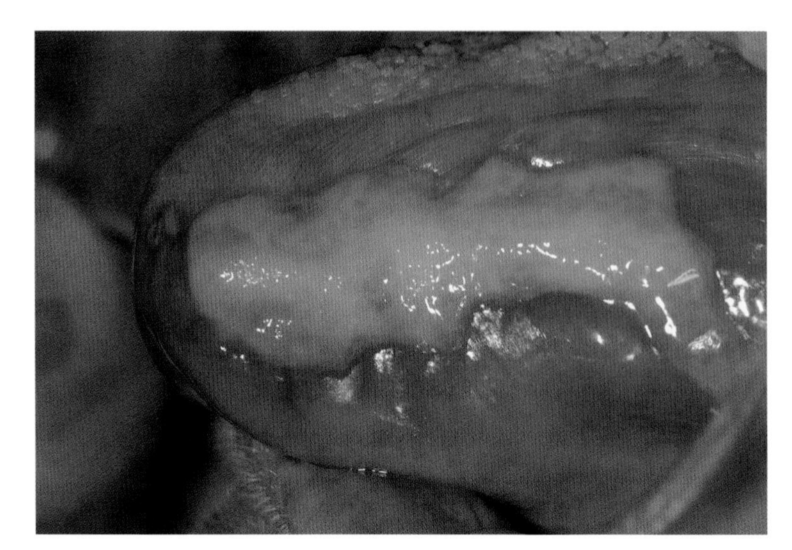

Fig. 11.1 Post-irradiation mucositis on the lingual mucosa.

negative aerobic and facultatively anaerobic bacteria such as *Escherichia coli*, pseudomonads, *Klebsiella* spp, and *Acinetobacter* spp.. Irradiation mucositis can be largely alleviated by selective decontamination of the oral cavity before and during irradiation therapy by applying topically a combination of non-absorbable antimicrobials onto the tissues to be protected. The usual combinations of antimicrobials are polymixin and tobramycin, and an antifungal is added to prevent yeast overgrowth. Two antimicrobials are used in order to prevent the selection of resistance in Gram negative bacteria. This combination can be used to ameliorate the effects of the mucositis.

BISPHOSPHONATE-ASSOCIATED OSTEONECROSIS

Bisphosphonates are drugs used in the treatment of osteoporosis, a condition in which calcium is gradually lost from bone. Osteoporosis is a serious condition in which there can be spinal compression, long bone fracture and bone pain. The bisphosphonates are pyrophosphate analogues that can prevent osteoporosis by inhibiting osteoclast activity. Unfortunately some patients who take bisphosphonates can suffer from a failure of bone to heal especially after extractions. The bone around the socket dies and may remain exposed to the oral cavity and get secondarily infected particularly with anaerobes. The exact cause of this condition is not known, but it is likely that this may be similar to the hypovascularity seen in osteoradionecrosis. One other suggestion is that bisphosphonate-associated osteonecrosis is due to anaerobic infection of the bone, but this is unlikely to be the primary cause as it is not cured by antimicrobials or surgery. The risk of this condition developing is small and has been estimated to be about 1:100,000 in those taking bisphosphonates. The risk of the condition developing however increases with the length of time the bisphosphonates are taken. This condition may become a serious problem in the future as a total of 70 million people were taking bisphosphonates worldwide in 2008.

STAPHYLOCOCCAL MUCOSITIS

Recent surveys of data from oral samples processed in microbiology laboratories have shown that *Staphylococcus* spp. are frequently isolated. The predominant species isolated is *Staphylococcus aureus* with a minority of these being methicillin-resistant (MRSA). Many of these isolations have been obtained from patients who are debilitated, or are terminally ill. In addition, staphylococci have been isolated from orofacial granulomatosis, in particular within fissures of swollen lips (Fig. 11.2). The presenting features of orofacial granulomatosis are identical to those of Crohn's disease, which is a chronic inflammatory condition of the gut. There is debate

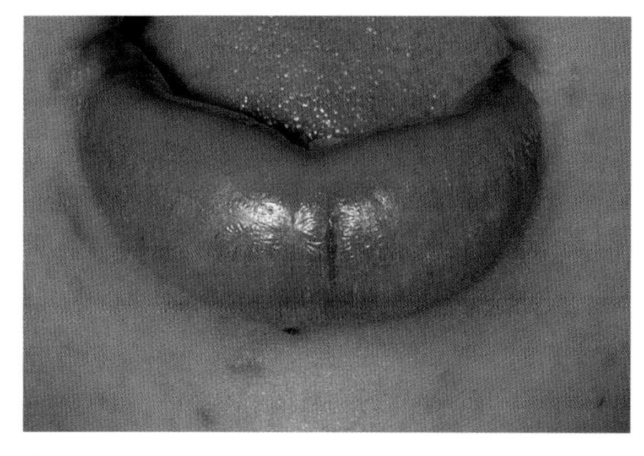

Fig. 11.2 Lip swelling in orofacial granulomatosis with midline split secondarily infected with *Staphylococcus aureus*.

as to how frequently staphylococci infect or colonize the mouth. Recently, it has been proposed that there is a discrete condition called staphylococcal mucositis which occurs in debilitated individuals.

PYOSTOMATITIS VEGETANS

This condition is associated with the presence of active inflammatory bowel disease, in particular, ulcerative colitis or Crohn's disease. The oral mucosa is diffusely inflamed, with fissured ulcers separating papillary projections (Fig. 11.3). Histological examination reveals suprabasal separation of the epithelium with the formation of eosinophilic abscesses. The severity of pyostomatitis vegetans often mirrors the bowel disease activity. Interestingly, the provision of metronidazole can relieve oral symptoms. Healing occurs when the underlying inflammatory bowel disorder is brought under control.

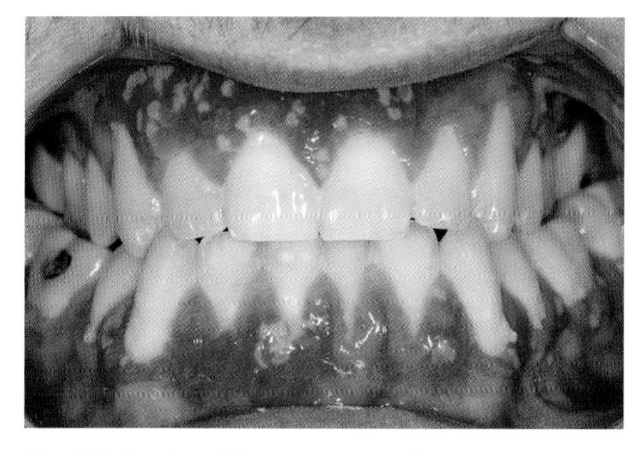

Fig. 11.3 Pyostomatitis vegetans presenting as mucosa erythema. This patient also had secondary infection of the mucosa with methicillin-resistant *Staphylococcus aureus* (MRSA).

CANCRUM ORIS (NOMA, GANGRENOUS STOMATITIS)

This is a severe form of necrotizing periodontal disease, and is seen occasionally in developing countries, in particular, sub-Saharan Africa (Ch. 6). The sufferer is characteristically less than 10 years of age, malnourished and has a history of a recent viral infection, such as measles (Ch. 10). The initial lesion spreads into the cheek, face and neck causing extensive tissue loss. Treatment is with a combination of antibiotics, such as benzylpenicillin with metronidazole, but each combination should include agents active against both Gram negative and Gram positive microorganisms.

NECROTIZING FASCIITIS

Necrotizing fasciitis is a serious rapidly progressive infection that can result in death, particularly in immunocompromised individuals. The majority of cases of necrotizing fasciitis that occur in the cervical region of the neck are of dental origin, in particular, subsequent to an acute dentoalveolar abscess. Microbiological studies of this rare condition have implicated members of the anginosus group of streptococci as the most frequent pathogens, often in combination with strict anaerobes such as *Prevotella* spp.. Management involves provision of antibiotic therapy intravenously and surgical debridement; hyperbaric oxygen is also used.

STROKE AND PARKINSON'S DISEASE

Loss of control of oral musculature can occur following cerobrovascular accidents (strokes) and in conditions such as Parkinson's disease. Loss of the oral musculature can result in changes in the oral microflora, but the reasons for this are not clear. The microflora becomes predominantly Gram negative with *Enterobacter* spp. and *Acinetobacter* spp. predominating. This change in the oral microflora is clinically significant as often the patient cannot swallow properly; oral microorganisms can also be aspirated into the lungs and cause pneumonia.

XEROSTOMIA

Xerostomia means literally dry mouth and can be caused by a variety of conditions or treatments (Table 11.2). One of the consequences of xerostomia is overgrowth of dental plaque, with acidogenic oral streptococci and lactobacilli predominating within the biofilm. This can induce a dramatic increase in dental caries if teeth are present. Xerostomia predisposes to the development of mucositis and opportunistic *Candida* infections of the oral mucosa.

GINGIVAL HYPERPLASIA AND IMMUNOSUPPRESSIVE AGENTS

Following organ transplantation it is necessary to take immunosuppressive agents to prevent the immune system causing rejection of the transplant. One of the curious consequences of taking these antirejection agents is that the gingivae enlarge due to overgrowth of fibrous tissue (Fig. 11.4). The gingival overgrowth is worse if the oral hygiene of the mouth is poor. No plaque bacteria have been associated with this condition, which was thought to be directly due to the systemic action of the immunosuppressive agents. If the patient is treated with low doses of macrolide antimicrobials (e.g. azithromycin), then the overgrowth can be prevented or reduced. This evidence supports the contention that gingival hyperplasia is an infective inflammatory process but the infecting bacteria have still to be identified.

Table 11.2 Causes of xerostomia
Drug therapy (in particular antidepressants)
Sjögren's syndrome (immunological destruction of salivary tissues)
Damage to salivary glands following radiotherapy
Undiagnosed or poorly controlled diabetes
Dehydration
Congential absence of salivary glands

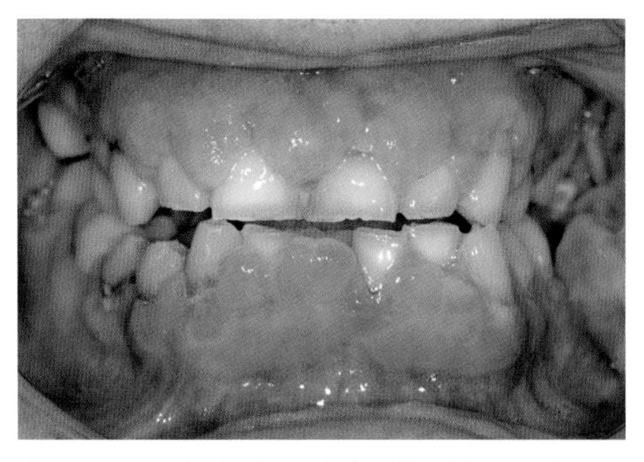

Fig. 11.4 Hyperplastic gingivae induced by ciclosporin therapy.

SUMMARY

A range of non-infective disorders and health conditions can cause changes in the oral environment that in turn predispose to localized orofacial infections. Such situations include alterations in the host defence as a result of the underlying illness or as a result of treatment. The principle problems usually arise due to opportunistic infections caused by commensal members of the oral microflora.

HUMAN IMMUNODEFICIENCY VIRUS (HIV) AND AIDS

The impact of HIV on the world's population is immense. AIDS, the acquired immune deficiency syndrome, now accounts for millions of deaths each year, especially in African countries. HIV infection is thought to affect at least 40 million people worldwide and it has been suggested that HIV infects a new person every 5 minutes. AIDS is a huge problem for both developed and developing countries.

The human immunodeficiency virus (HIV) was first described in the early 1980s and is classified as part of the Lentoviridae (subfamily Retroviridae). The virus has a core complex of double-stranded RNA together with an enzyme called reverse transcriptase (Fig. 11.5). Surrounding the core are matrix proteins and a coat of complex glycoprotein. The coat glycoprotein contains a receptor protein, gp120, which is thought to be involved in attachment of the virus to $CD4^{+}$ lymphocytes. The virus is approximately 100–120 nm in size and delta-icosohedral in symmetry.

The virus has a strange life cycle (Fig. 11.6). It infects predominantly $CD4^{+}$ lymphocytes, but can also infect macrophages, through the interaction of gp120 with co-receptors on the host cells. Following entry into the cell, the viral RNA genome is converted to complementary double-stranded DNA using the HIV enzyme, reverse transcriptase.

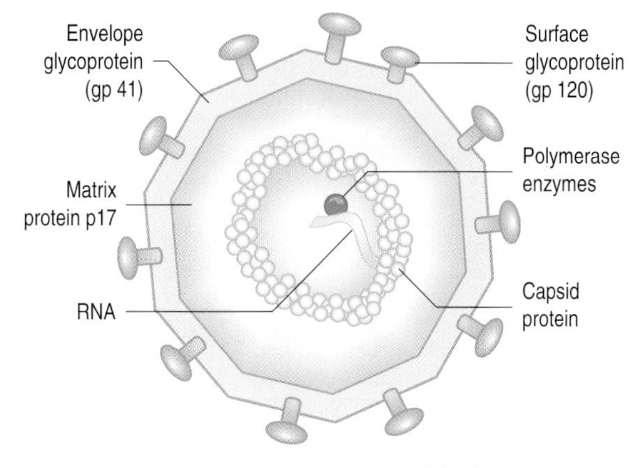

Fig. 11.5 Diagrammatic representation of the human immunodeficiency virus.

This new HIV-derived DNA is integrated into the host cell nucleus and is transcribed using the host cell's enzymes, leading to the formation of the components necessary to form new virus. New HIV is assembled at the host cell membrane at specialized sites which allows budding of the new virus and its eventual release into the blood stream. The process of HIV replication results in death of the lymphocyte when the virus is released.

The process of conversion of RNA into DNA by HIV is very wasteful and often is not successfully completed resulting in incomplete formation of HIV. Part of this may be due to mutations occurring which do not allow the virus to reproduce. This is in part responsible for the low transmission rate of the virus, which is around 4% if infected blood is transmitted to an uninfected person. The high rate of mutation also allows HIV to respond to attempted therapy by mutating to become resistant. One of the earliest attempts at preventive therapy was by the use of azothymidine (AZT), a DNA analogue. Within one month of the first use of AZT, HIV mutants were reported that were resistant to the drug.

AIDS results from a depletion of CD4$^+$ lymphocytes (T-helper cells) so there is no functional immunity, particularly to infection. T-helper cells mediate both humoral and cellular immunity, and are able to direct the host response to different infectious agents to give predominantly either humoral or cell mediated immunity. The loss of CD4$^+$ lymphocytes results in an inadequate host response to a range of frank or opportunistic pathogens.

A huge variety of infections, lesions, signs and symptoms are associated with HIV infection and some of the oral manifestations are listed in Table 11.3. It is important to realise that AIDS is a syndrome, which is a collection of potential signs and symptoms which may occur. In contrast, a disease is a collection of signs and symptoms that always go together.

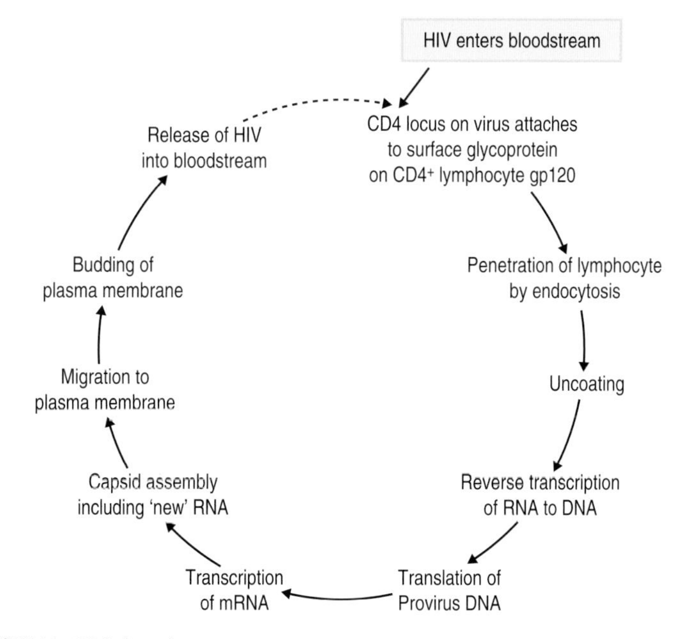

Fig. 11.6 The life cycle of HIV in CD4$^+$ lymphocytes.

Table 11.3 Lesions associated with HIV infection

Group 1	Group 2	Group 3
Lesions strongly associated with HIV	**Lesions less commonly associated with HIV**	**Lesions sometimes associated with HIV**
Candidosis: Erythematous Pseudomembranous	Bacterial infections: *Mycobacterium tuberculosis* *Mycobacterium avium-intracellulare*	Bacterial infections: *Actinomyces israelii* *Escherichia coli* *Klebsiella pneumoniae*
Hairy leukoplakia Periodontal disease Linear gingival erythema Necrotizing periodontal diseases Kaposi's sarcoma	Melanotic hyperpigmentation Necrotizing stomatitis Non-specific ulceration	Cat scratch disease Drug reactions Fungal infections: *Cryptococcus, Geotrichium* *Mucor, Aspergillus*
Non-Hodgkins lymphoma	Salivary gland disease Thrombocytopenic purpura	
	Viral infections: Herpes simplex type 1, Human papilloma virus, Varicella zoster virus	

HIV can easily penetrate the blood–brain barrier and one of the early signs of AIDS may be mental deterioration of the patient due to infection of the brain. Such neurological deterioration can be misdiagnosed as dementia.

HIV can be found in a wide range of body fluids including blood, saliva, sputum, semen, vaginal secretion, peri-anal secretion and breast milk. The virus can be grown in tissue culture, but this is not the usual method used for HIV detection. The main test used for detection of HIV uses the antibody produced in response to infection by the virus. The HIV antibody test is relatively simple utilizing an enzyme linked immunosorbent assay (ELISA). The detection of this virus relies on HIV generating an antibody response, which can take between 22 days and 11 months. There are periods, therefore, when the virus has infected lymphocytes and macrophages and is not being released into the blood stream. In this time period the person infected would give a negative antibody test, but still be infectious.

In the early stages of infection, HIV releases a protein, present in its core, called p24. This protein can be detected sometimes within one week of infection, but always within one month. This is a direct test which confirms the presence or absence of the virus, but it is more complex and expensive than the detection of antibody.

The screening of individuals for HIV is subject to varying legislation in different countries and involves civil liberties. In some countries no precise records are kept of HIV infection rates as the number of individuals infected is not registered. In such circumstances, the prevalence of the disease can only be estimated from the number of those who seek treatment, develop AIDS, or indirectly by screening blood donations. Testing for HIV infection is a highly emotive issue which, because of the seriousness of its consequences, both socially and personally, has to be done carefully and sensitively. One of the most difficult situations is the testing of patients who have been treated by HIV-infected healthcare workers, where there could have been blood contamination; these are often called 'exposure prone procedures'. In order to assess whether HIV or other infection has been transmitted, all the patients who have been treated by the healthcare worker are contacted and offered counselling, or HIV tests. The value of such retrospective surveys has been questioned, as the risk of transmission is often low and not worth the anxiety generated in the population who are offered the counselling or the tests.

There have been very few proven transmissions of HIV by healthcare workers, the most notable being an orthopaedic surgeon in France and a dentist in Florida (Dr Acer – see later).

The value of such retrospective surveys is also scientifically questionable as the test may be taken when no HIV markers are detectable and false negative results will be obtained. The risk of transmission of HIV by healthcare workers is very low, unless a significant amount of blood is transferred directly into the recipient's blood stream. Even if this occurs the risk of transmission is thought to be only 0.4%.

One of the most significant advances in the treatment of HIV is the use of highly active antiretroviral therapy (often given the acronym HAART). The use of a combination of a DNA analogue and two protease inhibitors has been found to stop HIV replication. The agents penetrate the HIV infected cell and the DNA analogue integrates into the elongating DNA chain stopping further replication. Some of the proteins necessary for the assembly of new HIV are made in chains and are separated and made functional by HIV-generated proteases. Protease inhibitors stop the newly synthesised HIV proteins from becoming functional by inhibiting the HIV proteases. A combination of a DNA analogue and two proteases are necessary to inhibit HIV replication. It is important to stress that this is not a cure for HIV infection; the person remains infected but does not progress to develop AIDS.

The use of HAART therapy is not without its problems. Such anti-HIV therapy has significant side effects and must be continued for the life of the infected person without any interruption. Such treatment regimens present an enormous health economic problem which can be an insuperable barrier in poorer countries of the world.

Anti-HIV therapy can also be used to prevent the transmission of HIV. If a healthcare worker suffers a significant injury and exposure to HIV-infected blood, then the prompt use of anti-HIV therapy can prevent infection. The therapy has to be instituted as soon as possible and always within 4 hours; it needs to be continued for 4–6 weeks. This use of anti-HIV therapy is often described as post-exposure prophylaxis (PEP) and is very effective at preventing transmission of the virus.

The dental management of HIV infected individuals is no different to any non-infected person. The aim is to get rid of any incipient sepsis and to ensure good periodontal health. Patients on HAART can be managed in general dental practice, even though they may be on a large number of other antimicrobial agents.

The only instance of transmission of HIV after dental procedures is associated with a Florida dentist called Dr Acer. He managed to infect at least six of his patients with HIV including a young lady called Kimberly Bergalis, for whom he extracted two teeth under local anaesthetic. The death of Kimberly Bergalis from AIDS raised enormous questions, among which was whether HIV could be transmitted by dental operations. There was intensive investigation of Dr Acer's mode of practice, but this failed to reveal how the transfer of infection had occurred. Epidemiological surveys of dental procedures in nearly two decades since the death of Kimberly Bergalis have failed to demonstrate any other putative transmissions through dental procedures. HIV does not normally get into the mouth in large enough numbers to cause infection. It can be detected in the mouth where it has entered by gingival bleeding or injury, but the numbers present would be insufficient to cause cross infection. The Dr Acer case is still unresolved. However, one alleged explanation is that Dr Acer may have mixed his own blood with local anaesthetic solutions given to his patients in an act of homicide.

SUMMARY

Acquired immune deficiency syndrome (AIDS) represents a cell-mediated immunodeficiency, principally T lymphocytes, due to infection by an RNA retrovirus known as the human immunodeficiency virus (HIV). Once infected an individual may remain HIV positive for many years, particularly since the development of antiretroviral drugs, before progressing to AIDS. The conditions that define AIDS include a reduced $CD4^+$ lymphocyte count accompanied by a number of orofacial signs and symptoms, including candidosis, hairy leukoplakia, Kaposi's sarcoma and herpetic ulceration. Since oral manifestations of HIV infection are relatively common, changes in the mouth may be the first indication of infection. Although it is unlikely that HIV is spread in saliva, it is relevant to dentistry due to the potential for contact with blood during the provision of dental treatment. Universal infection control procedures are required on all instruments (Ch.12). At the present time, an HIV-positive dental healthcare worker should not provide treatment to patients. All dental students must show evidence of being HIV negative on entry to dental school.

TRANSMISSIBLE SPONGIFORM ENCEPHALOPATHIES

The last 25 years has been quite remarkable for the discovery of novel microorganisms. There can be none more remarkable than **prions**, the agents thought to be responsible for the transmissible spongiform encephalopathies (TSE). Prions are thought to be responsible for a variety of unusual, lethal neurological conditions, which are listed in Table 11.4. All of the TSE produce the same range of pathological changes, which include progressive and often rapid loss of voluntary and autonomic function (non-voluntary), resulting in loss of vital processes (e.g. breathing) and eventual death. The signs and symptoms may vary, as does the rapidity of the degeneration, but the result is always death. The most common forms of TSE are those called Creutzfeldt–Jakob disease (CJD).

Prions can enter the body through contaminated surgical instruments, surgical grafts, hormones, blood or through the food chain. The mechanism and exact site of entry of prions through the food chain is not precisely known, but is thought to be in the first part of the small intestine. Once in the body, the prions migrate to the brain either through the lymphoid system, or by passage along nerves. Once in the brain, whether they cause disease appears to depend on whether another protein is present which has the acronym PRP^{sc}. It is the interaction of prion proteins (PRP) and the PRP^{sc} that triggers the pathological change. The pathological process, which is still not fully understood, causes gross destruction of brain tissue and can lead to vacuolation ('holes' in the brain, hence spongiform neuropathies; see Fig. 11.7). Another possible change is replacement of brain tissue with amyloid (a globulin-like material; Fig. 11.8A). Susceptibility to prion disease is thought to be congenital or acquired, but requires the presence of the PRP^{sc} protein in the host. The destruction of the brain appears not to be an immunological process, so it is unlikely that there will be a vaccine against prion disease.

Table 11.4 Prion-induced diseases
Kuru
Creutzfeldt–Jakob disease (CJD)
Variant Creutzfeldt–Jakob disease (vCJD)
Fatal familial insomnia
Gertmann–Straussler–Scheinker syndrome

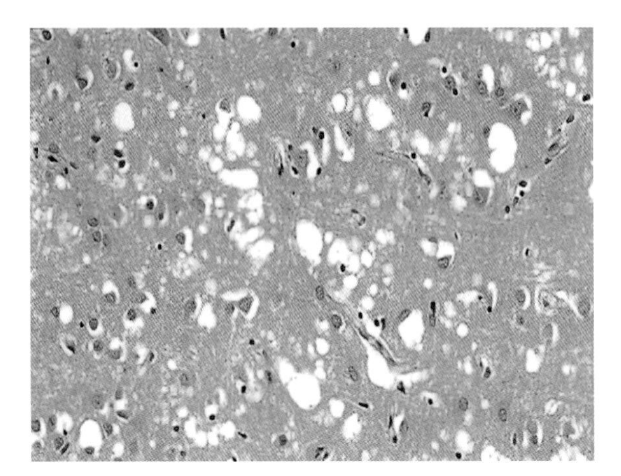

Fig. 11.7 Section of human brain showing typical degeneration caused by prion disease.

Prions are quite remarkable proteins that exist in two forms, the alpha helical form which is thought to be the cause of disease and as a beta-pleated sheet. When prions are found in the brain they are in the alpha helical form and it is this change in conformation that is thought to allow binding to PRP^{SC} and the initiation of disease.

There are four forms of CJD-sporadic, variant, genetic and iatrogenic. The most common form of CJD is the sporadic form and, fortunately, this is rare. Sporadic CJD has been found in every country in the world where it has been sought. Approximately sixty deaths each year occur in the UK from sporadic CJD and similar numbers of people die annually in the USA, Australia and Canada. This form of CJD occurs in vegans and people who have not been exposed to meat. It is thought to be due to a spontaneous change in a protein in the brain which initiates CJD onset but this is theoretical and as yet unproven.

During the epidemic of 'mad cow' disease in the 1990s in the UK a new variant of CJD was identified. Sporadic CJD tends to affect people in their sixth and seventh decades of life and takes a few months to be fatal. In mid-1995, a new variant of CJD which affected people in their 20s was recognised in the UK. This was initially called new variant CJD, but this was later shortened to variant CJD with the acronym vCJD. Not only did this new clinical type of CJD affect younger individuals than previous forms of CJD but it also had a longer clinical

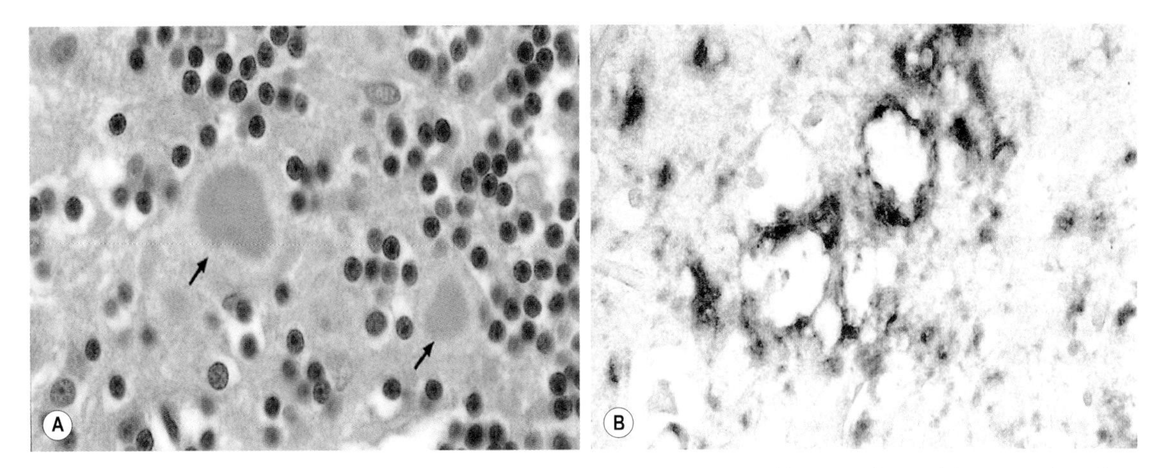

Fig. 11.8 (A) Section of human brain stained to show amyloid tissue (arrowed) caused by prion disease. (B) Same section of human brain as shown in (A) but stained brown to show the presence of prions. Note that the prions are concentrated mainly around the amyloid deposits.

course, with affected persons taking about a year to die. After extensive research, it was concluded that vCJD arose as a result of the consumption of prion-infected beef products.

Genetic forms of CJD are very rare and due to an abnormal gene; it is not caught but tends to affect families. This form of CJD can be found in families which have not been affected before.

Iatrogenic transmission, which is caused by treatment of prion disease, sent shock waves through microbiological circles. It was first reported following neurosurgery to remove a central brain tumour. The neurosurgeon removed the tumour successfully, but the patient was subsequently found to be also suffering from CJD. The instruments used in the operation were sent to the central sterile services in the hospital where they were decontaminated using the usual processes and re-used. Four patients on whom the instruments were re-used also developed CJD.

Prions are resistant to strong disinfectants, heat, autoclaving and enzyme activity. This means that the emphasis in infection control of prions has to be on effective cleaning of the instruments prior to sterilization. The normal processes of cleaning and sterilization had failed to remove the prions from the instruments used in the first operation and this had allowed transmission of the disease. This happened because prions stick tenaciously to stainless steel instruments and are not fully removed by normal cleaning methods. These properties of prions have practical implications for the cleaning, sterilization and re-use of dental instruments.

CJD is still a rare condition, with only 1245 deaths being reported between 1990 and November 2007. By far the most common form of CJD is the sporadic form with variant CJD being approximately eight times less. Figures are not available before 1990 but the disease was first described separately by two German neurologists in the early 1920s. Ironically, reviews of the early cases of CJD described by both Creutzfeldt and Jakob show that they were not the prion type disease but other neurological disease, but the name has remained. Best estimates of the prevalence of this disease suggest that it is responsible for one death in every million, so it is rare. The incubation period of CJD is unknown as is the number of people who may be affected by it in the future. The incidence of CJD rose substantially in the mid-1990s during the epidemic of bovine spongiform encephalopathy (BSE) in the UK following the consumption of contaminated beef products. In turn, CJD probably arose from a genetic change in the scrapie protein. Scrapie is a form of prion disease that affects sheep. The practice of feeding meat to herbivorous cows which was widespread in the early 1990s probably facilitated the change in the prion. The changes to the prion that caused BSE also seemed to allow it to infect man.

There are no simple tests for the identification of prions in a particular body location. Prions are detected by taking samples from the location and seeing what pathological effects they have on an experimental animal; this process can take as long as six months. Prion disease can also be detected *post mortem* by the pathological effects it has on neurological tissue. The presence of prions can also be detected in tissue by certain histological stains derived from animal prions (Fig. 11.8B). These are, however, all indirect methods and require tissue to detect the prion presence. This makes the accurate detection of prions in specific locations in living people difficult without biopsies.

The presence or numbers of prions in the mouth is still a subject of debate. One group have successfully transmitted CJD using gums and tooth pulps from hamsters infected with a sheep or scrapie prion. This experiment used sheep-derived prions which do not completely mimic human prions, but it still raised the possibility of CJD transmission by oral tissues. This piece of work together with the lack of knowledge of the number of prions necessary to cause an infection had serious consequences for dental practice. It was advised at that time that instruments used on patients had to be disposable, incinerated after use, or buried in deep land-fill sites. This advice has now been rescinded as it has been found that a large number of prions may be necessary for infection. In addition, *post mortem* examinations of gingival tissue and dental pulps from people who have died of CJD have failed to detect prions in any of the few samples examined. It is likely, therefore, that prions do not get into the mouth or oral tissues in large quantities. However, there is no doubt that prion-related disease has changed clinical practice for ever, particularly in relation to decontamination. There has been particular attention on the problem of adequately decontaminating endodontic instruments and matrix bands, both of which come into direct contact with neural tissue of the dental pulp and gingivae, respectively. It has been proposed that such dental instruments be considered as single-use items and disposed of after use.

SUMMARY

Prions are self-replicating low molecular weight proteins (PrP) that are the cause of rare and fatal transmissible spongiform encephalopathies (TSE), the most important being variant Creutzfeldt–Jacob disease (vCJD). The relevance of the possible presence of prions in dental tissues and provision of dental healthcare is uncertain. However, in view of the difficulty in inactivating and removing prions from equipment, there have been recommendations for single usage of some types of dental instruments.

HEPATITIS B

This virus can be found in the blood of patients who are infected. It consists of a double-layered coat which contains an important glycoprotein called hepatitis B surface antigen (HBsAg), which is often used to detect whether or not a patient has been exposed to the virus. Inside the coat is another glycoprotein called the hepatitis core antigen (HBcAg). There is another antigen from the virus called hepatitis B e antigen (HBeAg) which is used to assess whether a patient has active disease. The period taken from inoculation of this virus to the development of symptoms is long and can be up to 8 weeks. The majority of patients (over 60%) who contract hepatitis carry it asymptomatically and eventually overcome the disease. Even though they may be asymptomatic, HBsAg and HBeAg can be detected in their blood. Patients who develop symptoms may become chronic carriers, develop cirrhosis or have acute illness and, in a minority of cases, die. There are no precise figures as to how many people carry hepatitis B worldwide but in some countries as many as 5% are known to have been exposed to this virus. Patients who have hepatitis will release intact hepatitis B into saliva where it could potentially be a source of cross infection. It has been estimated that 0.0001 ml of blood could transmit the disease. The primary route of transmission of hepatitis B is sexual, but blood to blood transmission in unvaccinated persons has a 40% transmission rate. An effective vaccine against this disease is available.

HEPATITIS C

Hepatitis C is another virus which is transmitted primarily by the sexual route. There is some controversy as to whether this virus could be transmitted by dental procedures and although as much as 0.1 to 5% of the population may carry it, depending on the individual country, no transmission from the mouth has ever been definitively described. The virus is detected by serology by detection of antibodies to the virus (HCV antibodies) and confirmed by direct detection of the virus using the polymerase chain reaction (Ch. 10). No completely effective vaccine against this disease has been developed.

Recent work on a large number of dental personnel who may have been exposed to the hepatitis C virus from inoculation injuries have shown that the risk of transmission is in the region of 3%.

SUMMARY

Hepatitis B virus (HBV) is a double-shelled DNA virus that can be spread by extremely small volumes of blood and, as such, is a potential risk during the provision of dental treatment. Markers of infection include intact virion (Dane particle), surface antigen (HBsAg) and a breakdown product of core antigen termed e antigen (HBeAg).
An effective vaccine against HBV is available and dental students on entry to dental school must show evidence of protection by adequate antibody titres. Similarly, dental healthcare workers should maintain an adequate level of protection. Dental healthcare workers who are found to have HBeAg should not provide dental treatment.
Hepatitis C virus (HCV) is an enveloped RNA virus that is mainly spread in blood. The risk of transmission of HCV during dental treatment is unknown but unlikely. The presence of HCV is detected on the basis of serological markers of the virus. An effective vaccine is not available at the present time. Dental students have to show evidence of being HCV negative at entry to dental school. Dental healthcare workers who are found to become infected with HCV must not provide treatment.

TUBERCULOSIS

Tuberculosis (TB) is one of the most prevalent infectious diseases in the world. There are nearly two million deaths and eight million new cases of TB each year; it has been estimated that one third of the world's population is latently infected with TB, and this can reactivate in later years or following immunosuppression (e.g. following HIV-infection). Although the incidence of tuberculosis declined during the 20th century in Western countries, it has increased in recent years due to changing migration patterns from the developing to the developed world, and co-infection with HIV. Although principally caused by the acid fast bacillus, *Mycobacterium tuberculosis*, other species such as *M. bovis*, *M. africanum* and *M. kansasii* can also cause disease. Infection is spread in droplets of sputum from patients with active pulmonary tuberculosis. In some patients infection also produces lesions within the oral cavity. The classical intra-oral presentation is of an ulcer on the dorsal surface of the tongue but lesions may affect any site. The ulcers are irregular with raised borders and may resemble deep fungal infection or squamous cell carcinoma.

A mucosal biopsy should be taken to demonstrate the characteristic granulomatous inflammation with well-formed granulomata, Langhans giant cells and necrosis. Ziehl–Neelsen stain may be used to detect tubercle bacilli. Microbiological culture of suspected clinical material may also be useful to establish the diagnosis of tuberculosis. It is important to inform the microbiologist that tuberculosis is suspected because specialized media (Löwenstein–Jensen's) and prolonged incubation (2–3 weeks) is required for recovery of the organism. Molecular microbiological methods are being used increasingly to establish the diagnosis. A Mantoux (tuberculin) skin test will be positive as a result of previous infection in patients who have not received prior BCG immunization. Previous infection may occasionally be seen as incidental radio-opacities on radiographs due to calcification within lymph nodes.

Oral lesions will resolve when systemic chemotherapy consisting of rifampicin, isoniazid, pyrazinamide and ethambutol is administered. Typically, combinations of these drugs are given initially for 2 months after which time the therapy is reduced to isoniazid and rifampicin for a further 4 months. Longer and different regimens are required for the management of patients found to have resistant strains of *Mycobacterium tuberculosis*. Strains of *M. tuberculosis* that are resistant to the majority of the drugs that are used to treat this infection are referred to as multi-drug (MDR) or extensive (or extreme) drug resistant (XDR) strains. In the future, there may be difficulty in treating this condition. Vaccination with BCG is only partially effective in preventing TB.

GONORRHOEA

Gonorrhoea is caused by *Neisseria gonorrhoeae* and is a sexually transmitted disease that principally affects the genital mucosa, although it may also produce a range of non-specific oral changes including erythema, vesicule formation and pseudomembrane development, as a result of orogenital contact. These symptoms are usually preceded by generalized oral burning or itching and submandibular lymphadenopathy, which make speaking and swallowing difficult. In view of the vague symptoms, diagnosis can only be made by examination of a smear of a lesion, which will show Gram negative pairs of cocci (diplococci) within neutrophils. Culture of a swab on chocolate agar or Thayer–Martin agar will yield typical translucent oxidase-positive colonies. Identification of *N. gonorrhoeae* can be confirmed by carbohydrate utilization or fluorescent antibody tests. Treatment has historically involved a single dose of intramuscular penicillin or high-dose oral amoxicillin. The 3 gram sachet of amoxicillin was originally developed for the treatment of gonorrhoea. However, the emergence of resistance to amoxicillin has resulted in the need to use alternative antibiotics, such as ceftriaxone or ciprofloxacin. Clinical trials are also being undertaken to assess the efficacy of a single dose of 1 g or 2 g azithromycin.

SYPHILIS

Syphilis, which is caused by the spirochaete *Treponema pallidum*, has four distinct stages, the first three of which (primary, secondary and tertiary) can affect the orofacial tissues. In addition, since *T. pallidum* is one of the few microorganisms that can cross the placenta, this condition may manifest as congenital disease in childhood. Primary syphilis characteristically develops on the genitalia but can also present initially as a highly infectious indurated red painless ulcer on the lip or oral mucosa. Secondary syphilis appears approximately six weeks after the primary infection and, in addition to generalized symptoms, may produce oral lesions described as snail track ulcers. Finally, if unsuccessfully treated, syphilis can become latent and produce tertiary lesions many years after initial infection that manifest as an area of ulceration (gumma) in the palate or leukoplakia affecting the dorsal surface of the tongue.

A provisional diagnosis of syphilis may be made by use of dark-field microscopy to demonstrate numerous structures consistent in size and form with *T. pallidum* in a smear taken from either primary or secondary lesions. The causative spirochaetes cannot be cultured routinely *in vitro* and therefore serological investigations are used to diagnose syphilis from the late stage of primary infection onwards. *T. pallidum* haemagglutination (TPHA) and fluorescent treponema antibody absorbed (FTAabs) tests should be undertaken. The most effective treatment of syphilis is intramuscular procaine penicillin. However, patients should be followed up for at least 2 years, and serological examination repeated during this time.

SUMMARY

A range of human infections may rarely either primarily infect the orofacial tissues or have secondary manifestations of infection at these sites. Examples of these are tuberculosis, gonorrhoea and syphilis. Appropriate diagnostic tests should be arranged in a patient with orofacial signs and symptoms of such infectious diseases.

CHAPTER SUMMARY

Changes in general health and the treatment of disease can alter the composition of the oral microflora. A good example of this is the treatment of head and neck cancer which can cause Gram negative enteropathogens to colonize the mouth and cause destructive changes in bone following extractions. Drugs such as bisphosphonates can also cause similar effects on the jaw bones. Bacteria which are part of the normal commensal oral microflora can cause infection and destruction of facial tissue in conditions such as cancrum oris, particularly if they are not treated and there is associated malnourishment. Hepatic infections such a hepatitis B can result in the release of large quantities of viruses into the saliva which could be potentially transmitted to health care workers. In contrast, hepatitis C probably does not get into the oral cavity to cause an infectious risk. Similarly, on present evidence, prions, the agents thought to be responsible for CJD and other transmissible spongiform encephalopathies, probably are not transmissible through saliva, but may be present in other oral tissues necessitating some dental instruments being single use items and disposed of after use. Sexually transmissible diseases such as syphilis and gonorrhoea can cause oral lesions, as can tuberculosis, and are potentially transmissible through saliva. Thus, effective infection control strategies are needed (Ch. 12).

FURTHER READING

Arrain Y, Masud T 2008 Recent recommendations on bisphosphonate associated osteonecrosis of the jaw. Dent Update 35:2238-242.

Fihman V, Raskine L, Petitpas F et al 2008 Cervical necrotising fasciitis: 8 years' experience of microbiology. Eur J Clin Microbiol Infect Dis 27:691-695.

Gibson J, Wray D, Bagg J 2000 Oral staphylococcal mucositis: a new entity in orofacial granulomatosis and Crohn's disease. Oral Surg Oral Med Oral Pathol Oral Radiol Endod 89:171-176.

Guidance for clinical health care workers: Protection against infection with blood-borne viruses. Recommendations of the Expert Advisory Group on AIDS and the Advisory Group on Hepatitis. http:/ www.open.gov.uk/doh/chcguid1.htm.

Lewis MAO, Jordan RCK 2004 A colour handbook of oral medicine. Manson Publishing, London.

Lyons A, Ghazali N Osteoradionecrosis of the jaws: current understanding of its pathophysiology and treatment. Br J Oral Maxillofac Surg 46: 653-660.

Ramalho VL, Ramalho HJ et al 2007 Comparison of azithromycin and oral hygiene programs in the treatment of cyclosporine-induced gingival hyperplasia. Ren Fail 29:265-270.

Scully C, Cawson RA 2005 Medical problems in dentistry, 5th edn. Churchill Livingstone, London.

Walker JT, Dickinson J, Sutton JM, Marsh PD, Raven ND 2008 Implications for Creutzfeldt-Jakob disease in dentistry: a review of current knowledge. J Dent Res 87:511-519.

Chapter 12

Infection control

INFECTION CONTROL

The term infection control is defined as all the processes and precautions that can be taken to control the spread of infection. The type of processes and precautions that are used in infection control are described as high, medium or low level. The classification of infection control procedures are based on the risk of transmission of the diseases that are being encountered and the procedures being done. High level infection control is where a patient is isolated from all contact with professional or family members and every procedure is done with appropriate barriers in place. High level disinfection is employed when patients contract highly infectious disease such as the haemorrhagic fevers which if transmitted are fatal. Medium level infection control is where barrier protection is used, but the risk of contracting the disease is not high but still possible. Low level infection control measures are used where the risk of transmission is low and only normal cleanliness is required.

There are problems in categorizing which level of infection control is appropriate for dentistry. Many of the patients who attend dental surgeries may asymptomatically carry potentially infectious diseases but they do not know they are infected (e.g. hepatitis B or C). The risk of transmission could be high in dentistry if there is blood to blood contact through, for example, an inoculation (sharps) injury. In addition, the major fluids encountered in dentistry are blood and saliva and these could potentially transmit infectious disease. The risk for most of the surgical procedures done in dentistry, therefore, is in the medium category. Since most dental patients who asymptomatically carry disease are unaware of their infectious status it is wise to treat everyone with the same precautions; these are often described as **Standard** or **Universal Precautions**.

WHICH INFECTIOUS DISEASES ARE TRANSMITTED BY DENTISTRY?

The number of proven cases of infectious diseases that have been transmitted by dental personnel, treatment or patients is very limited and the diseases are listed in Table 12.1. The pathogens include *Mycobacterium tuberculosis* (the causative organism of the majority of cases of tuberculosis in humans), methicillin resistant *Staphylococcus aureus* (MRSA), *Pseudomonas* spp., and the hand, foot and mouth virus (Ch. 10), and their transmission has resulted in serious, but not life-threatening infections. The list also includes infections caused by *Legionella* spp. and hepatitis B virus which have resulted in death of dental personnel. The most infectious agent that is constantly present in the oral cavity of at least 30% of the population is herpes simplex type 1 (Ch. 10). This virus has not caused death, but it has been responsible for blindness, usually in dental personnel who do not wear protective spectacles. Some authors have reviewed the low number of transmissions of infection in dentistry and have questioned whether many of the precautions used are necessary or justified, based on a risk assessment. Whether infection control measures in dentistry are necessary cannot now be answered as it would be impossible to revert to anything but standard precautions. Public pressure and ethical responsibility would prevent any diminution in the standard of precautions or to test a reduced level of protection. In addition, most regulatory authorities now demand standard precautions are taken in dentistry and have used litigation to ensure that it is done.

Table 12.1 Proven cases of infection transmitted by dentistry.

Infectious agent	Route of infection
HIV	Use of infected instruments or direct injection of blood
Hepatitis B virus	Sharps injury
Herpes simplex type 1 virus	Contact of infected material with skin or eyes
Coxsackie viruses	Contact with skin
Legionella spp.	Inhalation of contaminated dental unit water supplies
Pseudomonads (e.g. *Pseudomonas aeruginosa*)	Contact with contaminated dental unit water supplies
MRSA (Methicillin resistant *Staphylococcus aureus*)	Contact with skin
Mycobacterium tuberculosis	Inhalation of infected droplets

PERSONAL PROTECTION

Personal protection is an important part of infection control. Important elements of personal protection in dentistry are immunization, protection of hands, eye and face, protective clothing and management and avoidance of inoculation (sharps) injuries.

Immunization

The protection of dental personnel by immunization before they engage in dental procedures is an important part of infection control. Nowadays, many regulatory authorities require that dentists, nurses, hygienists and therapists are not carrying any potentially infectious disease before they undertake or assist with any dental procedures. Freedom from infectious disease and satisfactory records of immunization should be a contractual prerequisite before dental personnel are employed. The vaccinations required are listed in Table 12.2 and many of these are done routinely in adolescence. The exception to this is hepatitis B vaccination which needs to be satisfactorily completed before any exposure to surgical procedures is done.

Hand protection

Hands of dental personnel are potentially one of the most vulnerable areas of the body to infectious disease and also may be a potential vector for infection.

Table 12.2 Recommended vaccinations for all dental personnel.

Vaccine	Route	Length of protection
Diphtheria	IM*	Probably life-long
Hepatitis B	IM	At least 5 years but probably life-long
Pertussis (Whooping Cough)	IM	Probably life-long
Poliomyelitis	IM	Probably life-long
Rubella	IM	Probably life-long
Tetanus	IM	At least 10 years but probably life-long
Tuberculosis (BCG)	IM	Probably less than life-long in most recipients

*IM = intramuscular

The maintenance of an intact layer of epithelium, although difficult to achieve, is an important part of protection. The problem is that procedures such as handwashing in soap and water, and covering hands with gloves, can have a serious and deleterious effect on the integrity and pliability of the skin. Both glove wearing and handwashing can have a hyperosmotic effect on the hands and cause the skin to crack and lose its pliability, thereby rendering it susceptible to microbial ingression. Handcreams used after every session restore essential oils to the skin and help retain pliability.

Handwashing has to be done systematically ensuring that all surfaces are washed and rinsed. The technique devised by Ayliffe (Fig. 12.1) ensures that all surfaces are washed and rinsed. If the hands are not visibly contaminated after patient treatment then the use of combined alcohol and disinfectant handrubs are recommended. These handrubs are applied using a systematic technique and have been found to be as effective as handwashing with soap and water. The advantage of handrubs is that they are less injurious to the integrity of hand skin and many contain emollients that help protect the skin from drying.

Gloves

Gloves are an essential part of infection control in dentistry. They provide a physical barrier which protects the hands from the ingress of microorganisms and should be worn for all dental procedures. They are a single use item and a new pair should be used for each patient. Most gloves are made out of natural

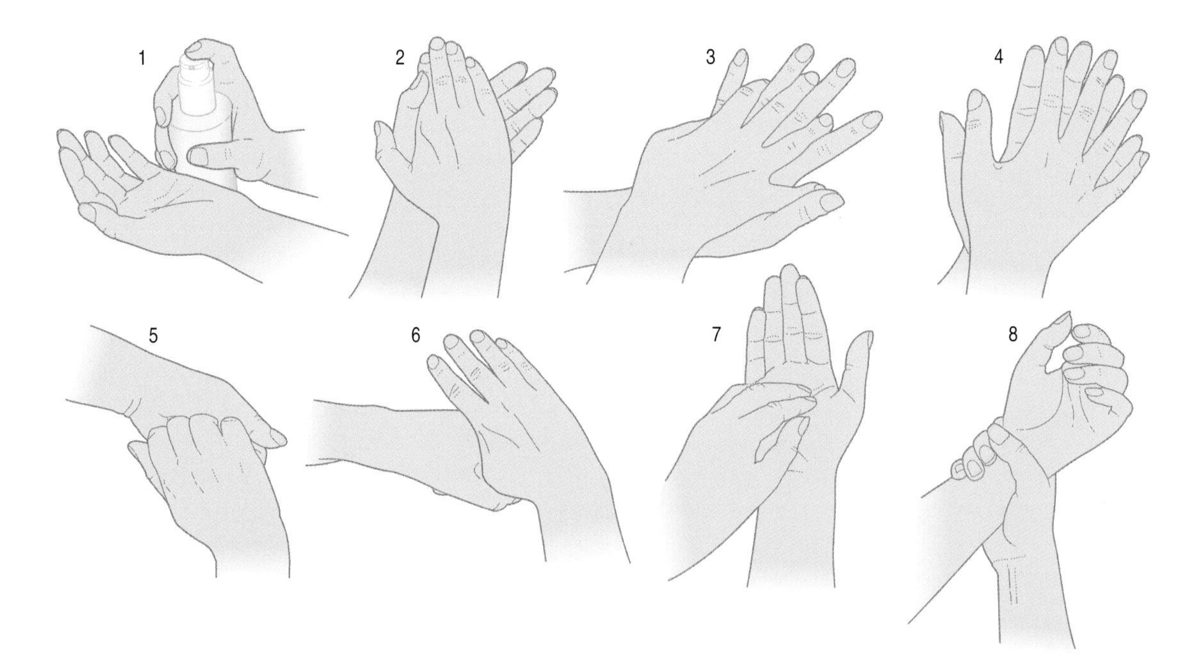

Fig. 12.1 The systematic handwashing technique of Ayliffe.

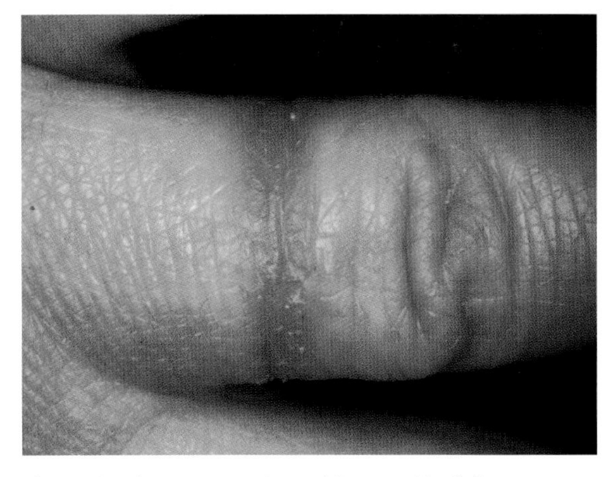

Fig. 12.2 Irritant contact dermatitis caused by failure to remove a ring prior to glove washing and glove wearing.

latex rubber and contain low molecular weight proteins that can be immunologically active. These low-molecular-weight proteins can penetrate the skin and induce inflammation; this condition is called irritant contact dermatitis. All rings and watches should be removed prior to handwashing or donning gloves otherwise irritant contact dermatitis can ensue (Fig. 12.2). Poor handwashing technique with soap and water can also cause irritant contact dermatitis and this condition can be cured by changing the make of gloves and careful attention to handwashing. Topical steroids may help alleviate the condition in more severe irritant contact dermatitis cases. In one major survey of hand problems in dental personnel, approximately 20% were shown to suffer intermittently from irritant contact dermatitis.

Immunological reactions to latex proteins are more serious and can be life-threatening if they progress to anaphylaxis. Sensitivity to latex proteins is fortunately still rare, but in the USA it has been estimated that 40% of medical personnel have detectable antibodies to latex proteins. Immunological contact dermatitis is immediate and the inflammation spreads well beyond the glove wearing area (Fig. 12.3); it is not controlled by handwashing and always requires steroid or other systemic therapy. Concern about latex proteins is now so serious that latex gloves are slowly being phased out from healthcare procedures in Europe.

Many gloves contain donning agents which help them to be put on dry hands. One agent that has been extensively used as a donning agent is starch but it should not be used because it causes latex allergens to be dispersed in the atmosphere when the gloves are donned. If allowed to contaminate wounds, starch can cause granulomas (excessive fibrous tissue) to form and it can prevent veneers from adhering properly to teeth.

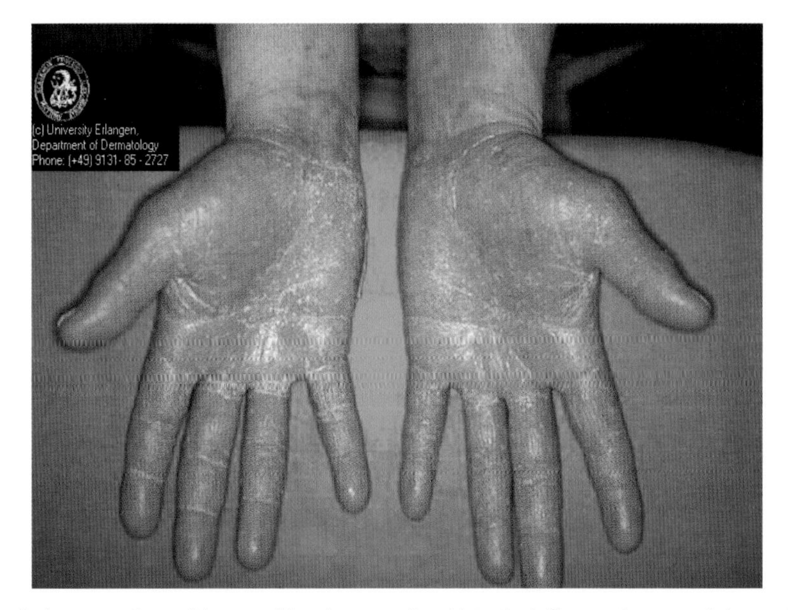

Fig. 12.3 Immunological contact dermatitis caused by glove wearing. Note the inflammation spreads beyond the glove wearing area (courtesy of the University of Ehlingham).

Eye and face protection

Eye protection is mandatory for all dental operators. The eye can be contaminated by patients coughing pooled saliva and blood from the floor of the mouth into the face of the operators (this is called 'splatter'). Eyes can also be contaminated from aerosols generated from the mouth when high speed instruments are used with coolants (Fig. 12.4). Since 30% of patients will have significant numbers of herpes simplex type 1 virus in the mouth, the risk of infection is high. Herpetic infections of the eye have a significant chance of causing blindness and this has happened to a number of dental personnel in the UK. Protective or prescription glasses should always be worn; these require washing and drying after use. An alternative form of eye protection is a visor and often these have a mask incorporated in them.

The type of mask worn in dentistry does not confer microbiological protection. Motile bacteria can penetrate masks once masks are wet. They are a single-use item and should be thrown away after use. Masks are a protection against splatter, but only initially protect against aerosols. The best protection against aerosols is high-vacuum suction which should be switched on before any coolants are used. The role of aerosols in the transmission of infection in dentistry is still unproven, but it is well established that many diseases such as tuberculosis, Legionnaire's disease and infectious mononucleosis are spread by this route.

Surgery clothing

There is a wide variety of surgery clothing available. There is no doubt that clothing does become contaminated during operative procedures. Surgery clothing should be capable of being washed at temperatures of greater than 60 °C as this kills many potentially pathogenic microorganisms. The debate about whether surgery clothing should have long or short sleeves is still unresolved. Many argue that long sleeves protect the arms from microorganisms. Others argue that bare arms can be washed and this is more hygienic. The choice of long or short sleeves awaits resolution and at the moment is still a matter of personal preference.

Inoculation injuries

Inoculation injuries (often called sharps or needlestick injuries) have a high potential for the transmission of serious infection as they can involve blood to blood contact. They must be avoided by careful

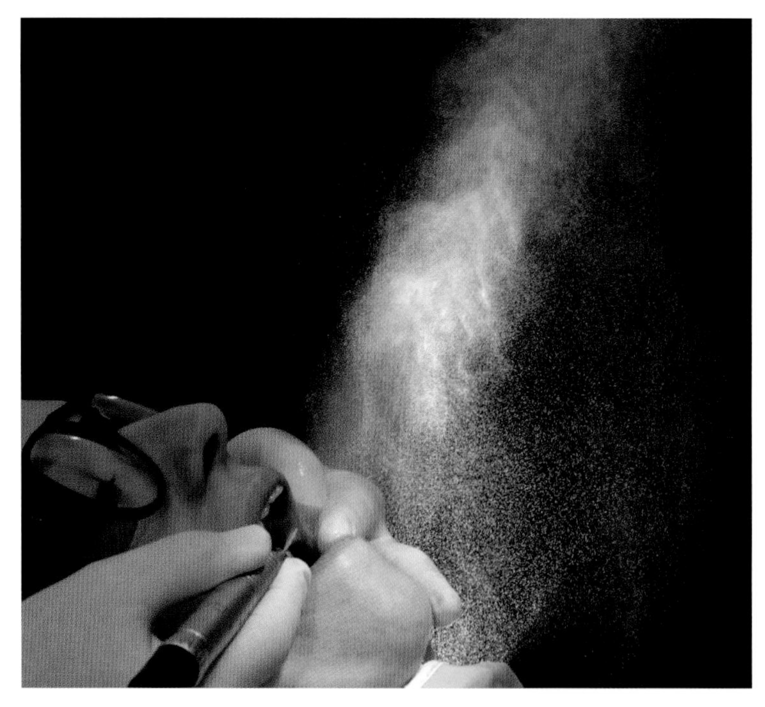

Fig. 12.4 Aerosol generated by high speed dental handpiece.

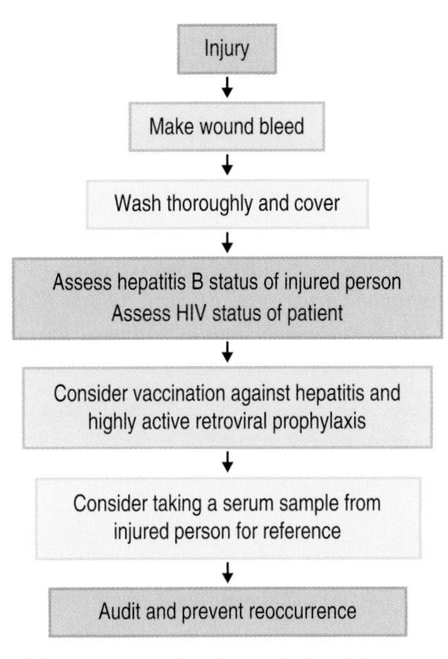

Fig. 12.5 Management of an innoculation injury.

needle resheathing techniques and safe disposal of sharps. The two occasions when they are most likely to occur are during the resheathing of local anaesthetic equipment and the removal and decontamination of used dental instruments. A schema for dealing with sharps injuries is shown in Fig. 12.5. After immediate first aid the injured person should be assessed and hepatitis B and/or HIV prophylaxis should be considered. An audit of the reasons for the sharps injury should always be done and surgery protocols modified to prevent it happening again.

SURGERY DESIGN

In order to reduce the risk of cross infection most surgeries incorporate three distinct areas or zones: an operator's zone, an assistant zone and a decontamination zone. The first two zones should have wash hand basins in them which should not be used for decontamination. All equipment should be capable of simple disinfection and easily kept clean. Surgeries should be tidy and uncluttered.

SURGERY DISINFECTION

Disinfection is the removal or killing of some microorganisms but not usually spores. Disinfection is reserved for four distinct places; these are (a) surfaces, (b) drains and spittoons, (c) dental unit water supplies, and (d) impressions and appliances.

Surface disinfection

The most important element of surface disinfection is cleaning. Surfaces should be thoroughly cleaned ideally with a combination of a detergent and a disinfectant. Although a large number of types of surface disinfectant are available, it is how they are used that is probably more important than their disinfectant action. The aim of surface disinfection is to remove the maximum number of microorganisms by dilution and cleaning; when this is complete then the disinfectant will kill the remainder. Disinfectant should be applied to surfaces, wiped off using a lot of energy and the process repeated. This is a progressive dilution technique with each application of disinfectant further reducing the number of microorganisms present.

Drains and spittoons

These are heavily contaminated areas as they collect saliva, blood and other material. These areas are prone to the formation of tenacious biofilms on the surfaces of their tubes. Biofilms are formed on the inner surfaces of tubing and are held together by extracellular slime-like materials secreted by the constituent microorganisms (Ch. 5). Microorganisms in biofilms are highly tolerant of disinfectants and very difficult to remove. A combination of a bactericidal disinfectant and a detergent should be used on drains and spittoons and this should be done after every session to prevent biofilm accumulation.

Dental unit water systems

Water delivered from dental unit water systems (DUWS) is not sterile and can contain high numbers of bacteria (sometimes exceeding one million colony forming units/ml), including opportunistic pathogens such as *Legionella pneumophila*, *Mycobacterium* spp., *Pseudomonas aeruginosa* and *Candida* spp.. The source water is often tap or deionized water, and this should have low microbial counts. The high microbial load in the outflowing water is due to the rapid development of biofilms (Ch. 5) on the inner surfaces of tubing in dental unit water systems (Fig. 12.6), from which large numbers of microorganisms are shed into the water. The water in DUWS is static for long periods of time, and is constantly

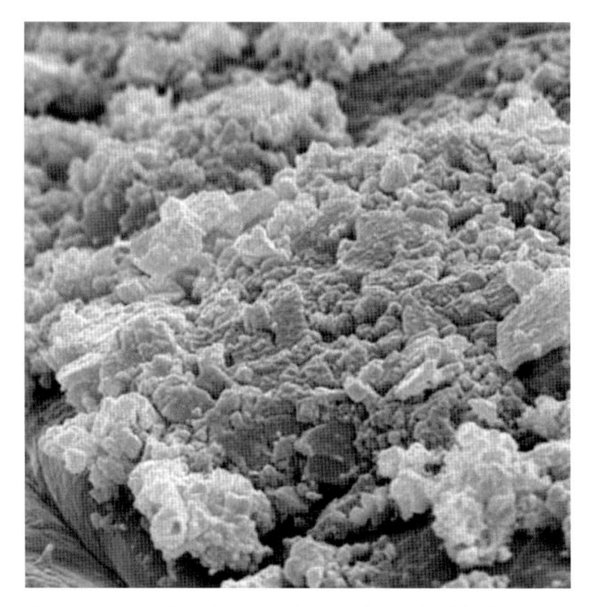

Fig. 12.6 Scanning electron micrograph of a biofilm formed on the inner surface of tubing in a dental unit.

heated to a temperature of between 22°C (room temperature) and 37°C (body temperature), which also encourages microbial growth. DUWS can also be contaminated with microorganisms derived from the mouth by back-siphonage. The latter occurs because when the turbine drill is deactivated, to prevent splashing the patient, a small amount of water contaminated with saliva is sucked-back into the turbine tubing; this inoculates the dental unit water with oral microbes, which can be passed on to subsequent patients.

Contamination of dental unit water supplies has been responsible for the death of a dentist in the USA from legionellosis, and also for amoebic eye infections and infections due to *Pseudomonas aeruginosa* in immunocompromised patients. Evidence of occupational exposure to such pathogens has come from the finding that dentists have higher antibody titres to *L. pneumophila* than other employment groups. Contamination has also been implicated as a cause of late onset asthma in dental personnel from endotoxins released from the Gram negative bacteria present in aerosols of dental unit water (Fig. 12.4). Guidelines are being introduced to set standards for the maximum microbial load delivered by water from dental units. In the USA, this is 200 CFU/ml, and other countries are setting equivalent standards. To achieve these levels, DUWS need purging with disinfectants that are effective not only against microorganisms in the liquid phase, but which are also active against established biofilms, as these are inherently more tolerant of antimicrobial agents (Ch. 5). Products containing hydrogen peroxide and silver ions have been found to be particularly effective. Care has to be taken to ensure that any disinfectant is used according to the manufacturer's instructions (e.g. frequency of application and concentration), and is compatible with the materials used in the construction of the particular dental unit.

Disinfection of appliances and impressions

Before leaving the surgery, appliances and impressions should be washed to remove debris and then disinfected by immersion. Spraying of disinfectants onto the surface is ineffective. A number of immersion disinfectants are now available which cause minimal changes to impression materials.

DECONTAMINATION OF INSTRUMENTS

The word decontamination is often misused; it is defined as the treatment of an instrument to make it fit for re-use. Decontamination therefore involves both cleaning and sterilization of the instrument and its safe storage.

Critical and non-critical instruments

Only instruments that are to be used in surgical areas where they will become contaminated need sterilization; these are called critical instruments. When critical instruments are purchased, the manufacturer must provide a statement of how they are to be cleaned and sterilized. Often critical instruments are difficult if not impossible to sterilize and disposal of them is the best option; a good example of this is saliva ejectors. Equipment such as patient spectacles and bib chains are not heavily contaminated and so are not critical instruments and are best disinfected by washing.

Unless critical instruments are cleaned they cannot be sterilized. This presents a particular problem because none of the methods used in dentistry can be guaranteed to remove prion contamination, but may reduce it. All the methods used for cleaning must be validated (shown to work), and be regularly checked. There are three methods currently used for instrument cleaning in dentistry; they are manual washing, ultrasonics and washer/disinfectors.

Manual cleaning

This is by far the commonest method of cleaning instruments, but it is not recommended. Inherently it is dangerous as there is always the danger of sharp's injuries and it is not reliable. Studies have shown that manual cleaning is inefficient with a high likelihood of residual material remaining.

Ultrasonic cleaning

This method of cleaning involves placing the instruments into a bath containing detergent and using an ultrasonic generator to clean the instruments. The ultrasonic generator creates vacuums within the liquid which collapse on the surface of the instruments and release energy. The energy dislodges material adherent to the instrument. Ultrasonic baths have to be properly commissioned and periodically validated if they are to be effective. The correct detergent has to be used in the bath and the instruments must be separated so the liquid can flow round them. The bath also has to be used for the manufacturer's recommended length of time without interruption. Ultrasonic baths need periodic testing and the easiest test to use is the foil ablation test in which pieces of foil are placed in the bath and are destroyed by the ultrasonics. Another test that is recommended for ultrasonic baths is a residual protein test. This test employs a test soil which is placed on an instrument; the test checks for removal of the protein. The reader is recommended to textbooks and guidelines on infection control that are cited in the Further Reading section at the end of this chapter. Ultrasonics are effective if used properly and checked regularly.

Washer/disinfectors

These machines are designed to clean and disinfect instruments to a high and reproducible standard. They first rinse the instruments in cold water which removes most of the debris. The machine then washes the instrument in hot water and detergent, rinses them and then heats the instruments to a temperature between 80–90°C for 1–3 minutes. The instruments are then dried. The length of the cycles of these machines is between 20–60 minutes. They also require a good standard of water which can be produced by cleaning mains supplies with ion exchange resins or by reverse osmosis. Washer disinfectors need monitoring daily to check that the manufacturer's parameters for the machine are met. They need periodic residual protein tests as described for ultrasonic machines.

STERILIZATION OF INSTRUMENTS

An instrument has to be clean before sterilization, otherwise residual material can protect microorganisms in biofilms retained on the surface and they can remain viable. Sterilization is defined as the complete killing of all forms of life including prions. In practice, sterility is probably never achieved as the type of process used does not kill or inactivate prions.

In dentistry, the commonest process used for sterilization is the autoclave which uses the latent heat of steam to achieve its killing of microorganisms. Water is heated under pressure beyond its boiling point and circulates around the instruments in a pressure-resistant chamber. The steam condenses on the instruments until they are heated to the temperature of the steam. This temperature is then held until the instruments are sterile. The temperature–time combinations that are necessary for sterility in autoclaves are shown in Table 12.3. The efficiency of killing in an autoclave is partly dependent on the amount of air that is driven out of the chamber. The more air that is driven out of the autoclave chamber, the more efficient the penetration of steam. The penetration of the steam is important when instruments with small diameter tubes in them are being sterilized (e.g. dental handpieces). The most common form of autoclave is called a type N where the air is pushed out of the chamber by the steam; this type of autoclave is only suitable for solid instruments. Type S autoclaves pump the air out and a large amount of residual air is removed; these autoclaves are suitable for some

Table 12.3 Recommended temperature, time and pressure combinations for sterilization.

Temperature (°C)	Time (min)	Pressure (bar)
134	3	2
115	30	1
121	15	1

instruments with tubes as specified by the manufacturer. Type B autoclaves repeatedly pump out the air from the chamber and the amount of residual air remaining is small; these autoclaves are recommended for any instrument. The autoclaves recommended for dental instruments are type B or S.

Autoclaves need periodic testing and this is best done by thermocouples. In some countries the mandatory testing of autoclaves is done by assessing the killing of a heat-resistant bacterium, *Geobacillus stearothermophillus*. The spores are contained on strips in the autoclave for one cycle and then incubated; if the autoclave works then no growth should occur.

Storage of instruments

Once sterilized, instruments are best stored in dry cassettes, bags or pouches. They can remain sterile if kept airtight and dry for considerable periods of time.

WASTE DISPOSAL

Clinical waste is material which has been exposed to blood, saliva, tissue or other bodily fluids. It has to be disposed of separately from other non-clinical waste by incineration or by burial in deep land-fill sites. Different countries have varying regulations for the disposal of this material. Sharps must be kept in rigid containers until disposal.

CHAPTER SUMMARY

Infection control in dentistry is important and standard precautions must be used for all patients. Care must be taken with personal protection, disinfection, decontamination and disposal of waste. Personnel must be successfully vaccinated against infectious disease and avoid sharp's injuries. Protective spectacles, masks and surgery clothing capable of being washed at above 60 °C should be worn. Instruments need complete cleaning preferably in validated washer disinfectors then steam sterilized in appropriate autoclaves. Disinfection is best reserved for surfaces, drains, impressions and appliances and dental unit water supplies.

Waste, particularly from clinics, must be separated from other material and disposed of according to local regulations.

FURTHER READING

Martin MV, Fulford MR, Preston AJ 2008 Infection control for the dental team. Quintessence Publications.

Walker JT, Dickinson J, Sutton JM, Raven ND, Marsh PD 2007 Cleanability of dental instruments- implications of residual protein and risks of Crutzfeldt-Jakob disease. Br Dent J 203:395-401.

Walker JT, Marsh PD 2007 Microbial biofilm formation in DUWS and their control using disinfectants. J Dent 35:721-730.

Index

A

D

E

I

J

K

L

M

N

O

P

Q

R

S